Rick Carlton

Rick Carlton

Producing
Quality
Radiographs

Producing Quality Radiographs

Second Edition

ANGELINE M. CULLINAN
R.T. (R), F.A.S.R.T.
Henrietta, New York

JOHN E. CULLINAN
R.T. (R), F.A.S.R.T.
Henrietta, New York

Illustrations
Arnold L. Gomez
Rochester, New York

J.B. Lippincott Company   *Philadelphia*

Acquisitions Editor: Andrew M. Allen
Coordinating Editorial Assistant: Miriam Benert
Project Editor: Tom Gibbons
Indexer: David Amundson
Design Coordinator: Kathy Kelley-Luedtke
Interior Designer: Susan Hess Blaker
Cover Designer: Robert Freese
Production Manager: Helen Ewan
Production Coordinator: Kathryn Rule
Compositor: G&S Typesetters, Inc.
Printer/Binder: Walsworth Publishing Company

2nd Edition

6   5   4   3   2   1

Library of Congress Cataloging-in-Publication

Cullinan, Angeline M.
    Producing quality radiographs / Angeline M. Cullinan, John E.
  Cullinan; illustrations, Arnold M. Gómez—2nd ed.
      p. cm.
    Includes index.
    ISBN 0-397-55031-6
    1. Radiography, Medical.   1. Cullinan, John E.   II. Title.
  RC78.C84   1994
  616.07′572—dc20   93–1621
                                                       CIP

The authors and publisher have exerted every effort to ensure that
drug selection and dosage set forth in this text are in accord with
current recommendations and practice at the time of publication.
However, in view of ongoing research, changes in government regulations, and the constant flow of information relating to drug
therapy and drug reactions, the reader is urged to check the package insert for each drug for any change in indications and dosage
and for added warnings and precautions. This is particularly important when the recommended agent is a new or infrequently employed drug.

Lovingly dedicated to

Angela
Adam
Elizabeth
Christopher
Kevin
Melissa
Leah
Jaimie

Preface

Professional skills must be continually refined to take advantage of new improvements in image recording media and techniques in order to produce quality radiographs.

Producing quality radiographs requires selection of proper exposure factors and control of processing conditions. The skill of the radiographer has the greatest effect on the final image; even a minor technical adjustment can affect image quality.

Radiographic technique is not a simple topic. We hope that we have presented this material in a manner that makes it easy to read and understand. Topics such as modulation transfer function are introduced in one page or less. Since entire books have been devoted to sensitometry, only sensitometric illustrations of practical value are used in this book.

The terms found in the Glossary of Related Terminology are defined only as they relate to radiography. Simple definitions are used whenever possible.

Radiation physics, radiation protection, and quality assurance concerns influence radiographic exposure. Considerable space is devoted to the description and operation of radiographic equipment. A full operator control panel and the schematic functions of the x-ray circuit are illustrated in Chapter 2. Almost 400 line art illustrations, radiographs, and tables are used to support the text. Related technical concepts are presented as composite illustrations.

Diagnostic medical imaging has changed dramatically in recent years; newer imaging modalities are now in common use. A portion of Chapter 12 highlights some of the more widely accepted imaging techniques that are not essentially radiographic in nature. Although newer imaging modalities such as ultrasound, computed tomography, and magnetic resonance imaging have become the primary imaging techniques for selective examinations, conventional radiography is still widely used for most medical imaging. Technologies using optical disks, video tape recorders, computers, and laser printers coexist with conventional radiography. New dual-receptor, zero-crossover screen film systems that revolutionize conventional imaging can be found in Chapter 6. New grid technology is introduced in Chapter 5. The image evaluation material in Chapter 10 should help radiographers judge their work.

We have tried to follow the content recommendations in the Curriculum Guide of the American Society of Radiologic Technologists and the guidelines for the certification examination set by the American Registry of Radiologic Technologists.

Angeline M. Cullinan
John E. Cullinan

Acknowledgments

We find the writing of these acknowledgments a most pleasant task, for it gives us the opportunity to recognize those who contributed to this textbook. Sometimes it is difficult to identify exactly where one has learned specific information. Many educators, physicists, radiologists, radiographers, professional colleagues, and students have been our teachers.

We acknowledge the following for their advice and suggestions: Dawn Beck and Roseann Jackura, Health Sciences Division, Eastman Kodak Company; Jeanne Anne Cullinan, MD, of Vanderbuilt University Medical Center; Russell A. Hall of Elema-Schonander; Lars-Ake Isaksson of Seimens-Elema AB; Hy Glasser, Martin J. Ratner, and Al Zirkes of Nuclear Associates; Diana M. Ladd, R.T.(R), CNMT of The Genesee Hospital; and Mike Peterson and Ronald S. Sciepko Jr. of Picker International.

Gómez of Sizzle-Ink, whose quick grasp of the material presented to him helped express our thoughts visually.

Most of the photographs used in this book are the work of Dave Welker and his staff at Campos Photography, especially Ruth De Boer. We want to thank them for the time spent faithfully reproducing our artwork and radiographs.

A special thank you to Andrew M. Allen, Allied Health Editor at J.B. Lippincott, for his encouragement and attention to the development of this book. The editing and production staff involved in this work should also be recognized.

Thank you to the educators, radiographers, radiologists, and commercial equipment and film companies for their acceptance of the first edition of this book. Your kind comments and professional criticisms are reflected in this second edition.

Contents

14 Quality Assurance Guidelines   *240*

Glossary of Related Terminology   *263*

Appendix I *Abbreviations, Symbols, and Professional Organizations*   *277*

Appendix II *Technical Formulas and Related Data*   *280*

Index   *301*

Producing Quality Radiographs

Chapter 1

Energy, Atomic Structure, and Electromagnetic Radiation

The problems encountered in the production of quality radiographic images cannot be addressed without a working knowledge of how x-radiation is produced. The purpose of this chapter is to review and to summarize basic physics principles and their relation to radiography.

Energy and Work

Energy is involved when objects are moved, heated, caused to emit light, and caused to take part in chemical reactions. Work occurs when a force is exerted on the mass of an object over a given distance. The force on a body is referred to as *work*, and it must overcome the inertia, or tendency of a body at rest to remain at rest, that is inherent in all matter. The mass of a body is the determining factor of its inertia.

The terms power, work, and energy are closely related but should not be used interchangeably; they can be expressed as follows:

$$\text{Power} = \frac{\text{Work}}{\text{time}} \qquad \left(P = \frac{W}{t} \right)$$

$$\text{Work} = \text{force} \times \text{distance} \ (W = F \times d)$$

Energy, defined as the ability to perform work, exists in nature in many forms, such as kinetic energy, potential energy, thermal energy, chemical energy, electromagnetic energy, and molecular energy (Fig. 1-1).

According to the Conservation of Energy Law, the total energy of a system isolated from its surroundings remains constant, but the energy can be changed from one form to another. For example:

Angeline M. Cullinan and John E. Cullinan:
PRODUCING QUALITY RADIOGRAPHS, 2ND ED.
© 1987, 1994 J. B. Lippincott Company.

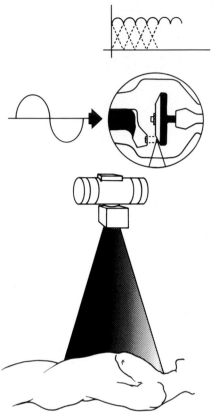

Figure 1-1
Electrical Energy Conversion to X-radiation

Electrical energy is converted into x-radiation in the x-ray circuit. In the United States, 110-volt or 220-volt current is supplied by commercial power companies in the form of alternating current (60 Hz per second). The alternating current is transformed into direct current, which is put in motion (kinetic energy) from cathode to anode in the x-ray tube to produce heat (thermal energy) and x-radiation (radiant energy).

Electrical energy can be converted to light, radio waves, heat, and kinetic energy (motion) and can cause chemical changes.

Mechanical energy can be converted to heat and electrical energy or to motion of objects.

Chemical energy can be converted to light, heat, mechanical energy, and electrical energy.

Radiant energy can be converted to heat and electrical energy, can cause chemical changes, and can be used to transmit messages.

Nuclear energy can be converted to light, heat, motion, and electrical energy.

Electrical and mechanical energy can be converted into electromagnetic energy such as light, radiowaves, and x-radiation. X-rays and gamma rays, parts of the electromagnetic spectrum, are capable of ionizing matter and are forms of ionizing radiation (see section on Ionization and Excitation of the Atom).

Atomic Structure

Matter

Matter is any substance that is composed of atoms and occupies space. The amount of matter contained in an object is assessable by means of its mass. Depending on its surroundings, mass can change in size, shape, and form. For example, water, ice, and vapor have the same atomic number but are represented in different forms.

Matter is made up of relatively few kinds of elementary particles. All known substances are made up of a combination of these elementary particles. The number and arrangement of the elementary particles determine the atomic structure of an elemental atom. Three of the particles of the atom—the proton, neutron, and electron—are the basis of simple atomic structure (Fig. 1-2). Elements are classified according to their atomic number, which is the number of protons in their central nucleus.

Each element has characteristics that distinguish it from other elements. These characteristics determine whether the element can participate in certain chemical reactions, whether it is a good or bad conductor, whether it is a nonconductor or insulator or a superconductor, and so on.

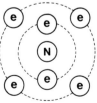

Figure 1-2
Atomic Structure

A typical atom consists of a nucleus (N), which contains positively charged photons and neutrons (no charge) and negatively charged electrons (e). The electrons orbit around the nucleus. This representation of the carbon atom is not in scale. In actuality, neutrons and protons each constitute 1838 times more mass than electrons.

IMPORTANT

Matter and energy are interchangeable in form. This was demonstrated by Albert Einstein in his famous derivation $E = MC^2$, where E = energy, M = mass, and C, a constant = the speed of light. The speed of light is about 186,300 miles per second.

Atomic Number and Mass Number

The nucleus contains both neutrons and protons and comprises almost all of the mass of the atom—1838 times more mass than the electron. The number of protons in the nucleus is called the atomic number, (Z). The total number of protons and neutrons in the nucleus is called the atomic mass number, (A).

IMPORTANT

The diameter of an atom is about 100,000 times greater than the diameter of its nucleus. A high-speed electron interacting with matter can go through the mostly empty space of many atoms before interacting with any part of an atom.

Electrical Charges

The atom has been described as a miniature solar system, with its nucleus as its sun and electrons orbiting around it (Fig. 1-3). However, there is an important difference: Planets are held in orbit around the sun by gravitational forces. Electrons, which are negatively charged, revolve around the nucleus of the atom at high speed and are held (bound) in orbit by a balance in attraction of the positive charges of the protons and the centripetal and centrifugal repulsion forces created by the velocity of the rapidly spinning and revolving electrons.

The charges of the nucleus come from its protons, which possess a positive electrical charge, and these are balanced by an equal number of negative electron charges in the outer portion of the atom. The charges of the protons (+) and the charges of the electrons (−) are equal in quantity. Neutrons, which do not have net charge, also reside in the nucleus in quantities sufficient to stabilize the nuclear forces. The number and arrangement of the electrons in a neutral atom establish

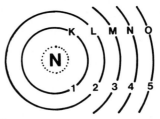

Figure 1-3
Electron Shell Arrangement and Binding Power
The binding force on the electron shells holding the electrons in orbit around the nucleus weakens as the number of shells increase. The five electron shells shown are labeled K, L, M, N, and O. The K shell possesses the strongest binding power. The electrons in the K shell require the most energy to dislodge from orbit, whereas the electrons in the peripheral shells are easier to displace.

the chemical and electrical properties of the atom. The number of protons in the nucleus establishes how many electrons an atom must have to remain electrically neutral and stable.

Energy Levels

The electrons in atoms are arranged in energy levels or shells in a complex system derived from quantum theory. The shells are labeled K(1), L(2), M(3), N(4), and so on, with the K shell being closest to the nucleus and possessing the greatest binding force (see Fig. 1-3).

The number of shells present in each atom is dependent on the atomic structure of the atom. There is a maximum number of electrons permissible in each shell. Up to 2 electrons are permitted in the K shell, 8 in the L shell, 18 in the M shell, 32 in the N shell, and 50 in the O shell. The number of permissible electrons in a given energy shell can be determined by multiplying the number of the square of the given energy level by 2 and is expressed as $2(N)^2$.

IMPORTANT

Electrons may move or be made to move from one energy shell to another. Whenever a vacancy occurs in an energy shell, movement of an electron to a lower energy shell is almost always accompanied by emission of energy.

Ionization and Excitation of the Atom

An atom in its normal non-ionized state contains an equal number of protons and electrons. If an electrical change occurs in an atom as the result of a gain or loss of an electron, the atom will become ionized. Ionization occurs when an interaction causes a transfer of energy to an orbital electron sufficient to remove the electron from orbit, thereby converting the atom to ions. The removed orbital electron and the atom from which it was displaced are called an *ion pair*. The removed orbital electron is the negative ion, and the atom the positive ion.

There are several interactions of significant importance to radiology that can cause an atom to gain or lose an electron. For example, atoms can be ionized

By electron bombardment of matter
By x-ray bombardment of matter
By reaction with the emissions from radioactive substances
By release of electrons by thermionic emission
By bombardment of specific elements by light
By nuclear capture of a K electron
Chemically

Excitation occurs if, in the interaction with the orbital electron, the electron receives enough energy to move it to a higher energy shell location within the atom. The atom is then raised to an excited stage. An ionized or an excited atom will remain in this state for only a very short period of time. The removed orbital electron of an ionized atom may unite with a neutral atom to form a neutral ion or recombine with a positive atom to form a neutral atom. In an excited atom, the gap in the orbit either is quickly replaced as the original electron returns to the orbit or is replaced by another electron. The original energy acquired by excitation will be released as a single photon of energy.

I M P O R T A N T

If an atom absorbs extra energy this energy can be released as photons of electromagnetic energy, heat, or chemical energy.

These energies are typically photons of electromagnetic energy or light.

Electromagnetic Radiation

Wave and Particle Theories

Electromagnetic energies that are present in space as bundles of electrical and magnetic fields are arranged in nature in an orderly fashion according to the wavelength of their energies.

I M P O R T A N T

When we speak of long and short wavelength in the portion of the x-ray spectrum in which medical x-rays are found, we are limiting our discussion to a range from approximately 0.1 angstrom to 0.5 angstrom (0.01–0.05 nm) (Fig. 1-4).

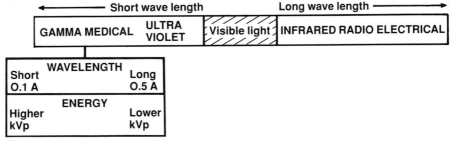

Figure 1-4
The Relationship of Medical X-ray to the Electromagnetic Spectrum
In this abbreviated illustration the electromagnetic spectrum runs from gamma radiation (short wavelength) to electrical waves (long wavelength). Within the medical x-ray portion of the spectrum, wavelengths may be short (0.1 Å) or long (0.5 Å). In the medical x-ray range, a short wavelength will be produced with high kilovoltage values, whereas a long wavelength will be generated by low kilovoltage values.

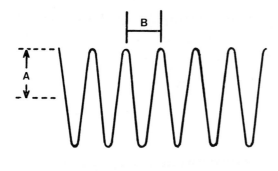

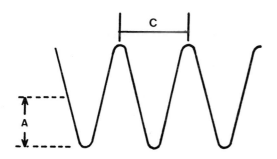

Figure 1-5
Sinewave

Electromagnetic energy is transported through space in the form of sinewave-like oscillations. This energy travels at the speed of light, about 186,300 miles per second, and can be schematically illustrated. Components of the sinewave include amplitude, wavelength, and frequency. Amplitude refers to the height of the wave from crest to mean value (A). Wavelength describes the distance from one crest of the wave to another and represents the distance between two corresponding points on the wave (B and C). Frequency is determined by the number of crests or valleys passing through a specific point in a given time. There are more wavelengths in B compared with C. Shorter wavelengths (B) will result in increased frequency of the wave.

When this energy is transported through space, it is referred to as *electromagnetic radiation* and travels in the form of sinewave-like oscillations at the speed of light (Fig. 1-5).

Electromagnetic radiation includes cosmic rays, gamma rays, x-rays, ultraviolet rays, visible light, infrared rays, radio waves, and electrical field waves.

The sinewave oscillation can be characterized by the following:

1. Amplitude—the height of the wave from crest to average or from valley bottom to average.

2. Wavelength—the distance from one crest to another; the distance between two corresponding points on the wave. Wavelengths in the diagnostic x-ray spectrum are measured in Angstrom units (Å) and are expressed as lambda (λ). An angstrom is equal to 10^{-10} meters.

3. Frequency—the number of crests or valleys passing by a specific point in a given unit of time. It is measured in Hertz (Hz) or cycles per second and expressed as Nu (ν).

The smallest particle of any type of electromagnetic radiation is called a *photon* or a *quantum* and is thought of as a small bundle of energy having no mass and no charge. These particles are radiant energy that has been released from the atom and, like all electromagnetic radiation, travel at the speed of light (Table 1-1). Photon energy can be reduced by transfer to or absorption by an object with which it interacts.

The velocity of a wave can be determined by the formula:

$$\text{Velocity} = \text{frequency} \times \text{wavelength}$$

where the velocity, a constant, equals the speed of light ($C = \lambda\nu$).

The speed of light and other electromagnetic energies is equal to 3×10^8 meters per second or about 186,300 miles per second.

I M P O R T A N T

The energy of the photon emitted from a radiation source is directly proportional to the frequency or inversely proportional to the wavelength of the radiation. Energy is increased with increased frequency and shorter wavelengths.

Production of X-radiation

X-rays are produced when rapidly moving electrons interact with the nucleus of the atoms of the

Table 1-1. X-ray Photon Characteristics

Wavelength	Frequency	Velocity
Short	High	Constant
0.1(Å)–0.5(Å)	10^{18}–10^{21} Hz	3×10^8 meters/sec*

Equal to the speed of light.

anode of the x-ray tube. The x-ray tube is discussed in Chapter 3.

X-rays, discovered by Wilhelm Conrad Roentgen on November 8, 1895, are a part of the electromagnetic spectrum. Professor Roentgen, a physicist, working with a vacuum tube in his darkened laboratory at Würzburg University, Germany, noted that a plate on his workbench coated with barium platinocyanide fluoresced even though it was some distance from a completely covered Crookes' tube. Investigating this phenomenon, Roentgen discovered and recorded several properties of this new ray, which he called "X" because it was previously unknown. The phenomenon recorded by Roentgen had been observed by others but had not been documented or investigated further.

The source of the electrons is the filament (cathode) of the x-ray tube, which, when heated to incandescence, causes electrons to "boil off" in a process known as thermionic emission. The potential difference (voltage) between the terminals of the cathode ($-$) and the anode ($+$) pulls the "free" electrons from the vicinity of the filament across the tube to strike the anode. The electrons' energy is converted into heat and x-ray energy when the electrons strike the anode. The milliampere (mA) setting selects the tube current and determines the heat of the filament and, therefore, the number of "released" electrons available for interaction with the target. The range of the applied voltage (kVp) determines the wavelength and thus the energy of the x-ray photons. X-ray beam intensity is influenced by both mA and kVp.

Electron Interaction with the Anode of the X-ray Tube

When electrons interact with the atoms of the anode of the x-ray tube (Table 1-2), the following occur:

1. More than 99% of the energy is converted to thermal energy (heat). The remaining energy is divided among bremsstrahlung and characteristic radiation. Heat is produced by the energy derived from the movement of the atoms and their quick return to a normal state. The greater the kinetic energy (energy of motion or vibration), the greater the temperature.

2. Production of bremsstrahlung radiation, a braking action, that occurs as the electrons interact with the anode. This process involves electrons that grazingly pass by the heavy nuclei of the metallic atoms in the target material. The attraction between the negatively charged electrons and the positively charged nuclei cause the electrons to be deflected and decelerated from their original path and to lose some of their energies. Since energy cannot be destroyed, the energies lost by the electrons are transformed and emitted as x-ray photons (Fig. 1-6).

   This radiation is known as general radiation, the continuous spectrum, white radiation, or, most commonly, bremsstrahlung radiation.

   The considerable rate of deceleration causes the emission of short wavelength radiation in the form of x-rays. As this braking action var-

Table 1-2. Electron Interaction with the X-ray Target

Action	Effect	Amount
Incident electrons collide with atoms in target	Heat	99% or greater
Electrons approach strong positively charged nucleus	Bremsstrahlung (braking radiation); electron deviated from its path; loses some kinetic energy into equivalent x-ray energy of varying intensities	90% of remaining 1%
Interaction of inner orbital electrons	Characteristic radiation; produces radiation characteristic of the energy level differences of the target atoms	10% of remaining 1%

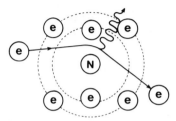

Figure 1-6
Bremsstrahlung Radiation

When an electron moves into the proximity of the nucleus of an atom, the attraction between the negatively charged electron and the positively charged nucleus causes the electron to be deflected from its original path. A "braking" action occurs when the electron collides with the target atom of the x-ray tube. The electron will lose some of its energy. The fact that energy cannot be destroyed results in the lost energy of the electron being transformed to and emitted as an x-ray photon. This radiation is commonly called bremsstrahlung radiation. In German, bremsstrahlung *means "braking radiation."*

ies, so does the intensity of the resultant x-ray energy. In the 80 to 100 kVp range, using a tungsten anode, these bremsstrahlung rays constitute about 90% of the radiation emitted as x-rays.

 Increasing the voltage generates an increased number of x-rays with shorter wavelengths and, therefore, produces a more penetrating beam.

3. Characteristic radiation. Characteristic radiation occurs as electrons emitted from the hot filament collide with the atoms of the target and displace structural electrons from any inner shell of the target atom. Approximately 10% of the radiation emitted at 80 to 100 kVp is characteristic radiation. The incoming electron must be of sufficient strength to dislodge any inner shell electron by overcoming its binding force. Electrons from other shells move in to fill this lower level vacancy. The x-ray photons emitted by this action have wavelengths equal to the differences in energy between the various shells involved in the interaction. The excess energy resulting from the electron transition to a K shell is usually emitted as an x-ray photon (Fig. 1-7). If this interaction occurs in the innermost shell (K), the wavelength of the characteristic radiation is determined by the composition of the target material and the binding power of the K shell over the atoms in the target. For example, to produce characteristic radiation with a tungsten target, at least 70 kVp is required for K-shell interaction, because the K-shell electron of tungsten is held with 69.53 keV (effective kilovoltage).

IMPORTANT

Characteristic radiation can be produced in the production of x-rays when the electrons interact with the target material and can also be produced as a secondary effect when x-rays interact with any matter. Characteristic radiation produced in the interaction of x-rays with matter is usually referred to as secondary radiation and is a form of scatter.

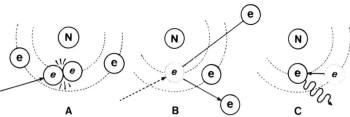

    A   B   C

Figure 1-7
Characteristic Radiation

When an electron is emitted from the cathode of the x-ray tube, and it collides with any inner shell electron of the target atom (A) and overcomes its binding force (B), an electron from another shell will fill this vacancy (C). The x-ray photon generated by this action has wavelengths proportional to the difference in energies of the various shells involved in this interaction (C).

Characteristics of X-rays

The following characteristics of x-ray photons can be demonstrated by experimentation:

Possess no mass

Are electrically neutral

Are invisible

Travel at the speed of light in a vacuum

Cannot be focused by a lens

Are highly penetrating. The degree of penetration depends on the mass density of the object, its chemical composition, and the kilovoltage range and type of x-ray tube filtration used.

Travel in straight lines, in a divergent beam when emanating from a focal point

Produce secondary and scatter radiation when they interact with matter

Can cause certain substances to fluoresce

Can expose photographic or radiographic film

Have an extended diagnostic, medically useful range of wavelengths and energies, from 20 to 30 kVp (long wavelength/low energy for soft tissue studies such as mammography) up to 150 kVp (short wavelength/high energy for latitude imaging techniques such as chest radiography)

Can convert themselves to heat when passing through matter

Can ionize gases and remove orbital electrons from atoms. This is known as ionization.

Can produce biologic changes by means of induced molecular alterations

X-ray Interaction with Matter

The interaction of x-rays with matter is significant in radiology. Every effort must be made to reduce the amount of non-useful ionization of patient tissue by x-ray bombardment. This can be accomplished by the careful use of highly specialized equipment, radiographic accessories, state-of-the-art radiographic techniques, and radiation protection methods.

The following types of x-ray energies are important to diagnostic radiology:

Primary x-rays or photons emitted by the x-ray tube

Scattered x-rays or photons produced when primary photons collide with electrons in matter

Remnant radiation, or the x-rays that pass through the patient, striking the image detector

When x-rays pass through matter, the interactions continue until the primary energy and the energies of the secondary and characteristic radiation are spent. Theoretically, there are many possible x-ray interactions with matter, five of which are usually described in x-ray physics textbooks (Table 1-3).

Table 1-3. X-ray Photon Interaction with Matter

Energy Range	Where	X-ray Photon (wavelength, direction)	Effect
Low	Interacts with target atom	No change	Classical scattering (Thompson, coherent)
Moderate	Interacts with inner shell electron, which is quickly absorbed	X-ray absorbed; generally not scattered	Photoelectric effect—absorption of x-ray; production of photoelectron. The photoelectric effect is responsible for differential absorption. Secondary effect—characteristic radiation also produced
Moderate	Interacts with outer shell electron	Change in direction with reduced energy	Compton effect—ionizes atom, produces scatter radiation
High (E > 1.1 MeV)	Incoming photon in the vicinity of the nucleus	Photon disappears	Pair production—positive and negative electrons are created from the energy transformation
High	Photon escapes electron interaction	Absorbed by nucleus	Photodisintegration; nuclear fragments emitted; great variety available

I M P O R T A N T: *Only photoelectric effect and Compton effect are significant in the production of diagnostic radiographic images.*

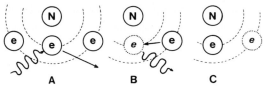

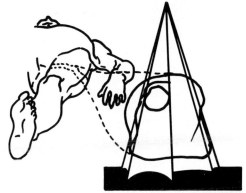

Figure 1-8
Photoelectric Effect

(A) When an inner shell electron of an atom is struck by an x-ray photon, the photon may give off all of its energy. This photon collision causes photoelectric effect (absorption). The electron struck by the x-ray photon is emitted as a photoelectron and is quickly absorbed. (B) The electron ejected as a photoelectron is quickly replaced by another electron from any outer shell or any "free" electron. The x-ray energy (characteristic radiation, a secondary effect) emitted is determined by the binding energies of the shells participating in this event. (C) The vacancy created in the outer shell by the movement of an electron to fill the inner shell results in an atom with a deficiency of one electron (ionized).

Figure 1-9
Differential Absorption

There are five basic medical radiographic densities: air, fat, water (soft tissue), bone, and metal. Air, a negative contrast agent, is the most radiolucent and will result in the blackest image. Bone, metal, or positive contrast agents absorb all or most of the x-radiation and are seen as lighter radiographic densities.

Any interaction depends on the x-ray photon energy and the atomic number (Z) of the absorber.

Two x-ray interactions with matter that are of significant importance in the production of radiographic images are listed:

1. Photoelectric effect (absorption). When the x-ray photon collides with the inner shell electron of an atom, the photon may give off all of its energy, and the collision causes the photoelectric effect along with ionization. The photoelectric effect occurs mainly when low to moderate x-ray energies interact with high atomic absorbers such as bone or barium. The x-ray image results from the radiation being absorbed totally, partially, or not at all. This effect is known as *differential absorption* and is a contributing factor to contrast on the recorded image (Figs. 1-8 and 1-9).

2. Compton effect (scatter). If the incoming x-ray photon has increased energy, resulting from increased kilovoltage applied to the x-ray tube,

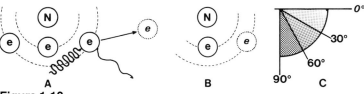

Figure 1-10
Compton Effect

When the kilovoltage value is increased, the incoming x-ray photon has increased energy. (A) This photon can strike an electron in an outer shell and be deviated from its original path with a reduction in energy. The photon (x-ray) will then travel in a different direction, but with less energy (Compton effect). The process can be multiplied if the incident photon retains part of its energy and the remaining energy becomes a recoil electron. This interaction is called Compton effect of scattering, and many secondary collisions may occur with additional Compton and recoil electrons being generated. (B) If the incoming photon is of sufficient energy to dislodge the electron, in addition to giving up some of the photon energy, the recoiled (ejected) electron causes a vacancy in the outer shell and the atom becomes unstable (ionized). (C) Energy decreases as the deflection angle of the scattered photon increases.

the x-ray photon as it strikes an electron gives up part of its energy and is deviated from its original path with a reduction in energy. Part of the incident x-ray energy is retained, and the remaining energy goes to a recoil electron as kinetic energy. This interaction is called *Compton effect*, or scattering. The scattered photons may have other secondary collisions and eject more Compton or recoil electrons until their energy is finally spent (Fig. 1-10).

Photons are scattered, in all directions, at low energies, with the most scattering occurring in a forward direction at high energies. With an increase in kVp, the production of scatter radiation rapidly increases.

The scattered photons retain most of their energy and frequently reach the film screen system, producing mostly undesirable supplemental radiographic densities.

In the diagnostic energy range, Compton scattering is the most common type of x-ray interaction with matter.

IMPORTANT

To produce a quality radiograph, scatter radiation must be controlled by the radiographer.

Production and control of scatter radiation is discussed in Chapter 5.

Basic Components of an X-ray Generating System

Electrical energy conversion into electromagnetic energy occurs in the x-ray generator and tube system. The radiographer should be aware of the basic components and functions of these systems, since the function of the x-ray circuitry and the application of the technical factors of kilovoltage, milliamperage, and time are closely interrelated. In this chapter, electrical and magnetic principles are reviewed in a simplified manner. Schematics of a typical x-ray circuit are presented as an aid to understanding what occurs when technical factor selections are made.

Basic Components of an X-ray Generating System

Electromagnetics

Electromagnetics entails the physical relations between electricity and magnetism.

Electrical charges may be static (at rest) or dynamic (in motion). Electrical current is always surrounded by a magnetic field, which exists only while the current is flowing. By the process of electromagnetic induction, current can be induced in a second wire if the wires cut through the magnetic field lines produced by an electrical current. Since both coils are not electrically connected, placing a second coil of wire adjacent to the first coil induces an electrical current in the second coil by mutual induction. The force in the second wire loop is directly proportional to the number of turns in the first wire loop.

When the wire of a conductor is coiled, a helix is formed. A helix with current flowing through it is called a *solenoid*. The solenoid, an electromagnet, has a strong magnetic field in its center when current is flowing through the coiled wire.

Angeline M. Cullinan and John E. Cullinan:
PRODUCING QUALITY RADIOGRAPHS, 2ND ED.
© 1987, 1994 J. B. Lippincott Company.

Electrical Current

There are two basic types of current alternating and direct current.

Alternating current of sinusoidal waveshape results from the application of an alternating voltage with its polarity and values reversing direction at regularly occurring intervals, typically 60 times per second (60 Hz) in the United States (Fig. 2-1). Electrical energy in the form of voltage and amperage is usually supplied by commercial power companies and delivered as alternating current, because it is easier to produce and transfer from place to place in this form. Alternating current can be greatly increased or decreased by employing a simple device called a transformer (see Transformers).

Direct current may be steady or may be intermittent. The direction of flow does not change with direct current.

Electrical Circuits

An electrical circuit is used to gather, carry, or use flowing electron energy. Electrical energy is carried through the circuit by electrical current (electrons in motion). The measurement of the amount of electrons flowing from the source is called *amperage*, or the number of electrons per unit of cross-sectional area.

A circuit must have the following:

1. A source of electrical power capable of doing work. Electrical energy can be stored for future use in condenser plates or capacitor discharge devices. Batteries can also be a source of electrical current, converting chemical energy to electrical energy.
2. Ability to use the electrical energy to perform work. An electromotive force (EMF) causes the electrons to flow in a particular direction along the surface of a conductor. The EMF is defined and measured between two points or terminals by a unit known as the *volt*. Often the terms *potential difference* or *voltage* are substituted for the term electromotive force. Potential difference exists because there is an excess of electrons maintained at one end of the conductor and a deficiency of electrons at the opposite end. This situation makes electrons available for flow whenever a voltage drop is put across the material.

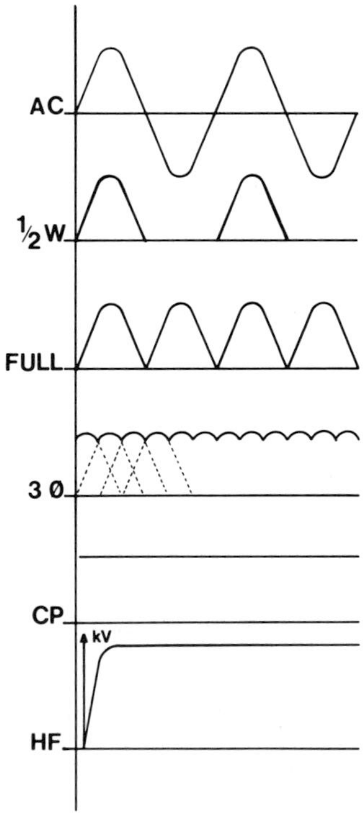

Figure 2-1
Waveforms

Alternating (oscillating) current is the electrical energy form supplied by commerical power companies. Alternating current (AC) is depicted as a sinusoidal wave shape. Alternating current reverses its polarity at regularly occurring intervals—typically, 60 times per second (60 Hz) in the United States.

Since only the positive impulses of an alternating current can be stepped up to kilovoltage for use in a radiographic tube, the negative impulses must be suppressed or rectified in some manner. Half-wave rectification (½W) uses the x-ray tube as a rectifying source to suppress the negative impulse of the alternating current. Full-wave rectification uses four rectifiers and converts negative impulses to positive impulses to produce 120 positive impulses per second. The alternating current is changed to direct current. When three separate but interconnected power sources are used instead of a single source of electrical current, three-phase (3Ø) current is supplied. Multiphase generators use either 6 or 12 rectifiers to convert three-phase current into almost ripple-free direct current. High frequency is almost ripple-free, similar to 3 Ø (12 rectifiers) current. Constant potential has 0% ripple.

Voltage is measured with an instrument called a voltmeter. In radiography, high voltage is measured in terms of kilovoltage, where 1 kV = 1000 volts.

3. A path to carry the electron flow from the source to where it will be used (load). When a conductor is made into an uninterrupted, closed path, a circuit is formed and electrical current will flow. A simple electrical circuit carries current in a closed path and must possess the following:

   a. Potential difference, measured in volts (V) from start to end of path

   b. Current (I) or electron flow, measured in amperes (A). There is resistance (opposition) to the electron flow in all circuits, with some absorption and thus loss of energy. Current must overcome the opposing force of resistance. Resistance comes about from the impeding effects of conductor atoms to the flow of the electrons. An ammeter is used to measure current. Small amounts of electrical current are measured in milliamperes (1/1000 of an ampere).

   c. Electrical resistance (R), measured in ohms (Ω). The term resistance is used in reference to a simple direct current. Impedance denotes resistance in alternating current. The resistance of a conductor is directly proportional to the resistivity of the material of which the conductor is formed. Resistance is also directly proportional to the length of the conductor, but inversely proportional to the width (cross-sectional area) of the conductor.

   Resistance is also affected by changes in temperature of the conductor. Resistance is inherent in all conductors at normal temperatures. Some materials are good conductors and will conduct when they receive even a small amount of energy. Some materials are able to conduct only when they receive a specific increment of energy; these are known as semiconductors. Some materials do not conduct and are thus referred to as insulators.

   Resistance is the cause of a conductor heating up when in use. Superconductors lose all their resistance at very low temperatures, close to absolute zero. Rheostats are controls used to add resistance to the circuit in order to adjust incoming voltage and amperage values. The relation of voltage and amperage to resistance can be expressed by Ohm's law, which states that

$$I = \frac{V}{R}$$

where I = amperage, V = voltage, and R = resistance.

A break in the circuit can be achieved with switches that are used to control the length of time that the current may flow. Fuses or circuit breakers are protective devices that open at preset levels of current and thus prevent circuit overloading and damage.

Types of Electrical Circuits

Current flows from one terminal to another in a simple circuit. In all circuits, at any given time, the current arriving at a given point in the circuit is equal to that leaving the given point.

When current flows through several components or terminals, these components can be arranged in a series or in a parallel fashion. In a series circuit, the current will pass consecutively through each individual component and can be expressed as $I = i^1 = i^2 = i^3$. With a parallel circuit, current flow is divided among the branches of the circuit and is expressed as $I = i^1 + i^2 + i^3$.

Some other circuit arrangements include combinations of series, parallel, or more complex configurations of Delta and star (Wye) patterns.

The X-ray Circuit

X-ray circuits using complex electrical and magnetic principles produce x-radiation suitable for diagnostic purposes. The x-ray circuit is divided into subsections called primary (low voltage) and secondary (high voltage) circuits (Figs. 2-2 and 2-3).

The primary circuit consists of the following:

1. The main switch. Power from an electrical source is turned off and on at this point.
2. A line voltage compensator. This is used to compensate for variations in power supply. It is important to monitor the incoming line voltage. Line voltage compensation is automatic in some units.
3. Fuses or circuit breakers. These are used to prevent equipment overload or tube damage.

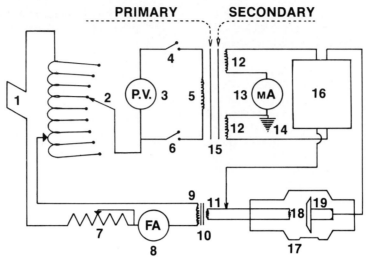

Figure 2-2
X-ray Generating System

The x-ray generating circuit is divided into a primary (low-voltage) and secondary (high-voltage) circuit. The primary circuit consists of (1) a main switch, (2) an autotransformer, (3) a prereading voltmeter, (4) fuses or circuit breakers, (5) the primary coil of the step-up transformer, (6) a timer that includes exposure switches, (7) a filament circuit and rheostat, used to vary current to the primary circuit of a step-down transformer to illuminate the filament of the x-ray tube, (8) filament ammeter, (9) the primary coil of the step-down transformer, (10) the step-down transformer, and (11) the secondary coil of the step-down transformer.

The secondary or high-voltage circuit consists of (12) the secondary of the step-up transformer, (13) an mA meter, (14) ground, (15) step-up transformer, (16) a rectification system, (17) the x-ray tube, (18) cathode of the x-ray tube, and (19) anode of the x-ray tube, including shockproof grounded cables to conduct high voltage from the secondary of the step-up transformer to the tube. The rectification schematic of this x-ray circuit can be found in Figure 2-7. The circuit is also displayed above the control panel in Figure 2-14. Solid state rectifiers are used to illustrate the rectification segment, since valve tubes (vacuum tubes with illuminated filaments) are no longer in common use. Valve tubes require step-down transformers.

4. An autotransformer. This is used to control voltage supplied to the primary of the step-up transformer, to allow for minimal variations in kilovoltage selection.
5. A pre-reading voltmeter. This indicates the amount of voltage being sent to the primary of the step-up transformer (Table 2-1). Kilovoltage is determined by the amount of voltage supplied to the step-up transformer and is present only when the exposure is being made. The kilovoltage value selected is indicated on the control panel.
6. Timer and exposure switches. Timers are used

Table 2-1. Voltage to Kilovoltage

Pre-reading Voltmeter	1:700 Step-Up Transformer	1:1000 Step-Up Transformer
50 V	35 kVp	50 kVp
80 V	56 kVp	80 kVp
100 V	70 kVp	100 kVp
120 V	84 kVp	120 kVp

Note: A pre-reading voltmeter displays the voltage selected by means of the autotransformer to be sent to the primary of the step-up transformer during the x-ray exposure. The voltage is stepped up to a kilovoltage value as determined by the ratio of the transformer.

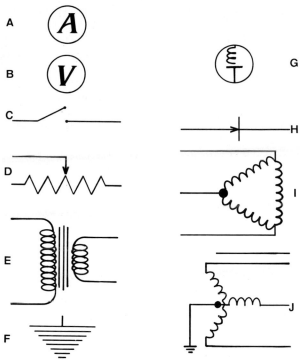

Figure 2-3
Schematic Representation of X-ray Circuit
Components

(A) The filament ammeter is usually designated in the circuit by a circular meter containing the symbol A. (B) A voltmeter is similarly indicated by the symbol V. (C) A circuit breaker or a timer is often represented as an open-ended switch. (D) A rheostat is used to vary electrical current to the primary circuit of the step-down transformer. (E) The step-down transformer shown has more turns in the coils of the primary than in the secondary windings. (F) The universal symbol for ground. (G) Vacuum tubes that contain a filament and flat anode can be used for rectification of alternating current to direct current. (H) A solid state rectifier.

Three-phase transformers used for three-phase equipment generate a more homogenous x-ray beam. Three separate circuits are required in an x-ray machine using three-phase power, one for each phase. Each circuit requires its own transformer, rectifiers, line voltage compensator, and so on. In the high-tension transformer the primary coils are wound around separate arms of a core common to all three transformers. (I) A "Delta" configuration depicts this arrangement of the coils. (J) The secondary high-tension coils have a common center, each coil radiating outward in a star ("Wye") pattern. (See Fig. 2-4.)

for manual or automatic exposure control. The timer is situated between the autotransformer and the primary of the step-up transformer.

7. A filament circuit. This provides thermal energy for the heating of the filament of the x-ray tube. A step-down transformer is used in the filament circuit (see Fig. 2-3E) . The filament circuit carries the relatively high amperage needed to heat the filament to produce thermionic emission. Resistance in the filament circuitry is varied by rheostats. These resistors can be used to vary the amount of current (milliamperage) so that the heating of the filament can be controlled.

8. A filament ammeter. This is used to measure filament current.

9. The primary coil of the step-up transformer. The step-up transformer is a part of both the low-voltage circuit and the high-voltage circuit. The primary of the step-up transformer is in the low-voltage circuit, whereas the secondary of the step-up transformer is located in the high-voltage circuit. The high-voltage transformer steps up the voltage from the autotransformer (Fig. 2-4).

The secondary or high-voltage circuit consists of:

1. The secondary coil of the step-up transformer, which is "center-tapped" to allow an mA meter to be installed at ground potential. In this center-tapped position, the mA meter can measure the actual current flowing through the x-ray tube (see Fig. 2-2). (See Transformers.)
2. The mA meter, used to measure tube current
3. A milliampere-second (mAs) meter, used to measure mAs values at short time intervals
4. Rectifiers. The x-ray tube is most efficient when unidirectional high-voltage current is used. Current is made unidirectional for use by the x-ray tube by means of a rectification system, which converts alternating current to direct current (DC), (see Fig. 2-3G,H). (See Rectifiers.)
5. Shockproof, grounded cables, which conduct high-voltage current from the secondary of the step-up transformer to the x-ray tube
6. The x-ray tube (described in Chapter 3)

Transformers

Transformers require alternating current for their operation. When alternating current is applied to one coil of a transformer, it induces a changing magnetic field within the iron core. This, in turn, induces an alternating current in the second coil. A transformer does not produce energy; it transforms voltage and current by way of the ratios of their respective windings (Fig. 2-5). A transformer can be used to increase or decrease the voltage of alternating current.

There are several types of transformers:

AIR CORE TRANSFORMER. By placing a coil of wire with current flowing through it, called a solenoid, adjacent to a second coil of wire, an air core transformer is formed. This is the simplest type of transformer.

OPEN CORE TRANSFORMER. To form an open core transformer, soft iron bars are placed in both the primary and secondary coils. The cores are not electrically connected; they only conduct field lines.

CLOSED CORE TRANSFORMER. A continuous laminated iron bar forming a rectangular annulus is used to support the primary and secondary windings in a closed core transformer. Again, there are no electrical connections between the coils.

SHELL CORE TRANSFORMER. A continuous laminated iron bar forming a rectangular figure-eight, with the primary and secondary wires wound around the center support, is called a shell core transformer.

STEP-UP TRANSFORMER. A ratio exists between the primary and secondary currents and is related to the number of turns in the wires in the individual coils. If the number of turns in the wire of the secondary coil exceed the number of turns in the wire of the primary coil, the transformer becomes a step-up transformer and voltage will be increased (see Fig. 2-4).

STEP-DOWN TRANSFORMER. If more turns exist in the wire of the primary coil than in that of the secondary coil, the transformer becomes a step-down transformer and voltage will be reduced (see Fig. 2-4). The filament circuit uses a step-down transformer.

AUTOTRANSFORMER. An autotransformer is easy to recognize in a circuit schematic. The primary and secondary windings of the autotransformer are connected in series with no electrical insulation between the primary and secondary sides. A large number of contacts (taps) are attached to the different turns of the transformer. Voltage is changed to kilovoltage by a step-up transformer, which operates on the principle of mutual induction to change the voltage ratio. Voltage values are taken from these taps to be sup-

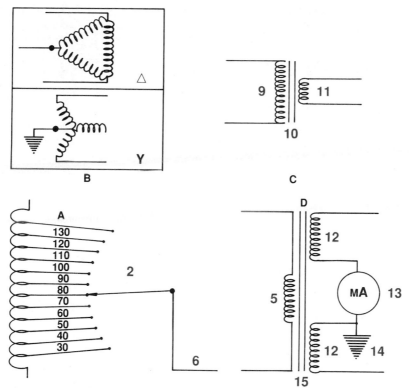

Figure 2-4
Schematic Representation of X-ray Circuit Transformers

The numerical designations are the same as those used in Figure 2-2. (A) A single coil with primary and secondary windings is required for an autotransformer (2). When kilovoltage is selected for a specific technique, differing amounts of primary voltage (30–130 volts in this illustration) are tapped from the contacts of the autotransformer. Each tap can provide a specific primary voltage to be sent to the primary of the step-up transformer (5) through the timer (6) where the voltage will be stepped up to a preselected kilovoltage level (see Table 2-1). Although kilovoltage selection is made on the primary side of the high-voltage transformer (5), kilovoltage is only produced during the actual x-ray exposure. (B) "Delta" and "star" (Wye) transformer windings are used with three-phase circuits. (C) A step-down transformer (10) is used to supply the voltage to the filament of the x-ray tube. This independent transformer steps down the preselected amount of current needed to illuminate the filament of the x-ray tube. A rheostat is used to vary the current to the primary of the step-down transformer (9) so that mA values can be adjusted for various radiographic techniques. In practice, multiple rheostats are included in the filament circuit to accommodate various mA settings. (D) The high-voltage, step-up transformer (15) steps up the voltage selected from the autotransformer (2 in A) to the required kilovoltage needed to generate x-radiation (see Table 2-1). The secondary of the high-voltage transformer (12) is center-tapped. One half of the voltage is generated by the upper portion of the high-voltage transformer and the remaining half by the lower portion. Because of this arrangement, an mA meter (13) can be maintained at near ground potential (14), making it possible to measure the actual current flowing through the x-ray tube.

The relationship of the transformers to the x-ray circuit can be better appreciated in Figures 2-2 and 2-14.

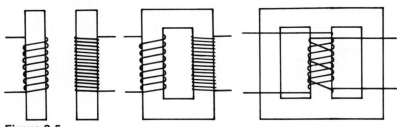

Figure 2-5
Transformer Types

(Left) Soft iron bars placed in both the primary and secondary coils form an open core transformer. The cores conduct field lines but are not electrically connected. (Center) A continuous laminated iron bar in the form of a rectangular annulus is used to support the primary and secondary windings of a closed core transformer. There are no electrical connections between the coils. This type of closed core transformer is commonly used in x-ray generating equipment. (Right) A continuous laminated iron bar that forms a rectangular figure-eight with the primary and secondary wires wound around the center support is called a shell core transformer.

plied to the primary of the step-up transformer (see Fig. 2-4, Table 2-1).

Three-phase equipment requires special transformer windings to accommodate three separate sources of alternating current. The primary circuit is triplicated: three autotransformers, three primary circuits to the autotransformers, and so on (see Fig. 2-3*I,J*).

There is some power loss in a transformer. Some types of power losses include:

Copper losses, arising from inherent resistance in the wire

Eddy current losses—heat losses resulting from swirling currents in the transformer core (solid iron bar). A laminated silicon steel sheet core will reduce eddy current loss.

Hysteresis losses. As the magnetic field constantly changes direction, it is physically impossible for the core's magnetic domain to continually align itself with the magnetic field. Hysteresis loss is the power lost in an attempt to resist the changes in magnetism.

A concise description of transformers can be found in *Practitioner Educational Package: Transformers and Autotransformers*, published by the American Society of Radiologic Technologists, Albuquerque, New Mexico.

X-ray Generators

X-ray generator ratings determine the maximal voltage and electrical power permissible with a specific unit. Voltage requirements are specified by the equipment manufacturer as to the power needed at the generator terminals. Types of generators include the following:

SINGLE-PHASE GENERATORS. An x-ray generator using electrical current from a commercial power source transforms this energy into milliamperage and kilovoltage values. A single source of power is known as a single-phase (S $\varnothing$) supply.

The x-ray generator must be capable of producing very short exposure times.

MULTIPHASE GENERATORS. Three separate but interconnected power sources produce a three-phase (3 $\varnothing$) supply (see Fig. 2-1). Multiphase generators use either 6 or 12 rectifiers with three-phase current to provide higher radiation output over a given time frame when compared with single-phase current (Fig. 2-6). Three-phase equipment, 6-pulse rectification, has an approximate 13.5% ripple factor, whereas a 12-pulse, multiphase unit has less than a 5% ripple factor and is almost ripple free (see Fig. 2-1).

The use of three-phase generators results in the following benefits:

Short exposures can be used with a significant increase in "film blackening" in a given time frame, since up to a twofold increase in film blackening occurs when compared with single-phase equipment. Shorter exposure times can be of value in angiographic procedures or when examining uncooperative patients. With three-phase equipment, there is a more even thermal loading of the x-ray tube when compared with the fluctuation or ripple of single-phase exposures.

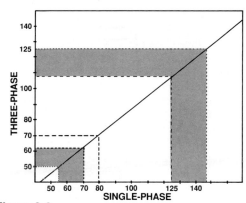

Figure 2-6
Kilovoltage Conversion,
Single-Phase to Three-Phase

When making technique conversions from single-phase to three-phase equipment, changes in kVp settings are usually needed to obtain similar radiographic results, since three-phase x-radiation is almost ripple-free when compared with single-phase x-ray (100% ripple). To match radiographic densities, kilovoltage values must be adjusted.

With higher kilovoltage levels, such as those used for chest radiography, three-phase 125 kVp (fine dotted line) must be raised to 147 kVp, single-phase. Single-phase 125 kVp (dashed line) must be lowered to 108 kVp, three-phase, for comparable densities.

When lower kilovoltage values are used, such as those used for osseous studies, three-phase 70 kVp (dashed line) must be raised to 80 kVp, single-phase (fine dashed line). Single-phase 70 kVp must be lowered to 62 kVp, three-phase, for comparable densities. Note that in the moderate kVp range, an approximate 10 kVp difference exists between current phases; in the high kilovoltage range there is a difference of more than 20 kVp.

A similar radiographic density can be obtained with 50 kVp three-phase and 55 kVp single-phase (dotted line).

If the kilovoltage values are adjusted as shown, comparable contrast is also maintained.

Less heating of the x-ray tube, thereby increasing the instantaneous tube rating
Higher effective kilovoltage when compared with that of single-phase generators (Table 2-2 and Fig. 2-6)

FALLING LOAD GENERATORS. With a falling load generator, for any given exposure, a very high milliampere value is initially applied to the x-ray tube. During the exposure, the mA is automatically reduced to avoid overheating of the anode.

Falling load generators are used with an automatic exposure device (AED).

Since the falling load generator starts the exposure with the maximal mA permitted, this level can be maintained for only a short time. If the needed mAs is not achieved, the mA is automatically reduced to lower levels until the predetermined AED exposure level has been reached.

HIGH FREQUENCY GENERATORS. Some high frequency generators operate at 7 to 30 kilohertz (kHz) (see Fig. 2-1). Newer units function at 100 kHz. At 100 kHz these generators produce twice the output of conventional x-ray generators. Exposure times are reduced by as much as 40%. Images produced with high frequency equipment are similar in radiographic contrast to those produced with three-phase equipment. Some high-frequency generators work on 110-volt current, eliminating the need for heavy duty 220-volt or three-phase power lines. High-frequency generators that do not require the large transformers and high capacity lines of low impedance make it possible to use this type of equipment in mobile vans and facilities with low power sources.

Constant potential represents a ripple-free current. Three-phase (12-pulse) current approaches constant potential (see Fig. 2-1).

CAPACITOR DISCHARGE GENERATORS. The capacitors are charged in parallel at low voltages and connected in series to place a high voltage across the x-ray tube. Capacitor discharge x-ray generators lose approximately one kVp for every mAs used during the exposure. These systems can be easily used in mobile units since they do not require a heavy duty transformer.

Note that x-ray tube ratings must be matched to the power output of the generator. X-ray tube rating charts used to determine total heat units

Table 2-2. Single vs. Three-Phase Kilovoltage: Comparison of Peak and Average (Effective) Values

Phase	Peak	Average
Single		
2 impulses per sec	100 kVp	70.7 kV (KeV)
Three		
6 impulses per sec	100 kVp	95.6 kV (KeV)
12 impulses per sec	100 kVp	98.9 kV (KeV)

Note the difference in peak vs. average (effective) kilovoltage between single- and three-phase output. For the same kilovoltage setting, three-phase generators will produce greater film blackening as well as longer scale contrast. Single-phase generators produce less density and a shorter scale of contrast. Technical factors must be adjusted when uniform (room-to-room) density and contrast are desired.

and instantaneous load characteristics of the x-ray tube are described in Chapter 3.

Rectifiers

Rectification changes alternating current from the secondary of a step-up transformer into direct current (Fig. 2-7).

In a single-phase cycle (60-Hz current) the voltage varies from zero to the maximal kVp selected. Using single-phase alternating current, every positive impulse produces x-radiation. When the tube current is in the negative phase, electrons cannot flow from cathode to anode; therefore, x-rays cannot be produced (see Fig. 2-1).

A single-phase, single-pulse x-ray generator can use the x-ray tube to suppress the inverse half cycle (negative impulse) of current, resulting in half-wave self-rectification. In this situation, the x-ray tube functions as the rectifier; it controls when electrons can flow from cathode to anode.

From one to four rectifiers are used in single-phase x-ray units. A single rectifier can be placed in the circuit to avoid using the x-ray tube as a rectifier, also resulting in half-wave rectification.

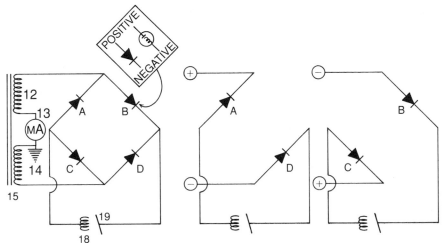

Figure 2-7
Schematic Representation of a Full-Wave Rectification System
The numerical designations are the same as those used in Figure 2-2.

(Left) A typical full-wave rectification system is shown. The rectifiers are labeled A, B, C, and D. Rectification occurs on the secondary side of the step-up transformer (12). Electrons must flow from cathode (18) to anode (19) through the x-ray tube. The alternating current used with a transformer changes polarity at regular intervals. Rectifiers are used to change alternating current into direct current. (Center) Current flows from the secondary of the step-up transformer (12) through A to the cathode and anode to D. In this time frame, the first half of the alternating cycle is completed. (Right) The current then goes through the second half of the cycle. Polarity reverses and current then flows from the secondary of the step-up transformer (12) to C through the cathode and anode to B, and so on.

Low-output generators often use a half-wave rectification system where the "negative" portion of the wave is suppressed (see Fig. 2-1). When a full-wave rectification system is used, the anode (19) is positive in relationship to the cathode (18) throughout the entire exposure.

Vacuum tube rectifiers (see Fig. 2-3G) were in common use for many years. A step-down transformer is required to illuminate their filaments. Most rectification systems now use solid state semiconductors, made either from selenium or silicon (see Fig. 2-3 H), which has an inherent low resistance to the flow of current in one direction and a higher resistance to current flow in the reverse direction. Three-phase systems require 6 or 12 rectifiers. When three-phase current is used with 12 rectifiers, 12 impulses per cycle are produced. The resultant current is almost ripple-free (see Fig. 2-1).

A full-wave rectification system uses both pulses of the cycle (+ and −). Converting the negative pulse to a positive pulse results in 120 positive pulses per second (see Fig. 2-1). With full-wave rectification, the anode remains positive in relation to the cathode throughout the entire exposure (see Fig. 2-7).

IMPORTANT

Full-wave rectification occurs only when four rectifiers are interconnected and operating complementarily in the circuit. If only one rectifier fails to function, rectification would be half-wave.

When current is rectified with a single-phase generator, the current output fluctuates from a zero point of the wave to a maximal peak and returns to zero. This fluctuation in output is called *ripple* (the percentage of difference from maximal voltage to the minimal voltage). When using single-phase equipment, a ripple of 100% occurs (see Fig. 2-1).

Valve tubes, or thermionic diode tubes, which permit current flow from cathode to anode, are rarely used in modern x-ray equipment. The filaments of valve tubes (see Fig. 2-3G) require a step down transformer.

Solid state rectifiers made of silicon or selenium are used in most radiographic equipment. Unlike valve tubes, silicon and selenium rectifiers do not require a power supply or filament transformer for their operation. Solid state rectifiers (semiconductors) have an inherently low resistance to the flow of current in one direction but can be made to strongly resist current flow in the reverse direction.

Specially doped silicon chips are classified into two types, P and N (+ or −), to form semiconductors. When placed in close proximity to each other, a P–N junction exists. When no external voltage is applied, there is practically no flow of current. When forward voltage is applied (1/2 of AC current cycle), there is a large forward current flow (forward bias). When a negative voltage cycle is applied, there is a very small reverse current flow (reverse bias).

Timers

A timer is used to initiate and terminate an x-ray exposure. Exposure timers include the spring-

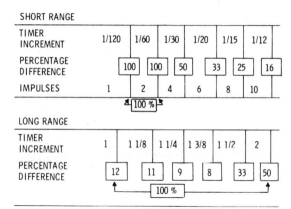

Figure 2-8
Timer Increment Variations
Many radiographic timers do not have sufficient increment steps, particularly in the ultra-short exposure range. A 100% change in exposure value is common (1/120th to 1/60th of a second) between steps. A single-step adjustment in time can result in 100% increase in exposure and doubling of film density (top). Timer increment values above 1/2 second are not as critical (bottom).

driven mechanical timer (limited to 1/10th of a second or longer), the synchronous or motor-driven timer (usually not reliable for exposures shorter than 1/20th of a second and thus not in common use), and electronic or impulse timers. Most electronic timers operate at 1/120th of a second or less.

Timer increment settings, while seemingly even spaced, can be erratic; variations as great as 100% can exist between timer increments (Fig. 2-8). A typical timer increment on a standard impulse timer varies from 1/120th of a second (one impulse) to 1/60th of a second (two impulses)—a difference of 100%.

The x-ray timer control can indicate elapsed time, but elapsed time does not always signify radiation output (see Fig. 2-1). With 12-pulse or high-frequency generators, radiation output and the length of the exposure (elapsed time) are almost identical.

Automatic Exposure Devices

An automatic exposure device (AED) should help to ensure the radiographer of exposures of consistent density. In theory, an AED eliminates the need to measure part thickness or to calculate milliampere-second values. Many automatic exposure technique charts use fixed kilovoltage values.

The exposure is initiated by the radiographer. The AED controls the length of exposure, which is affected by kilovoltage, milliamperage, focal film distance, and the size of the patient. Positioning skills are essential. Knowledge of surface anatomy and the relation of one organ to another help to avoid body part/sensor misalignment. The correct sensor must be selected for specific body parts (Fig. 2-9).

Characteristics and Action

The phototimer consists of a highly light-sensitive phototube, optically and electrically connected to a fluorescent pick-up screen. A signal to the photomultiplier tube is amplified by an associated electrical circuit and terminates the radiographic exposure when a predetermined quantity of fluorescent light has reached the photocell.

Another type of automatic timer uses an ionization chamber to detect ionization in the air produced by the x-ray beam. When a preselected quantity of charge has been collected, the exposure is automatically terminated by a complex electronic circuit.

An AED can be installed in front (entrance) or behind (exit) the grid in either the table or upright Bucky. Ion chambers are generally located in front of the cassette (Fig. 2-10).

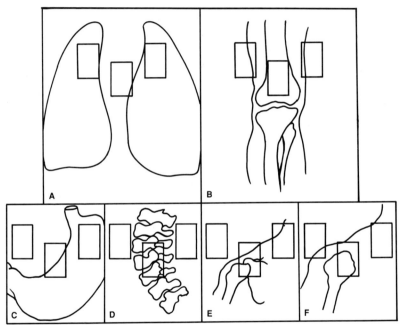

Figure 2-9
Automatic Exposure Device: Sensor Centering

The sensor of an automatic exposure device (AED) must be properly centered to the part under study to achieve a predetermined film density. Over- or underexposed images can result if a patient is not properly centered to the pick-up screen (fluorescent screen, or ionization sensor) (1). Ionization chamber sensors usually use three detectors (see Fig. 2-10 for sensor locations). Improper centering to the detectors negates the effectiveness of the AED.

(A) For a posteroanterior chest film, either lateral sensor can be used. (B) The central sensor is required for the knee in the anteroposterior position. (C) It is difficult to select a sensor for the barium-filled stomach. The lateral sensor, over the fundus, could result in an overexposed image. (D) A central sensor should result in proper exposure of the lumbar spine in the lateral position. (E) None of the sensors are properly positioned for the shoulder, and an underexposed radiograph should result. (F) The central sensor should be selected for proper exposure of the shoulder.

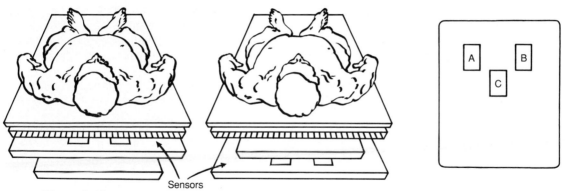

Sensors

Figure 2-10
Automatic Exposure Device: Sensor Placement

Two different types of AED sensor placements are shown. On the left, *the sensor is positioned beneath the grid but above the cassette (entrance-type sensor). In the* center, *the sensor is positioned beneath the grid and the cassette (exit-type sensor). The x-ray beam must pass through both the grid and the back of the cassette to strike this sensor. The use of metal strap-type cassettes with an exit sensor can result in overexposed radiographs. If the straps are inadvertently positioned over the AED, remnant radiation may be absorbed by the straps, resulting in a longer exposure time than is desired.*

A typical illustration of the sensor configurations used for automatically exposed studies is shown on the right. *See Figure 2-14 for control panel sensor selection options.*

Conventional radiographic cassettes have a sheet of lead foil behind the posterior intensifying screen to absorb backscatter. Phototimer cassettes were originally designed without lead foil to avoid problems with exit-type sensors. In practice, most cassettes contain posterior lead foil sheeting, and phototimers are appropriately adjusted.

A problem may result from using older style cassettes that have dense metallic closure straps in combination with the exit-type detectors. If the straps are inadvertently positioned over the phototimer pick-up cell, remnant radiation may be absorbed by the straps, resulting in longer exposure times and, therefore, overexposed radiographs (see Fig. 2-10).

The radiographer should be aware of other conditions that might cause an AED to malfunction:

If a patient is positioned for a table Bucky radiograph and the chest x-ray sensor is energized in error, the x-ray beam will exit from the radiographic tube through the patient to the table AED. Since the table Bucky sensor is not energized, the x-ray tube will give off x-radiation until the radiographer realizes the error or until the x-ray tube is destroyed (see Back-Up Time).

The reverse situation could occur—the patient is positioned for chest radiography and the table Bucky sensor is activated in error. In either situation, the patient receives unnecessary radiation.

If the AED is used for a cross-table, horizontal beam technique, the AED sensor is not able to terminate the exposure since the sensor is located beneath the x-ray table or in the upright cassette holder.

If a patient is protected with a lead shield or if sandbags are used to support an injured limb, and if the sensor is covered by these accessories, the exposure might not terminate properly.

A primary beam leak can undercut the image, causing the premature termination of the exposure (Fig. 2-11). Image undercutting is described in Chapter 5.

Two important principles associated with automatic exposure controls are minimal response time and back-up time.

Minimal Response Time

The minimal response time or minimal reaction time of an AED represents the time required for

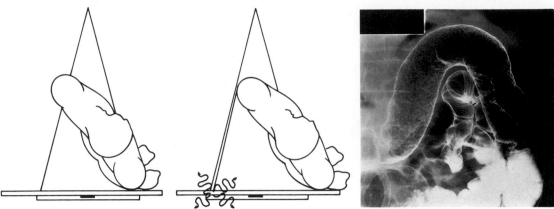

Figure 2-11
The Effect of a Primary Beam Leak on an
Automatic Exposure-Controlled Image

(Left) *When a patient is properly positioned to an AED sensor, remnant radiation as well as scatter radiation determines the amount of exposure to the radiographic film.* (Center) *If a patient is mispositioned so that a primary beam leak occurs, the AED may not function correctly. As the primary beam strikes the tabletop or upright holder, scatter radiation is generated in all directions. Some of this scatter strikes the sensor. Since an AED can only sense preselected densities, the scatter can cause the phototimer or ionization chamber to terminate prematurely. An underexposed radiograph would result. A primary beam leak, with image undercutting, could lead one to believe that the AED is not functioning properly. The AED is not able to distinguish between primary, remnant, or scatter radiation. In actuality, the AED is working as designed, since it is sensing a preselected density value.* (Right) *A fluoro spot film of an air-contrast study of the colon is shown with undercutting of the barium-filled colon owing to a primary beam leak.* (Sterling S: Automatic exposure control: A primer. Radiol Technol 59: 421–427, 1988.)

the shortest possible automatic exposure (Fig. 2-12). The use of faster screen film combinations that produce greater film blackening per unit of exposure can accentuate minimal response time difficulties.

IMPORTANT

The minimal response time is independent of the quality (kVP) or quantity (mA) of the x-ray beam.

When a patient requires less x-radiation than the minimal response time is capable of delivering at a predetermined kilovoltage and milliamperage setting, some type of technical factor adjustment must be made. Since the timer cannot terminate an exposure quicker than the minimal response time of the unit, mA or kVp must be lowered. A common error in chest radiography is the lowering of kilovoltage. When kvP is lowered, shorter scale contrast is produced. The lungs become blacker, whereas osseous structures and the mediastinum may appear chalk-like, resulting in a radiograph

suitable for examination of the ribs or thoracic spine. Lowering of the mA value is recommended to overcome this problem (Figs. 2-12 and 2-13).

An AED density adjustment control is present on the control panel console for use with most automatic exposure timers (Fig. 2-14). The density control is generally set on "normal" density to produce the accepted departmental standard for radiographic density. Changes in density should occur when the minus or plus density stations are used (Fig. 2-15).

IMPORTANT

If a radiograph is overexposed because a shorter exposure time is not possible, owing to minimal response time limitations, the use of the minus density station is not effective. No change in radiographic density can occur if the x-ray exposure time needed is less than the minimal response time.

Newer automatic exposure devices, whether light-sensitive (phototimers) or radiation-sensitive

	SMALL	MEDIUM	LARGE	EXTRA LARGE
	50 MA	100 MA	200 MA	400 MA
1x	0.5 MAS	1 MAS	2 MAS	4 MAS
2x	1 MAS	2 MAS	4 MAS	8 MAS

Figure 2-12
Lowest mAs Possible with a Minimal Response Time
of 1/100th Second at Two Different Screen Film Speeds

When a high mA station is selected for a radiograph, the minimal response time of an AED may result in too high an mAs value for a proper density. This is often a problem when examining the chest of a small patient in the posteroanterior or anteroposterior position. The AED is not able to terminate an exposure faster than the minimal response time of the unit. A minus density selection on the AED control cannot overcome minimal response time limitations in this situation (see Fig. 2-14).

Four representative patient sizes are listed: small, medium, large, and extra large. The radiographic density required for the largest patient would exceed 1/100th of a second exposure for proper density. Smaller patients require less mAs for proper exposure. Since the AED cannot terminate faster than 1/100th of a second, in this example, higher mA values will result in higher mAs values than may be needed for the smaller patients. The use of a faster speed screen film combination compounds this problem. By lowering the mA value, the proper mAs can be achieved by the AED, since it can remain activated for longer than the minimal response time. The AED can make the correct response regarding density.

Lowering kilovoltage will also help overcome the effect of minimal response time limitations, but shorter scale contrast may result. This may be desirable in some examinations, such as iodinated contrast studies or osseous examinations, but it can result in blackened lung fields and chalk-white ribs in a chest image. Low mA values with a large patient will increase the length of exposure and can result in patient or organ motion on the image. The mA values must be raised or lowered according to patient size if one is attempting to overcome minimal response time limitations when a fixed kVp technique is used.

(ionization chambers), are capable of exposures as low as 0.001 second (1 msec).

Automatically programed exposure controls are available with preselected appropriate baseline techniques for given body parts. Changes can be made in the program by the radiographer.

Back-Up Time

The back-up time represents the maximal exposure that an AED will permit for a given mA and kVp value. The back-up time is generally set by the manufacturer within the instantaneous load capacity of the x-ray tube. On some units, the back-up time can be manually selected on the control panel by the radiographer. The manual or automatic settings must fall within the tube recommendations for instantaneous loading set by the manufacturer.

Back-up timer settings help avoid additional x-ray exposure to the patient as well as damage to the x-ray tube.

Special Uses for Automatic Exposure Devices

Automatic exposure devices have several special applications.

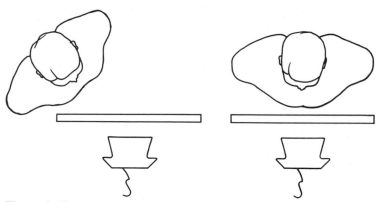

Figure 2-13
Minimal Response Time

The response time needed for the shortest possible exposure with an AED is known as the minimal response time (MRT). An average- or large-size patient (right) would require more exposure than with the typical MRT to achieve proper radiographic density. If the same patient were to step out of the x-ray field (left), the AED would attempt to terminate the exposure immediately; however, the MRT of the unit would control the length of the exposure.

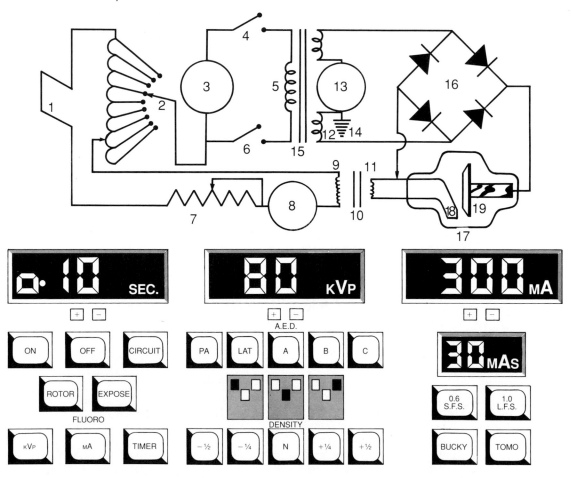

Mobile exposure control. An AED will help to maintain consistent image quality over a broad range of kilovoltages and patient sizes, when used with a mobile unit. Density variations that could require retakes can be reduced by the use of an AED. There is a saving both in the cost of x-ray film and in the radiographer's time. The most important benefit is the reduction in patient discomfort and radiation exposure.

Components of a typical AED used with a mobile unit include a control display module connected by a cable to an ion chamber detector paddle. This paddle is used on the exit side of the cassette and must be centered properly to the area of interest (see Chapter 9, Fig. 9-11).

Mammography. An AED on a dedicated mammographic unit will compensate for the density difference seen between atrophic, more radiolucent breasts requiring decreased exposure and dense, fibrocystic breasts requiring increased exposure.

Image intensifiers. The image intensifier uses a type of automatic control for fluoroscopy as well as cineradiography. This device, known as an *automatic brightness control (ABC)*, adjusts technical factors as areas of the body with large density differences are scanned. For example, when the right lower segment of the radiolucent lung is being examined and the fluoroscope is moved below the diaphragm into the radiodense right upper quadrant for evaluation of the liver, the brightness control will automatically adjust either milliamperage or kilovoltage, or both, to produce the desired fluoroscopic density.

The X-ray Tube

Within the x-ray circuit, the incoming electricity is passed through switches, timer, meters, transformers, rectifiers, and the x-ray tube.

The x-ray tube is a major component of the x-ray circuit, converting electrical energy into elec-

◀ **Figure 2-14**
Operator Controls of an X-ray Machine

This representation of a control panel is divided into the following segments: kilovoltage and related circuits (center), milliampere settings and focal spot size selection (right), and timer control (left). A representative schematic of the x-ray circuit is shown above the control panel. The numerical designations are the same as those used in Figure 2-2. Depending on the equipment design, these controls can be presented in many configurations. Additional meters such as tube load limits, heat displays, and a direct readout of the fluoroscopic examination time are often found on control panels.

Kilovoltage can be raised or lowered (center) as required to adequately penetrate the part being examined. A power "On" and "Off" button and a circuit breaker are shown. The rotor control as well as the expose button are on the left. At bottom are fluoroscopic kilovoltage and milliampere stations and a fluoroscopic timer that can be set to limit the length of the fluoroscopic procedure.

The milliampere readout is shown on the right. Milliamperage can be raised or lowered depending on technical needs. A high mA value combined with a short exposure time is sometimes needed to overcome motion. The selection of a moderate mA value often permits the use of a small focal spot. The focal spots represented in this panel are 0.6 mm and 1.0 mm in size. Directly above focal spot selection indicators is an mAs meter. This device is required when extremely short exposures are used so that an accurate reading of the mAs used can be obtained. Below the focal spot size selection are the Bucky "On" and "Off" buttons and a tomographic selector control.

At the top left of the control panel is the manual timing section. The time of exposure can be raised or lowered by the radiographer, or an AED can be selected. Specific AED sensor indicators for the chest (posteroanterior or lateral) or other Bucky stations are shown. Table Bucky is represented by A, the upright Bucky by B, and the radiographic spot-film component of the fluoroscope by C. The darkened sensors (left, right, or center) indicate the sensors selected for the part under study (see Figs. 2-9 and 2-10).

In the lower portion of the AED section on the control panel, density adjustment controls are shown. The center button, labeled N, is intended for use when a normal or preselected density is desired. The (−) control can be adjusted for a ¼ or ½ decrease in density. The (+) control can be adjusted in a similar fashion for an increase in density. When an examination must be repeated, image density should be adjustable by the use of the (−) or (+) settings.

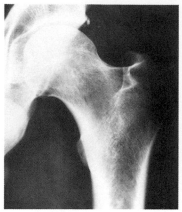 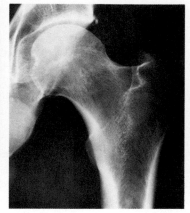 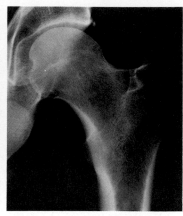

Figure 2-15
AED Density Adjustment

A density adjustment control (see Fig. 2-14, bottom of center panel) is used when an increase or decrease in radiographic density is required for a specific AED study at the same kVp level. These radiographs of the hip were photographically altered to demonstrate the effect of an AED density adjustment. (Left) An image at minus ½ density; (center) an image at normal density; (right) an image at plus ½ density.

tromagnetic energy. Several conditions are necessary for the production of x-radiation:

1. There must be a source of electrons: a heated filament.
2. The electrons: must be made to move rapidly across the x-ray tube from cathode to anode using applied kilovoltage.
3. The rapidly moving electrons must be stopped suddenly.

Selection of appropriate technical factors determines the quality and quantity of radiation needed to produce a quality image.

The x-ray tube is discussed in Chapter 3 and selection of technical factors in Chapter 9.

The Control Panel

Variation in power delivered by way of the x-ray tube permits the radiographer to control several technical factors. Selection of the factors required to produce a quality radiograph is made at the control panel (see Fig. 2-14), after consulting a technique chart. There are three major exposure factors under the control of the radiographer:

1. Milliamperage, which determines the number or quantity of electrons available to flow across the x-ray tube. This setting is needed to produce "free" electrons in a process known as thermionic emission and controls the intensity of the x-ray beam.
2. Kilovoltage, the high voltage applied across the x-ray tube, which determines, as a result, the speed of the incoming electrons and thus influences the energy or quality of the x-ray beam.
3. Time or length of exposure, which determines the total time during which x-radiation is produced, usually given in fractions of seconds.

Chapter 3
The X-ray Tube

The x-ray tube is an important link in the x-ray equipment chain. Its components are illustrated in Figures 3-1 and 3-2. The tube consists basically of a filament, a target or anode, a highly evacuated vacuum glass envelope, and a housing.

The filament, the source of "free" electrons in the x-ray tube, is a small tungsten wire, slightly greater than 0.008 inch in diameter, tempered and coiled to form a helix, and mounted in a metal focusing cup. Radiographic tubes have two filaments, usually mounted side by side to produce small and large focal spots. Some manufacturers mount these filaments one above the other rather than side by side in their focusing cups (see Figs. 3-1 and 3-2). The higher the temperature of the filament, the greater the rate of the electron emission.

The heat of the filament is controlled by the milliampere setting on the control panel. Filaments used in radiographic tubes are relatively thin and, when heated to very high temperatures, can evaporate. This evaporation can be a gradual process that causes metallic deposits on the glass envelope, usually near the port area, and can lead to erratic mA output during tube operation. Continuous high milliampere settings, which can produce evaporation of the filament, should be avoided. The focusing cup, used as a support for the filament, has a negative charge applied to it to "focus" the negative electrons using the principle of repulsion of like charges. Mutual repulsion of electrons would spread out the beam without this focusing action. High mA values can counteract the focusing effect of the focusing cup, spreading the electrons over a larger area of the anode.

The anode is usually made of tungsten or a tungsten alloy, such as rhenium tungsten. The electron stream from the filament strikes the target area of the anode in an area known as the actual focal spot.

In order to produce x-radiation the filament must be heated within the vacuum of the glass tube. Beryllium window tubes are used whenever a minimum of inherent filtration is required for studies such as mammography. The use of a beryllium window results in an essentially unfiltered x-ray beam.

Angeline M. Cullinan and John E. Cullinan:
PRODUCING QUALITY RADIOGRAPHS, 2ND ED.
© 1987, 1994 J. B. Lippincott Company.

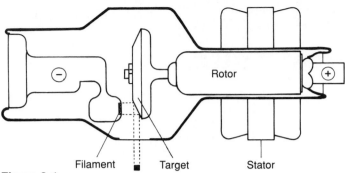

Figure 3-1
Basic Components of an X-ray Tube

A basic component of a radiographic tube is the filament, the source of electrons, at the cathode side of the tube. The cathode, a high negative potential, includes the focusing cup, which has a negative charge applied to it to "focus" the stream of electrons by the repulsion of like charges. The anode, a high positive potential, serves as a target for the focused electron stream. A stator rotor system that uses an induction motor rotates the anode at extremely high speed, usually 3000 rpm or 10,000 rpm. A Pyrex envelope houses the cathode and rotating anode and is placed in an oil-filled, lead-lined housing (see Fig. 3-8).

The x-ray housing, which acts as a mounting for the tube insert, is lined with lead for radiation shielding. Leakage radiation from the housing should not exceed 100 mR per hour when measured 1 meter from the source when the unit is operating at its maximal output.

The tube insert is grounded and surrounded by oil, insulating it from its metal shield. The oil used to cool the tube housing also provides high voltage insulation.

Basic Operation of an X-ray Tube

In a process known as thermionic emission, the electrons "boil off" from the filament surface. An electron cloud produces a "space charge" effect in the vicinity of the filament. This cloud of negative charges prevents other electrons from being emitted from the filament until a higher potential difference (kVp) is applied to the tube to overcome the force of the space charge. The electrons are attracted to the anode (+) side of the tube. As the electrons strike the metal surface of the anode, they are stopped abruptly. This interaction produces both x-radiation as well as considerable heat—a major yet undesirable byproduct. Less than 1% of the total energy produced is converted into x-radiation.

Increasing the kilovoltage increases the speed at which the electrons are pulled across the tube and decreases the wavelength of the resultant x-ray beam, making the beam more penetrating.

IMPORTANT

Careful consideration must be given to the production of heat to avoid damage to the x-ray tube. Tube rating charts and related terminology will be discussed in this chapter.

When the x-ray unit is "on," the filament is illuminated at a low level (standby illumination). When the anode is "boosted" to its proper number of revolutions per minute, the temperature of the filament is raised to the milliamperage selected for the study. If a delay occurs in the making of an exposure, prolonged rotation of the anode can produce excessive heat. When there is a delay in the making of an exposure, the radiographer should drop back to "standby illumination" by de-energizing the rotor of the anode. Prolonged rotation at high speed also produces severe strain on the bearings of the rotating anode.

Focal Spot Size Determination

The National Electrical Manufacturers Association (NEMA) lists several definitions with regard to acceptable tolerance of x-ray tube focal spot

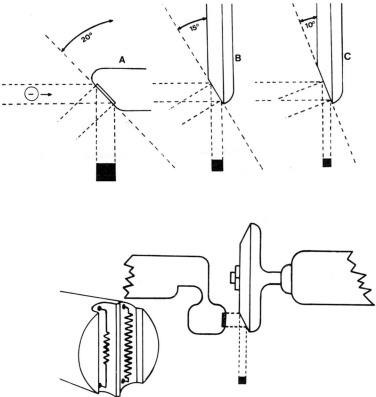

Figure 3-2
Focal Spot Size

The area of the angled (beveled) target surface bombarded by the electron stream is known as the actual *focal spot (top). It is larger in size than the effective focal spot, owing to the "line focus effect." The actual focal spot is rectangular in shape, whereas the effective focal spot is projected in an almost square configuration (black square). Whether the anode is stationary (A) or rotating (B, C), the line focus effect is the same. Note the change in the effective focal spot size due to different target angles: 20 degrees (A), 15 degrees (B), and 10 degrees (C). As the target angle becomes steeper, the effective focal spot becomes smaller, even though the electron stream used for A, B, and C is the same size. The focal spots, actual and effective, would be further reduced in size if a smaller filament were used to produce the electron stream (bottom left).*

Cathode assembly: A typical cathode has a small and large filament. The smaller filament produces a smaller electron stream on the anode (actual focal spot) when a potential difference (kilovoltage) is applied to the x-ray tube. Most x-ray tubes use side-by-side filament mountings in dual focusing cups (bottom left).

sizes.* The actual focal spot is defined by NEMA as the section on which the anode of the x-ray tube intersects with the electron beam. According to NEMA, the *projected focal spot* is the projection of the actual focal spot along the central ray, per-

pendicular to the x-ray port plane and passing through the center of the focal spot. This is often referred to as the focal spot (see Fig. 3-2).

The electrons, focused into a controlled stream from the filament, strike an area of the anode known as the *actual focal spot*, producing x-radiation and heat. The size of the electron stream is related to filament size. The smaller the electron

National Electrical Manufacturers Association Standard 1-8-1992.

stream, the smaller the actual focal spot and, therefore, the smaller the effective focal spot (see Fig. 3-2).

The projected x-ray beam exits from the tube to the area being radiographed. A quality assurance (QA) tool known as a slit camera can be used to measure the size of the projected focal spot in a specific direction (see Fig. 3-2). This measurement is known as the *effective focal spot.* The smaller the effective focal spot, the greater the potential for reduced image blur. Quality assurance tests are described in Chapter 14.

Effective focal spot size also depends, in part, on the angle of the anode. The smaller the angle of the anode, the smaller the effective focal spot. With the use of a smaller filament and a "steep angle" anode to produce a smaller actual focal spot, a correspondingly smaller effective focal spot is produced (see Fig. 3-2). The area of the angled anode surface bombarded by the electron stream, known as the actual focal spot, is larger in size than the effective focal spot to help dissipate heat over a greater area.

Focal spots are described in terms of their nominal size, for example, a typical x-ray tube with a 1.0-mm focal spot is rated as a nominal projected focal spot measuring 1.0 mm × 1.0 mm. The projected or effective focal spot may differ from its nominal size from 30% to 50% depending on the focal spot size under consideration, according to tolerances published by NEMA.*

Most modern x-ray machines are equipped with a rotating anode tube having a 0.6-mm (small) and 1.0-mm (large) focal spot (Table 3-1). Focal spots as small as 0.1 mm (microfocus) and as large as 2.0 mm are commercially available.

As focal spot size decreases, tube rating restrictions increase. The high temperatures (high mA

National Electrical Manufacturers Association Standard 1-8-1992.

Table 3-1. Milliampere Settings to Focal Spot Comparisons

mA	Older Tube	Modern Tube
100	Small 1.0 mm	Small 0.6 mm
200	Large 2.0 mm	Small 0.6 mm
300	Large 2.0 mm	Small 0.6 mm
500	Large 2.0 mm	Large 1.0 mm or 1.2 mm
1000	Not available	Large 1.0 mm or 1.2 mm

Up to 200 mA can be used with a modern fractional focal spot tube (0.3 mm or less at 10,000 rpm).

values) required to heat the filament can cause an increase in the size of the focal spot. Low kVp can similarly affect focal spot size. Unfortunately, longer exposure times may be required because of the lower mA values necessitated by the use of a smaller focal spot. In some examinations, motion may become a problem.

The Effect of Blooming

"Blooming" of the focal spot is described by NEMA as the change in values, usually an increase, in the focal spot dimensions when appropriate focal spot measurements are made. The specifications for making these measurements are outlined in the NEMA publication.*

Some focal spots can increase up to 50% in size. In theory, a 0.6-mm focal spot could approach the dimensions of a 0.9-mm focal spot. This can be discouraging to a radiographer if a small focal spot was selected with attention to radiographic detail, yet the image produced does not reflect the anticipated quality.

Radiographers, when comparing images, sometimes believe that there is no difference between the small and large focal spot. This may be the result of using a small focal spot at its highest mA setting, thereby promoting blooming. The use of the small focal spot at a maximal mA value may result in a focal spot that approaches the size of a large focal spot used at a moderate mA value.

IMPORTANT

Every effort should be made to ensure the integrity of the focal spot. One should avoid a combination of technical factors, such as a maximal mA/low kVp technique, that may contribute to focal spot blooming.

When performing direct roentgen enlargement techniques using a 0.3-mm or smaller focal spot, blooming must be considered. Most of the x-ray tubes used with magnification techniques are limited to less than 200 mA. This may appear to be a low mA value, but enlargement techniques do not require the use of a grid or Bucky. Film blackening effect is three to five times greater depending on the grid ratio needed for a conventional study of the same body part. For example, a fractional focal spot set at 100 mA in a magnification study

National Electrical Manufacturers Association Standard Publication XR-5-1984.

would produce a film blackening effect similar to the 300 mA to 500 mA value required for a conventional grid study. Direct roentgen enlargement is discussed in Chapter 11.

IMPORTANT

Angiographic technologists often use high mA values and short exposure times to minimize motion and increase the number of frames per second when using a serial film changer. The lowering of a mA value from its maximum and the use of a moderate kilovoltage, approximately 70 kVp or higher, helps to preserve the integrity of the focal spot by minimizing the blooming effect.

The Effect of Anode Angle

The electron stream emanating from the filament strikes the beveled outer edge of the face of the anode. The angle of the anode is measured from a 90-degree angle (Figs. 3-2 and 3-3). The beveled outer edge of anodes is manufactured with angles varying from 10 to 17 degrees. The use of a "steep angle" anode permits an increase in instantaneous loading when compared with a conventional anode angle (see X-ray Tube Rating Charts, heat limitations).

A benefit of the steep angle target is improved radiographic detail owing to the smaller effective focal spot. Early 10-degree steep angle targets were limited to field size coverage of 14 × 14

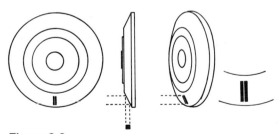

**Figure 3-3
Electron Stream Bombardment
of the Rotating Anode**

The electrons emitted from the cathode bombard the target area of the beveled rotating anode to produce x-rays and heat. The electron stream from the cathode strikes the actual focal spot as two separate energy sources to protect the center of the focal spot (right). As the anode rotates, the intense heat is moved away by conduction and heat radiation.

inches at a 40-inch FFD. A 10-degree angle target used at a 45-inch FFD will cover a 17 × 17 inch field. A 13-degree angle target is needed to cover a 17 × 17 inch field at a 40-inch FFD.

In selecting an x-ray tube for under-table fluoroscopic use, consideration should be given to what is the steepest target angle that will permit coverage of the input phosphor of the image intensifier and the largest radiographic film that will be used in the spot film device.

IMPORTANT

The steeper the target angle, the smaller the field coverage and the effective focal spot, but the greater the instantaneous load capability.

The Effect of Tube Vibration

Minor vibrations in the x-ray tube during an exposure can diminish the integrity of the focal spot. An improperly balanced tube or unstable tube stand or tube crane can add to vibration, with a corresponding degradation of the focal spot. A last-minute, often unnecessary, adjustment of the x-ray tube can produce an almost imperceptible vibration in the tube resulting in increased image blur.

The Line Focus Effect

The line focus effect, produced by the projection of the x-ray beam to the area being radiographed, results in an almost square effective focal spot, even though the electron stream strikes an area on the anode that is rectangular in shape (see Fig. 3-2).

Differences in sharpness across the field, cathode to anode, are related to the line focus effect. At the anode end of the tube, the projected focal spot is smaller than the effective focal spot measured at the central ray. The difference in sharpness produced from the line focus effect can sometimes be perceived on a segment of the image exposed by the beam at the cathode side of the tube (Figs. 3-4B and 3-5 to 3-7). In practice, variations in focal spot sharpness owing to the line focus effect may be masked by other sources of image blur.

The perfect focal spot would be round in configuration and could produce a homogenous intensity of distribution over the area to be examined.

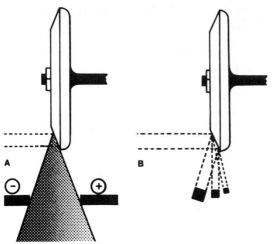

Figure 3-4
Heel Effect and Line-Focus Effect
of the X-ray Beam

The intensity of the x-radiation along the long axis of the tube, from cathode to anode, is not uniform. (A) The radiation is less intense on the anode (+) side of the tube than on the cathode (−) side owing to the absorption of x-rays within the anode. (B) Resolution differences can occur from cathode to anode as a result of the line-focus effect. The focal spot measured at the central ray is known as the effective *focal spot. As the x-ray beam diverges along the long axis of the tube, the focal spot becomes larger toward the cathode end and smaller toward the anode end.*

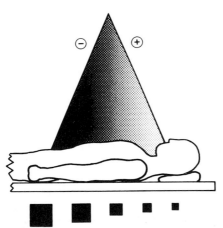

Figure 3-5
Heel Effect and Positioning Approach

Since the cathode (−) portion of the x-ray beam is more intense than the anode (+) side, thicker portions of the body should be positioned beneath the cathode side of the x-ray tube. There is an increase in image blur toward the cathode side.

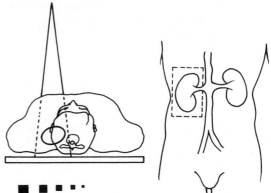

Figure 3-6
Line Focus Effect and Unilateral Image Blur

A tightly collimated field, restricted to the right kidney, is shown at right. If the x-ray tube is positioned crosswise, with the cathode over the lateral aspect of the kidney, some resolution of the peripheral arteries could be lost. Improvement in resolution would occur if the anode/cathode relationship were reversed, so that the focal spot effect on the anode side of the x-ray tube would be over the lateral aspect of the kidney. See Figures 3-5 and 3-7. The line focus effect on image blur is critical to magnification techniques.

The Heel Effect

The intensity of the x-radiation across the long axis of the tube is not uniform. X-radiation is not generated only at the surface of the target; it emerges from the target material, at varying depths, in a direction nearly parallel to the target face. This variation in x-ray intensity is called the *heel effect* (see Figs. 3-4*A* and 3-5). The radiation is less intense on the anode side of the tube than on the cathode side, owing to the absorption of some of the x-rays within the anode. The changes in beam intensity are significant only on the extreme cathode and extreme anode edges of the beam. Since the intensity of the beam nearest the central ray is more uniform, the heel effect is less noticeable when an increased FFD or a smaller field size is used. As the target angle is reduced, radiation intensity is less uniform across the field. The heel effect is more noticeable when using a steep angle target.

In theory, the thickest area of the part under study should be positioned beneath the cathode side of the x-ray tube to take advantage of the heel effect (see Fig. 3-5).

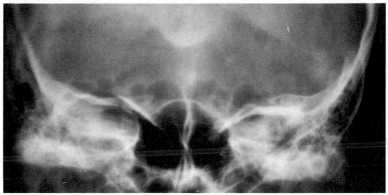

Figure 3-7
Line Focus Effect and Unilateral Image Blur
A clinical example of the line focus effect is shown. With the x-ray tube positioned transverse, the cathode over the right petrous ridge, there is an obvious increase in image blur. Note the difference in sharpness between the right and left sides of the skull. The difference in sharpness is more obvious when examining symmetric structures.

Filtration of the X-ray Beam

Any obstacle through which x-rays pass on their way from the focal spot to the object under study is called a *filter*. Filtration removes low energy photons from the x-ray beam (Fig. 3-8).

IMPORTANT

A filter should be installed in a permanent or semipermanent way so that it cannot be inadvertently removed.

Three types of filtration are of interest in diagnostic radiology. They are:

1. Inherent filtration
2. Added filtration, which includes compensatory filters
3. Total filtration

Inherent Filtration

All x-ray tubes are enclosed in shock-proof housings. A "window" in the housing permits radiation to exit from the tube.

Inherent filtration includes the window in the glass envelope of the tube and the insulation oil of the housing. Inherent filtration is intentionally kept very low by tube manufacturers. It is measured in terms of aluminum equivalent, that is, the thickness of aluminum that would be needed to produce the same degree of x-ray beam attenuation.

Added Filtration

Added or additional filtration increases the hardness of the x-ray beam, improving beam quality by removing the portion of the beam that consists of soft (long wavelength) x-rays. These soft x-rays do not contribute to the information on the radiograph, because they are not of sufficient strength to penetrate the part and are mostly absorbed by the patient. Unless these soft x-rays are absorbed by added filtration, they contribute to patient dosage. Added filtration should be inserted as close to the tube as possible in order to blur out any impurities that the filter may contain (see Fig. 3-8). A filter designed to reduce radiation dosage should not require a significant increase in x-ray tube loading.

Filtration can be described in terms of half-value layer (HVL). This refers to the thickness of aluminum that would be needed to reduce the intensity of the original x-ray beam to one half. Any filtration material may be specified as aluminum equivalent (equal to the thickness of aluminum that would produce the same filtering effect).

Scientists at the Mayo Clinic reviewed 200 x-ray tubes over an 8-year period for changes in half-

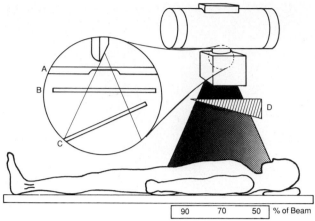

Figure 3-8
Filtration

Inherent filtration includes the glass window (A) of the x-ray tube and the insulation oil of the housing. Added filtration includes filters installed at the tube port (B) in compliance with federal, state, or local regulations. The mirror (C) in the collimator is considered part of the added filtration. The combination of inherent and added filtration is known as total filtration. When needed, a compensatory filter (D) can be added to the collimator to overcome variations in anatomic size or tissue density. The filter shown (D) is wedge-shaped and absorbs more primary radiation at its thicker end. Note the variation in x-ray intensity from the thinner to the thicker end (90% – 50%) accomplished by the filter used in this illustration.

A compensatory filter at port is recommended in place of underpart filters. The disadvantage of underpart filtration is that the part being examined receives the full x-ray exposure.

value layer.* HVL changes were previously attributed to the hardening of the x-ray beam caused by a build-up of tungsten on the x-ray tube glass window. Although tungsten build-up was seen as a source of change of x-ray emission and beam quality, it did not alter the HVL of the beam in this study. Glass thickness appeared to be the major factor affecting the HVL of the beam.

Composition of Added Filtration

Federal, state, and local regulations determine the amount of filtration necessary for specific equipment.

It would be helpful if variable filters could be used for various body parts, since no single filter

Gray JE et al: Half-value layer increase, owing to tungsten buildup in the x-ray tube Fact or fiction. Radiology 160: 837–838, 1986.

is optimal for every situation. Some collimators have variable filters on the overhead x-ray tube with different thicknesses of aluminum as well as a combination filter of 0.1-mm copper (Cu) combined with 1.0-mm aluminum (Al). Although each filter has a specific advantage, the use of a variable dial filter can be a disadvantage if an inappropriate filter is selected.

The most common material used for added filtration in diagnostic radiology is aluminum. Aluminum filtration reduces patient exposure but usually does not affect tube loading. A slight loss in contrast may occur when using additional aluminum filtration with pediatric extremities or when imaging small body parts.

Conventional filters with low K-shell binding energies usually absorb low-energy photons while they raise the mean energy of the beam. K-edge filters such as lanthanum (La), gadolinium (Gd), tungsten (W), and holmium (Ho) absorb photons with energies just above the K-shell binding energy of each element.

Combination filters such as 0.1-mm Cu with 2.0-mm Al are available for significant reduction in x-ray entrance exposure. There is a noticeable loss of contrast in extremity radiography when this filter is used. A 0.2-mm Cu with a 2.0-mm Al filter can be used above 100 kVp for chest or barium studies.

A twofold or greater increase in exposure factors is required when an erbium (Er) filter is used. Dosage to the patient, however, is decreased significantly without a loss in contrast. This filter can be helpful when imaging body parts opacified with an iodinated contrast medium. The use of 600-, 800-, and 1200-speed screen film systems minimizes tube loading concerns.

Compensatory Filtration

Compensating filters are used to overcome variations in patient anatomy, providing a more uniform density across the radiographic image. Over- or underpenetration of segments of the radiograph is reduced. Severe variations in patient thickness can be imaged with a single exposure (Figs. 3-8 to 3-12).

Some compensatory filtration materials in use include barium-impregnated clay, opaque plastic, aluminum, copper, and leaded acrylic. The use of compensatory filters is limited only by the innovative nature of the radiographer. Image quality is improved as a result of overall uniform film density (see Fig. 3-8).

Early attempts at high kVp, heavy filtration techniques of the larynx used 1.0 mm of brass at 130 kVp. Studies were made at even higher kVp values with increased brass filtration. The use of 3.0-mm brass filtration with linear tomography at 120 kVp to 140 kVp, depending on the size of the patient, results in a high-contrast laryngogram. The higher kilovoltage decreases the contrast between bone and soft tissue, while the air serves as a negative contrast medium.

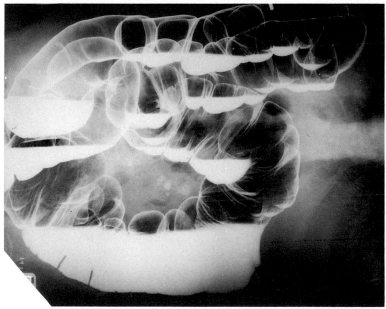

Figure 3-9
Leaded-Acrylic Wedge Filter for Lateral Decubitus Radiography
Often, severe differences in radiographic density occur when a patient is placed in the lateral decubitus position. There is a tendency for increased tissue thickness in the dependent portion of the anatomy. With double-contrast studies of the colon, barium may puddle in the dependent segments of the large bowel while air rises to the upper portions. A more overall uniform radiographic density is obtained with a compensatory filter. (Radiograph courtesy of Nuclear Associates, division of Victoreen, Carle Place, NY)

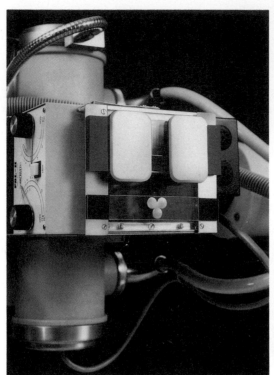
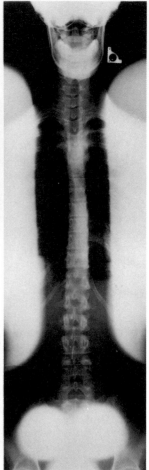

Figure 3-10
Scoliosis Evaluation of the Full Vertebral Column

It is impossible to uniformly expose the full vertebral column with a single exposure, since the cervical spine is thinner than the remaining vertebral column. The thoracic area is easy to overexpose because of the radiolucent nature of the lungs; the lumbar vertebrae require increased exposure. (Left) A compensatory wedge filter should be used when performing full vertebral column studies. Breast shields first are placed on the filter holder, and then the AP/PA wedge filter is placed on top of the breast shields. A gonadal shield is positioned below the AP/PA wedge filter. Built-up filters of this type provide additional filtration in the cervical area, compensating for the added exposure that is required in the lumbar area. By using a compensatory filter that holds back a considerable portion of the x-ray to the cervical area, holds back half or more of the exposure to the thoracic area, and permits full exposure to reach the lumbar area, a more uniform radiographic density can be achieved throughout the entire vertebral column. The compensatory filter selectively attenuates the x-ray beam, reducing patient dosage. (Right) Note the presence of a gonadal shield, as well as the shielding of the breast of this young female patient. The use of high-speed rare-earth screen film technology combined with breast and gonadal shielding and compensatory filtration significantly reduces dosage to the patient. When breast shields are not available for anteroposterior imaging, the patient can be radiographed in the posteroanterior position, avoiding unattenuated primary radiation to the breasts. Since the vertebral column is further away from the cassette (increased OFD), image blur will be increased. Image blur is not a problem since the examination is being done primarily for vertebral alignment. If vertebral enlargement is a problem, an increased FFD can be used to overcome the effect of the increased OFD. A 1200-speed rare-earth screen film system reduces dosage considerably. (Courtesy of Nuclear Associates, division of Victoreen, Carle Place, NY)

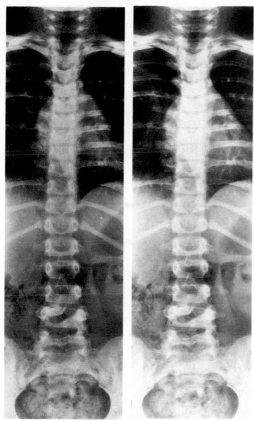

Figure 3-11
High Kilovoltage Technique
for the Full Vertebral Column

Kilovoltage levels from 100 kVp to 125 kVp can be used to evaluate the full vertebral column for scoliosis. High kilovoltage with 1200-speed screen film combinations will result in a moderate contrast image that is adequate for evaluation of the spinal curvature. (Left) An image made using 85 kVp. (Right) A photographically altered image made to simulate a 110-kVp exposure that would permit a significant reduction in mAs. If osseous details are required, conventional images should be made.

When using an anatomically programmed exposure control, it is conceivable that additional filtration could be automatically selected for each body part. For example, a copper filter could be added to an aluminum filter for high kVp chest radiography. A combination of yttrium and aluminum might be beneficial for most routine radiography in which significant patient exposure reduction is important.

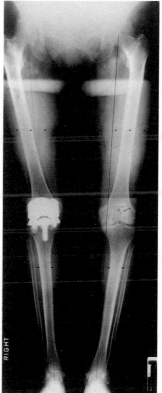

Figure 3-12
Full-Length Radiography of the Legs

Selective attenuation of the x-ray beam with compensatory filters achieves a uniform density from the hip to the ankle with a single exposure. This radiograph was made with the patient in the weight-bearing position. (Courtesy of Nucleur Associates, division of Victoreen, Carle Place, NY)

Anatomically Specific Filters

Anatomic compensatory filters are used in an attempt to overcome variations in patient size or anatomy and are designed to conform to the shape of the part being studied. They are usually attached to a thin sheet of plastic and inserted into the external tracks of the collimator. They are designed to minimize variations in anatomy to produce a more uniform radiographic density. For example, in the chest a significant amount of filtration is used over the lung fields with very little or none used over the mediastinum. An increase in exposure to overcome the filter helps to demonstrate mediastinal, retrocardiac, and retrodiaphragmatic structures that lie just outside of the toe region of the characteristic curve of a typical x-ray film.

Compensatory filters for chest radiography are often a compromise, since one size or type of filter cannot fit all sizes and types of patients or overcome variations in pathology or cardiac size. High-contrast screen film combinations, when used for chest radiography, usually result in short-scale contrast images, a chalk-like mediastinum, and blackened lungs. Specific technical information regarding chest radiography can be found in Chapter 10. New dual-receptor screen film technology, as described in Chapter 6, eliminates the need for a compensatory chest filter.

IMPORTANT

Some compensatory filters may produce edge markings in the lung fields that resemble a pneumomediastinum or a medial pneumothorax.

Transparent compensatory filters made of a leaded acrylic material are lightweight and easy to mount on x-ray equipment (Fig. 3-13). They replace machined or layered aluminum filters and are particularly helpful in imaging of the full vertebral column for scoliosis or for use with full-length angiography (see Figs. 3-10 to 3-12).

It is difficult to produce an optimal single radiograph of the abdomen, thigh, and lower leg.

When using a full-length cassette changer (14 × 51 inches), the use of different speed screens and film is cumbersome. An aluminum wedge filter, approximately 5 to 6 inches long, 3 inches in width, and 3/4 to 1 inch thick, tapered to a thin edge at one end, can be mounted on a piece of plastic, inserted into the tracks at the bottom of the collimator, and moved to accommodate patients of different sizes. (See Chapter 11, Fig. 11-25.)

IMPORTANT

The aluminum wedge filter should be attached to the collimator by a cord so that the filter cannot accidentally be pulled out of the track and possibly injure the patient. An acrylic filter of similar proportions is also acceptable.

An adjustable sliding aluminum wedge filter system described by Smith and Tidwell* overcomes the difference in thickness or composition of the body (Figs. 3-14 to 3-16).

The adjustable sliding aluminum wedge filter can be used in the following situations:

1. Imaging of the thorax, where there are considerable differences between the densities of the

Smith DC, Tidwell J: Adjustable sliding aluminum wedge filter: Device for angiographic enhancement. Radiol Technol 49: 459–471, 1978.

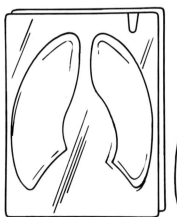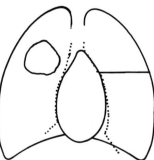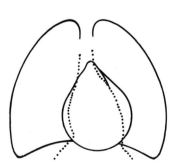

Figure 3-13
Compensatory Filtration for Chest Radiography

A transparent leaded-acrylic filter for chest radiography permits the penetration of the dense mediastinal area while holding back radiation from the aerated easy-to-overexpose lungs. Dual receptor screen film imaging eliminates the need for compensatory chest filtration. See Chapter 6. (Cullinan AM: Optimizing Radiographic Positioning. *Philadelphia: JB Lippincott Company, 1992)*

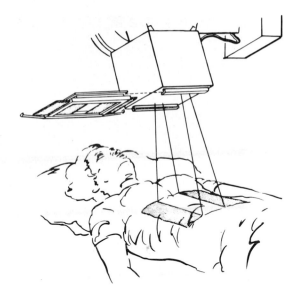

Figure 3-14
Transverse Mounting of the Sliding Aluminum Wedge

The adjustable wedge filter system overcomes the lack of uniform thickness or composition on both lateral aspects of the abdomen. Image burnout of the lateral aspects of the abdomen is avoided with this bilateral filtration technique. (Smith DC, Tidwell J: Adjustable sliding aluminum wedge filter: Device for angiographic enhancement. Radiol Technol 49:459–471, 1978)

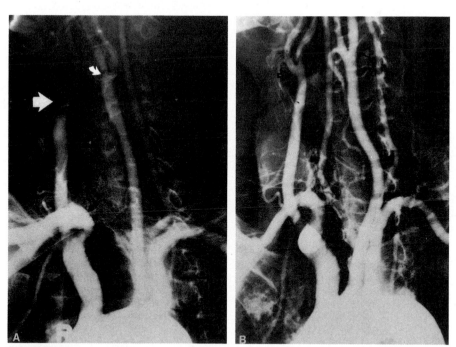

Figure 3-15
Right Posterior Oblique Arch Aortogram

(A) Conventional radiograph with overexposure of the upper cervical area obscures details of both common carotid arteries (arrows). (B) Exposure made using an adjustable wedge filter. Note uniform density throughout most of the image, with excellent visualization of the carotid arteries (arrows). (Smith DC, Tidwell J: Adjustable sliding aluminum wedge filter: Device for angiographic enhancement. Radiol Technol 49:459–471, 1978)

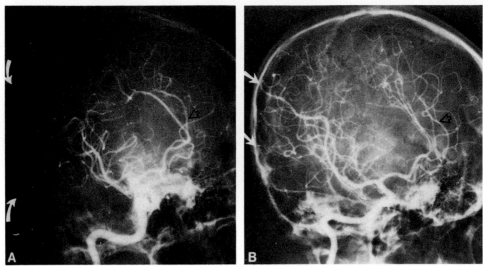

Figure 3-16
Left Posterior Oblique Carotid Arteriogram

(A) Conventional angiogram of the inner table of the skull (curved arrows) is greatly overexposed while the anterior cerebral arteries (open arrow) are optimally exposed. The middle cerebral arteries are slightly overexposed. (B) Using the adjustable aluminum wedge filter, note that the inner table of the skull (arrows) and the adjacent middle cerebral arteries, as well as the anterior cerebral arteries (open arrow), are all uniformly exposed. (Smith DC, Tidwell J: Adjustable sliding aluminum wedge filter: Device for angiographic enhancement. Radiol Technol 49:459–471, 1978)

radiolucent lungs and dense soft tissues of the mediastinum

2. Overcoming differences in anatomic thickness at the lateral aspects of the abdomen
3. Overcoming undercutting of the image by attenuating the primary beam
4. The lateral sternum, lateral lumbar, and lateral coccyx to attenuate a primary beam leak
5. The aortic arch study in an attempt to record on the same radiograph the aortic arch in the chest and the carotid and vertebral arteries in the neck (see Fig. 3-15)
6. The oblique carotid arteriogram (see Fig. 3-16)

The bilateral compensatory wedge filter has been further improved by the addition of a second set of wedge filters installed at a right angle to the first pair of filters so that four filters are available on a circular track to compensate for a wide variety of body segments.

Total Filtration

Total filtration is the combination of inherent and added filtration. When using a light beam collimator, the mirror must be considered as part of the total filtration (see Fig 3-8).

Underpart Filtration

Underpart filters such as sandbags or bags filled with cornmeal, flour, or rice are used in studies such as angiography or tomography to balance densities by restricting undercutting of the image.

The disadvantage of underpart filters is that the part being examined receives the full x-ray exposure. The use of a compensatory filter at or near the source of x-radiation is recommended in place of underpart filters.

Types of X-ray Tubes

There are two basic types of x-ray tubes: stationary anode and rotating anode tubes.

The Stationary Anode Tube

The term stationary anode is self-descriptive. A stationary anode is composed of a tungsten target embedded in a copper stem (see Fig.3-2A, top). These two metals are used for specific reasons: tungsten has a high melting point (about 3400° C) and an atomic number of 74, which increases the efficiency of bremsstrahlung production in the medical x-ray range. Copper is selected because it is a good conductor of heat.

Probably the only experience that the reader will have with a stationary anode tube is when operating a dental unit or a low-powered mobile device.

The Rotating Anode Tube

As in the stationary anode tube, the basic components of a rotating anode tube include cathode, anode, envelope, and an oil-filled, lead-lined tube housing. Additional components of the rotating anode tube assembly include an induction motor, used to rotate the anode, and a rotor and bearing assembly. As the anode rotates, unbombarded, cooler metal is brought into the path of the electron stream (Figs. 3-1, 3-3, and 3-17).

A tungsten disc, rotating about 3000 revolutions per minute (rpm), forms a circular focal track. The electron stream is delivered along the

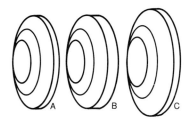

Figure 3-17
Rotating Anode Characteristics
The diameter and thickness of a rotating anode influences both the instantaneous and heat storage potential of an x-ray tube. The periphery of the target serves as its focal track. The greater the diameter of the target, the longer the focal track. The anodes represented by A and B are equal in diameter and therefore have focal tracks of equal length. The total mass of the anode determines its anode heat storage capacity; therefore, B, which is two times thicker than A, has greater heat storage capacity than A. Since the diameter of the anode has not changed, both A and B have the same instantaneous load capacity. The larger-diameter anode (C) has a longer focal track; therefore, instantaneous load capability is improved over A and B. It is possible that the total mass of C may be less than B, depending on the anode design. If so, B will have a greater heat storage capacity but a lessened instantaneous load capability.

lateral margins of the actual focal spot as two separate sources, protecting the center of the actual focal spot (see Fig. 3-3). The intense heat moves away from the focal track and is dissipated by radiation and conduction by the large metal anode.

Most rotating anodes vary in diameter from 3 to 5 inches. When using a radiographic tube with a 4-inch-diameter target instead of a 3-inch-diameter target, a 30% increase in the mA setting is possible. The larger the diameter or the greater the thickness of the anode, the greater the anode thermal capacity of a specific tube (see Fig. 3-17). (See X-ray Tube Rating Charts, heat units.)

Modern rotating anode x-ray tubes use an anode composed of either solid tungsten or molybdenum coated with a rhenium tungsten alloy. Rhenium is used to improve the thermal stress resistance of the relatively brittle tungsten. The use of a rhenium tungsten alloy results in an anode that is more resistant to surface roughening (pitting) (Fig. 3-18). A thin stem joins the anode to the rotor system, which drives the anode in a circular motion. The stem of the anode is usually made of molybdenum, which has a low thermal conductivity and can tolerate multiple temperature changes.

An induction motor is used to rotate the anode. The stator of the induction motor surrounds the tube on the external surface of the glass envelope. The rotor of the induction motor is held in place by bearings within the glass vacuum tube (see Fig. 3-1). Special thin-layered, soft metal lubricants such as silver or lead are used with the ball bearings to facilitate high-speed rotation. The rotating anode helps to dissipate the heat generated in the production of x-radiation over the surface area of the target (see Fig. 3-17).

High-speed rotors, which permit anode rotation up to 10,000 rpm, permit a significant increase in instantaneous load ratings and the use of extremely short exposure times. A rotating anode must be brought to a stop as quickly as possible after the exposure has been terminated to conserve the bearing life of the x-ray tube.

IMPORTANT

When a high-speed rotor is used, an electrical braking apparatus reduces the speed from 10,000 rpm to 3000 rpm almost immediately after the completion of the exposure. The energizing and de-energizing of the rotor can generate 3000 or more additional heat units per exposure.

The Grid-Controlled X-ray Tube

Conventional x-ray exposures begin and end at zero point of the sinewave (see Chapter 2, Fig. 2-1). The shortest possible single-phase exposure is usually 1/120th of a second.

In addition to the cathode and anode, the grid-controlled tube has another component called a "grid," not to be confused with the grid used for scatter control. The grid-controlled focusing cup is electrically isolated from the filament. During the operation of the x-ray tube, a negative bias voltage is applied to the focusing cup, making it negative with respect to the filament. As previously noted, the focusing cup is always negative to limit the electrons to an appropriate electron stream to form the actual focal spot. In a grid bias tube, a negative electrostatic field is set up, which acts as a gate to stop the electron flow to the anode by repelling the negatively charged electrons. A large-enough voltage will completely cut off the tube current; no electrons will flow from cathode to anode. When this bias voltage is removed, the electrons flow to the anode to produce x-rays. Extremely short exposure times are possible with grid-controlled tubes.

With a grid-controlled x-ray tube, exposures do not have to begin or end at the zero point of the wave. Exposures can be synchronized to a particular portion of the sinewave. Often the middle third or the peak of a single-pulse (1/120th of a second) is used, resulting in an exposure of 1/360th of a second. Since only the portion of the wave that produces high-energy photons is used, absorbed dosage from low-energy photons is reduced.

Grid-controlled tubes are used to advantage for cinefluorography and are synchronized to the cine camera shutters. Exposure to the patient occurs only when the camera shutter is open. Cineradiographic imaging is discussed in Chapter 13.

New X-ray Tube Design

In some new x-ray tubes, the center of the glass envelope has been replaced with a metal section, which provides a constant electrical field not influenced by tungsten deposits. The exit window of the glass tube is a thin, polished area whereas the metal tube has a beryllium window, which results in low absorption of the x-rays.

Electrons that rebound from the actual focal spot and strike other metal within the tube produce x-radiation similar to the primary beam, which is known as extrafocal radiation (described in Chapter 5). Since the electrons that rebound from the target are collected by the grounded center section, extrafocal radiation can be reduced with this new envelope design.

Anode Design

A new anode design reduces the overall mass and weight of the anode by about one half with the use of a graphite disc bound to a molybdenum anode. Graphite has a high thermal capacity, and new compound anodes are made with a graphite base to help dissipate heat faster than conventional anodes (see Fig. 3-18).

Conventional anodes are 90 mm in diameter. As the x-ray anode is increased in diameter, focal spot size remains the same but mass is increased; as a result, instantaneous load and anode thermal capacity increase. The heavier anode, however, can shorten bearing life.

A 200-mm diameter anode is available for high output tubes. These newer discs have multiple radial slits cut through the track to prevent cracking.

X-ray Tube Rating Charts

Tube rating charts are guides supplied by x-ray tube manufacturers to indicate tube heating and

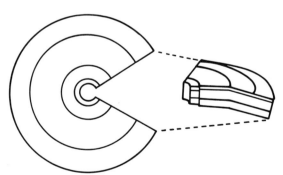

Figure 3-18
Compound Anode Disc

Since conventional x-ray tubes overheat with continuous operation, a compound anode disc made with a rhenium tungsten alloy bonded to molybdenum and graphite was developed. Heat storage capacity and heat dissipation are improved with this new technology. The total weight of the anode is less than a tungsten anode of the same size because molybdenum is half the weight of tungsten and graphite is 1/10th the weight of tungsten.

cooling characteristics, expressed in heat units or load ratings.

A tube rating chart is needed for specific information with regard to the tube in use, such as focal spot size, anode diameter, target angle, speed of rotation, heat storage capacity, and generator type.

IMPORTANT

Each specific tube has its own rating charts. Do not substitute one manufacturer's chart for another; they are not interchangeable.

Because of the effect of a series of exposures on an x-ray tube and concern for the maximal thermal capacity of the anode, the appropriate charts, including heat input/cooling charts, should be checked when performing complex technical procedures such as angiography or cineradiography.

When a high continuous load is required, special rating charts are supplied by the manufacturer of the x-ray tube. These procedures, with their higher ratings and multiple exposures, increase thermal stress.

IMPORTANT

When radiographers work together, studies are often quickly completed. However, heat units accumulate rapidly in these situations, with a greater potential for tube damage. For example, with follow-up fluoroscopy procedures of the gastrointestinal tract or with tomography, exposures can be made faster than the tube can cool.

Unfortunately, less than 1% of the energy used to produce x-rays is converted to x-radiation. More than 99% of the energy becomes heat, which is dissipated rapidly from the anode into the oil-filled housing. The heat is then dissipated from the housing into the surrounding room air. Some x-ray tubes have air circulators to facilitate housing cooling. Heavy-duty special-purpose tubes may require heat exchangers for faster heat dissipation. Heat exchangers circulate the housing oil to an air cooler at another location in the room to boost the housing heat dissipation rate.

A *heat unit (HU)* is defined as the energy produced in the form of heat by one kVp and one mA for one second, using single-phase, full-wave rectified radiographic equipment.

In the United States, almost all electrical energy is supplied as 60-cycle (60 Hz/second) current. The electron flow (current) is reversed (alternating current) 60 times per second. When three overlapping waves (separate currents) are used in a single circuit, three-phase current is generated. (See Chapter 2, Fig. 2-1.)

Multiphase radiographic equipment uses 6-pulse or 12-pulse current. To determine heat units when using three-phase equipment with 6-pulse rectification, multiply the single-phase heat unit factors by 1.35; for three-phase with 12-pulse rectification, multiply the single-phase factors by 1.41. To determine total heat units for a series of exposures, multiply the above factors by the number of exposures made in the series.

Three-phase generators produce higher-intensity x-radiation than single-phase generators at the same kVp and mA settings. For a similar film blackening effect, the three-phase, 6-pulse generator needs approximately two thirds of the exposure of the single-phase equipment. The 12-pulse generator needs half the single-phase exposure for a similar film blackening effect. For example, a single-phase, 80 kVp, 100 mA, 1-second exposure will generate 8000 HU. With 6-pulse, three-phase current, one must multiply this factor by 1.35 to calculate HU (10,800). In actuality, only 0.67 of a second would be needed with a three-phase, 6-pulse generator to produce the same film blackening effect as the previously described single-phase exposure. The heat units generated with a 6-pulse, three-phase current at 0.67 of a second would be 7236. A similar film blackening effect achieved with a three-phase, 12-pulse system using a time value of 0.5 of a second results in a total of 5640 HU (Table 3-2).

IMPORTANT

A similar film blackening effect is achieved at the same kilovoltage with less loading of heat on the anode with a three-phase generator as compared with a single-phase generator.

There are three types of tube rating charts:

1. Instantaneous load chart
2. Anode cooling chart
3. Housing cooling chart

INSTANTANEOUS LOAD CHART. This chart indicates the maximal kVp and mA values that can be

Table 3-2. Calculations of Heat Units with Compensation in Exposure Length for Three-Phase Equipment

Type	Heat Units	Compensating Factors (to approximate the film blackening effect of single-phase, full-wave exposure factors)
Single-phase, full-wave rectification (8000 HU)	80 kVp × 100 mA × 1 sec	
Three-phase, 6-pulse rectification	8000 HU × 1.35 (10,800 HU)	80 kVp × 100 mA × 0.67 sec × 1.35 (7,236 HU)
Three-phase, 12-pulse rectification	8000 HU × 1.41 (11,280 HU)	80 kVp × 100 mA × 0.5 sec × 1.41 (5,640 HU)

To achieve the same film blackening effect with three-phase equipment, approximately two thirds the time factor (or mAs) is needed for three-phase, 6-pulse equipment. For three-phase, 12-pulse equipment, the time factor (or mAs) can be reduced to approximately one half.

used for a given length of time for a single exposure (Fig. 3-19). Factors that determine the instantaneous load capacity (the heating effect of a single exposure) include:

Focal spot dimensions. These are determined by the size of the filament (small or large) or the angle of the anode (steep or conventional) (see Fig. 3-2).

Diameter of the anode. A larger-diameter anode improves instantaneous loading as well as heat storage capacity. As the diameter of the anode increases, more metal (increased mass) is available for heat storage. When two anodes of the same diameter but different thickness are compared, the thicker anode will have a greater heat storage capacity. Although the thicker anode has increased heat storage ca-

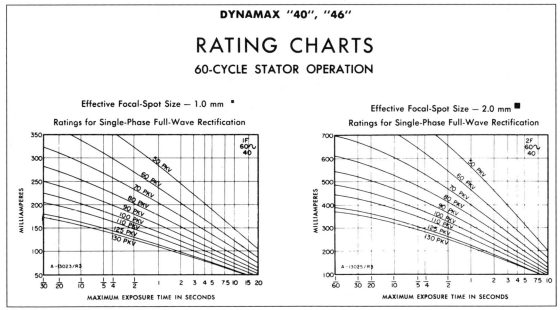

Figure 3-19
Tube Rating Charts

The small effective focal spot (1.0 mm; left) is compared with a large effective focal spot (2.0 mm; right). Tube ratings become more restrictive as high milliampere values are used with a given kilovoltage level. Specific tubes have their own rating charts. One manufacturer's chart should not be substituted for another, because they are not interchangeable. The tube rating chart used in this illustration is designed for a single-phase unit. (Courtesy of Machlett Laboratories, Stamford, CT)

pacity, its instantaneous load capability is not improved because both anodes are of the same diameter, therefore focal track lengths are equal (see Fig. 3-17). As the diameter of the anode increases, the focal track also increases in length, resulting in a dual benefit: instantaneous load improvement and increased heat storage capacity (see Fig. 3-17).

Rotation speed of the anode. The focal spot or focal track of a rotating anode tube receives direct electron bombardment. If the speed of the anode can be increased from 3000 rpm to 10,000 rpm, instantaneous load capacity will be significantly increased, as fresh, unbombarded tungsten is brought into the electron stream more rapidly than with conventional speed rotating anodes. Exposure times can be shortened and the use of a large focal spot can be avoided.

ANODE COOLING CHART. This chart documents the anode thermal capacity of the tube and is used

to determine the time required for the anode to cool either to zero heat units or to a level at which additional exposures are permissible (Fig. 3-20). The anode cools quickly; therefore, short time delays between x-ray exposures can be beneficial. Tube life can be extended if a radiographic tube is operated at a lower than maximal heat capacity.

If the tube is equipped with a heat sensor, it will operate up to approximately 80% of its anode thermal capacity before the sensor will prevent the radiographer from making an additional exposure.

HOUSING COOLING CHART. This chart is used to indicate the heat unit capacity as well as cooling characteristics of the housing (see Fig. 3-20).

Kilowatt Ratings

A watt is a measure of a current of 1 ampere under an electrical pressure of 1 volt. A kilowatt is equal to 1000 watts.

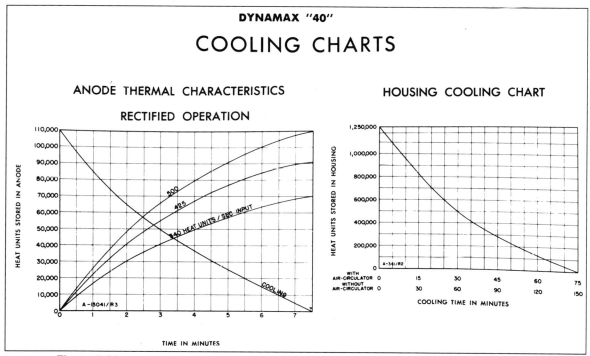

Figure 3-20
Cooling Charts

(Left) When radiographic studies such as tomography are performed, the anode thermal characteristic cooling chart should be consulted prior to the examination. Even though an individual exposure (instantaneous load) can be tolerated by an x-ray tube, the accumulation of heat units due to multiple exposures can damage the tube. (Right) Housing cooling is rarely a problem with conventional radiographic procedures because of the high heat storage capacity of modern tube housings. (Courtesy of Machlett Laboratories, Stamford, CT)

Radiographic tubes have specific kilowatt ratings. As focal spot size increases, higher kilowatt ratings are obtained. Kilowatt ratings vary with different mA settings.

Higher mA values with short exposure times are often needed for angiographic studies to stop motion or to increase the number of frames per second recorded with a film or cassette changer. This is a technical compromise, since the use of a small focal spot with greater potential for improved radiographic detail would require lower mA values and longer exposure times. The use of a rare-earth screen film combination should be considered to augment film blackening, particularly with a low-kilowatt-rated x-ray tube.

Angiography is described in Chapter 11.

Radiographic Tube Damage

Whenever possible, allow cooling time between exposures or a series of exposures. Two of the most common problems relating to tube damage occur simultaneously: the filament of the tube is heated to maximal incandescence while the anode of the tube is rotated at maximal speed.

Tube damage can be attributed to the following:

1. Evaporation of the filament. When an x-ray unit is turned on, the filament is illuminated to a standby level of heating. As the anode is rotated to maximal revolutions per second, the filament is boosted to a predetermined heat level and "free" electrons are boiled off. Minute particles of tungsten can evaporate from the filament and be deposited on the glass envelope of the tube. When tungsten build-up occurs, cracking of the glass envelope is possible owing to high-voltage arcing between the cathode, by way of the glass envelope, and the anode. The use of higher kilovoltage increases the possibility of arcing.

IMPORTANT

A prime cause of filament evaporation is the holding or delaying of the exposure after the filament has been heated to incandescence. Filament evaporation is accentuated by high mA values. Occasionally, tungsten can also be vaporized from the surface of an overheated anode.

2. Anode damage. Pitting of the anode can occur with high instantaneous exposures. Thermal stress can cause the anode to warp, crack, or erode. This roughening, grazing, or erosion usually occurs as the result of overheating by repeated rapid exposures on an already heated target. A damaged anode can cause a non-uniform beam, increased image blur, and reduced radiation output. Although a heat load on a cold target may cause the target to crack, the same high heat load or multiple exposures on a properly warmed-up x-ray tube should not cause anode damage.

IMPORTANT

Manufacturers' warm-up procedures for heating the x-ray target to ductile temperatures, without overstressing the anode, must be rigidly followed. This is particularly important whenever a long time might occur between examinations. A proper warm-up procedure results in a uniformly warm anode, minimizing uneven expansion and contraction of the anode. Warm-up technique data can be obtained from the equipment manufacturer or service engineer.

3. Damage to the bearings of the x-ray tube. Conventional anodes rotate at approximately 3000 rpm as opposed to high-speed anodes (10,000 rpm). Increased speed helps to dissipate heat from the anode. Unfortunately, x-ray tube bearings deteriorate more rapidly at high speeds. Overheating of the x-ray tube can affect the rotor and rotor bearings. When the anode thermal capacity is exceeded, considerable heat is conducted to the rotor and rotor-bearing structure.

IMPORTANT

Do not rotate the anode at maximal speed while attempting to communicate with a patient. Energize the high-speed rotor immediately prior to an exposure. Drop back to standby illumination if an exposure is delayed.

Prolonged rotation of the anode also produces heat units, which are impossible to calculate since technical factors are not involved.

IMPORTANT

Do not abruptly change the direction of the x-ray tube while the high-speed rotor is energized. The torque created on the anode and stem assembly can shear the anode from its stem and break the glass envelope. If the x-ray unit is turned off before the electronic braking action has occurred, damage can occur to the tube. Do not adjust the x-ray tube either by bumping or striking it with your hand. When moving a mobile unit, make certain that the x-ray tube is locked in position.

Chapter 4

Radiographic and Fluoroscopic Equipment and Related Accessories

Inherent limitations in imaging equipment can affect the selection of technical factors and patient positioning. In this chapter, emphasis will be placed on the image-producing characteristics of permanently installed and mobile x-ray equipment rather than the design of specific units.

IMPORTANT

Equipment calibration is essential prior to the use of any radiographic unit.

Before operating radiographic equipment, the radiographer should consider the following:

1. The manufacturer's recommendations for the x-ray tube "warm-up" procedures
2. The maximal permissible mA and kVp values permitted for an instantaneous single exposure
3. Heat unit limitations. This is particularly important when radiographers work together to perform a procedure. For example, gastrointestinal or tomographic studies can generate large amounts of heat, taxing the anode thermal capacity of an x-ray tube.
4. Focal spot size. One should know whether focal spot size is automatically determined for specific mA stations or whether the radiographer must make the selection.
5. Filtration. Federal, state, and local filter requirements must be followed.
6. Timer considerations. When an automatic exposure device is used the radiographer should be familiar with

both minimal response time and back-up time limitations. (See Chapter 2.)

7. Collimation. One should be aware of all beam-limiting accessories that can be used with the collimator.

8. Grid characteristics. Grid ratio, radius, and lines per inch for each grid in use should be known.

9. List of radiographic accessories. Adequate supplies and tools can help to expedite patient flow. With the aid of a checklist, the radiographer can quickly identify deficiencies in room supplies.

10. Availability of oxygen and suction. Emergency aids are often wall mounted, requiring only replacement of the disposable portions of the emergency equipment.

11. Availability of telephone and emergency code numbers

Permanent Installations

Radiographic equipment can be either permanently installed or mobile. Permanent installations include conventional radiographic rooms (Fig. 4-1) and radiographic/fluoroscopic rooms equipped with either a conventional fluoroscope

or an image intensifier (Fig. 4-2). Image-intensified fluoroscopic units usually include a spot film device or a spot film photographic camera in tandem with the intensifier. (For more specific information see Chapter 12.)

Permanently installed dedicated units include daylight film-loading equipment, chest imaging equipment, cassetteless x-ray tables, conventional head units, and mammographic equipment.

Mobile or bedside x-ray machines can be operated from a conventional power source, can be condenser discharge energized, or can operate from a self-contained battery system. Mobile image intensifiers are useful in the operating room or for special fluoroscopic-controlled procedures such as catheter placement. (See Mobile Radiographic/Fluoroscopic Units.)

Routine Radiographic Equipment

X-ray equipment varies in output. The selection of a specific type of generator (single-phase or three-phase) is determined by imaging needs and is often directly related to the cost of the equipment. Specific information on generator types can be found in Chapter 2.

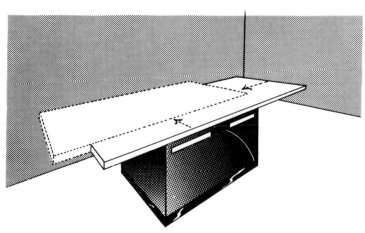

Figure 4-1
Permanently Installed Radiographic Table

A horizontal radiographic table with a movable tabletop makes patient positioning easier for both patient and radiographer. The table top is shown moved from its normal position, illustrated by dashed lines and arrows. After the patient is placed on the table, the floating tabletop is moved to center specific body parts to the table Bucky. Some tables can be elevated or lowered to facilitate patient transfer.

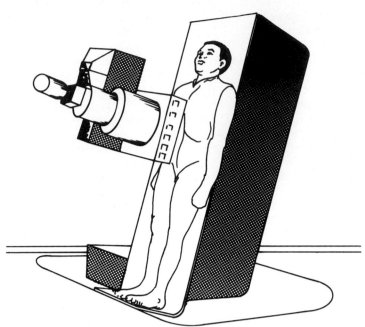

Figure 4-2
Radiographic/Fluoroscopic Unit
Some permanently installed radiographic/fluoroscopic units can be used in the horizontal position or can be motor driven to a full upright position. Most units can be adjusted to the Trendelenburg position (head lower than feet). Some tables have a dual 90-degree capability. In this illustration the table is almost upright as the patient is elevated for horizontal-beam fluoroscopic spot filming.

IMPORTANT

When a unit is rated at a high kilovoltage value as well as a high mA value, it is usually not possible to use both maximal values for the same exposure.

Radiographic Tables

A permanently installed radiographic room includes a table that can be fixed in the horizontal position, adjusted at any angle (motor driven) (see Fig. 4-2) up to a fully upright position, or placed in the Trendelenburg position (head lower than feet). Tables with dual 90-degree capability are associated with fluoroscopic/radiographic procedures.

Floating tabletops make the positioning of the patient easier for both patient and radiographer (see Fig. 4-1). Some tables can also be elevated or lowered for ease of patient transfer.

Of particular interest is the geometric relation of the tabletop to the Bucky tray (TT/BT). This distance can be as great as 13 cm, significantly increasing object–film distance (OFD). There is also a difference in OFD if a grid cassette is used instead of a table Bucky technique. Image geometry is discussed in Chapter 8.

Tube Cranes and Tube Stands

A birail tube stand often requires that the patient be placed on the x-ray table for an x-ray examination. This is a limitation in the emergency room. A ceiling-mounted tube crane can be moved over greater distances and, if the patient cannot be transferred to the x-ray table, can accommodate non-grid or grid cassette exposures on a litter (Fig. 4-3).

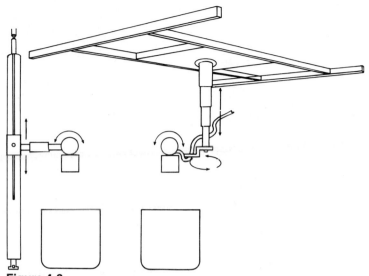

Figure 4-3
Radiographic Tube Holders

(Left) Birail, fixed tube stands limit the mobility of the x-ray tube. The tube usually can be moved back and forth in a single direction on its rails from one end of the table to the other. The tube may also be moved off-center to the Bucky, to the left or right, for non-Bucky radiographs. It is often difficult to examine a patient on a litter with a birail tube stand unless clearance for the litter is available at one end of the table.

(Right) A ceiling-mounted tube crane can be moved over a greater distance to accommodate non-Bucky exposures on a litter if the patient cannot be transferred to the x-ray table. The mobility of the tube crane is limited only by the dimensions of the ceiling-mounted tracks. Some of these cranes can be moved the full length and width of the radiographic room. This mobility can be particularly helpful when lateral horizontal beam radiographs such as skull, hip, or trauma examinations are requested. Decubitus examinations are also easier to perform with a ceiling-mounted tube crane.

Tomographic Attachments

Tomographic attachments can be installed on routine radiographic equipment. A fulcrum with a centimeter scale used to determine the x-ray focal plane can be attached to the x-ray table. An x-ray table with a tomographic attachment will produce acceptable linear tomographic images. Unfortunately, linear tomography will always exhibit linear parasitical streaks. (Tomographic equipment and techniques are presented in Chapter 11.)

Upright Cassette Holders

Most upright cassette holders can be used with several size cassettes. A typical upright cassette holder holds 14 × 17 inch cassettes for chest or abdominal radiography. These units can be equipped with either a fine-line stationary grid or a Bucky (Fig. 4-4). Some wall-mounted holders can accept a 14 × 36 inch cassette for upright radiography of the vertebral column or full-length weight-bearing for lower extremity evaluation.

Radiographic/Fluoroscopic Units

For some examinations, static imaging (radiography) must be supplemented by motion evaluation (fluoroscopy). A fluoroscope is used for this purpose.

The use of a conventional fluoroscopic screen

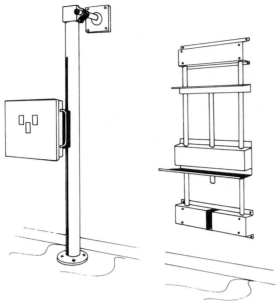

Figure 4-4
Wall-Mounted Cassette Holders

The basic types of wall-mounted cassette holders include a counterbalanced Bucky (left). This device houses either a moving grid or a fine-line stationary grid for upright radiography of the chest, skull, and abdomen. An AED sensor array is shown in this illustration. A standard cassette holder (right) uses tracks to hold the cassette in place. It is important that grid focal range be considered when using a grid with these cassette holders. Most abdominal or osseous studies are exposed at a 40-inch FFD, whereas most chest radiographs are made using a 72-inch FFD. If the focal range of the grid is not correct for the study, image cutoff can occur.

requires dark adaptation of the eyes and total room darkness because of the low light level of the fluoroscope. Modern fluoroscopic units use image intensifiers rather than a conventional fluoroscopic screen (Fig. 4-5). Image intensifiers with a television viewing system are operated in near to normal room-light conditions.

Conventional fluoroscopic screens are made of zinc cadmium sulfide (ZnCdS) crystals that phosphoresce yellow-green when excited by x-radiation. Similar in nature to the phosphors used in intensifying screens, fluoroscopic screen phosphors also absorb x-ray energy and convert it to visible light. The emissivity range of these phosphors match the color sensitivity of the human eye. ZnCdS phosphors exhibit lag or afterglow,

which persists for a short time after the activating source has ceased.

The fluoroscopic tube is usually mounted beneath the radiographic table. X-radiation passes through the tabletop, through the patient, and strikes the fluoroscopic screen. A fluoroscopic spot film mechanism that can hold a cassette is a major component of a fluoroscopic installation. When an area of interest is seen, the fluoroscopist can bring the cassette from the parked position into the x-ray field, make an exposure, and then return the cassette to its parked position (see Fig. 4-5).

Low mA values (1–5 mA) are used for fluoroscopy; conventional mA values (200 mA or greater) are used for spot film radiography.

The cassettes can vary in size; some are as large as 14 × 14 inches. The film can be exposed as a single frame or divided into several segments by a built-in lead masking system, making multiple sequential imaging possible.

Foot switches are sometimes used to activate the fluoroscope or to make radiographic images. Switches should be protected from contaminants that might cause them to stick in the closed position and produce prolonged fluoroscopy.

Most fluoroscopic/radiographic rooms use an image intensifier in place of a conventional fluoroscopic screen. Photographic cameras (70–105 mm) can be used with an image intensifier as a substitute for screen film cassettes. The field size of the input phosphor of the intensifier determines the size of the area to be recorded. (See Chapters 12 and 13 for more specific information.)

Specialized Units

Specialized units dedicated to specific examinations where there is high patient volume help to expedite workflow.

Dedicated Chest Units

The installation of a ceiling-mounted tube in a dedicated chest room (Fig. 4-6) permits an increased FFD for the examination of recumbent patients. A critically ill patient must often be examined in the supine position in a conventional radiographic room using a high-ratio 12:1 grid with a 36- to 40-inch focal range. The use of the increased FFD with a low 6:1 ratio grid and a 28- to 72-inch focal range to facilitate grid centering results in less magnification of chest anatomy. (See

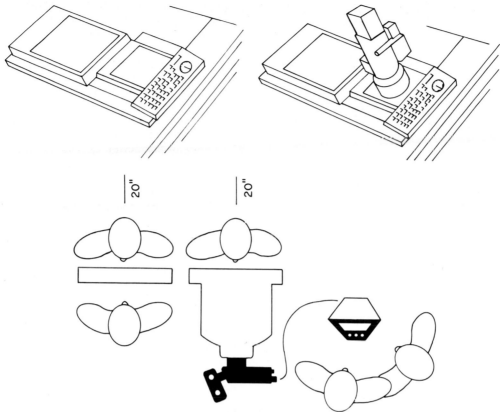

Figure 4-5
Conventional Fluoroscope Versus Image Intensifier

Prior to the advent of the image intensifier, fluoroscopic screens requiring dark adaptation of the eyes were used. The low light level of the fluoroscope produced a dimly illuminated image for the fluoroscopist (top and bottom left). The patient was examined in a darkened room, and radiographs were made using a spot film tunnel. When an area of interest was seen on the fluoroscopic screen, the radiologist brought the cassette into position and a spot film radiograph was made. Single- or multiple-frame studies per cassette were possible. Modern fluoroscopic spot film equipment (top right) is similar in design but uses an image intensifier for fluoroscopic guidance. Under almost normal room-light conditions, the radiologist can view the fluoroscopic procedure on mirror optical viewers or on a television screen (bottom right). For fluoroscopic spot film imaging, the cassette is brought into the x-ray field, an exposure made, and the cassettes is returned to its parked position. Because of the high light output of the image intensifier, photographic-type fluoroscopic spot films can be made using a strip or cut film camera (bottom right). The size of the image intensifier input phosphor (6–15 in) determines the area of the patient that can be imaged with a photographic spot film camera. Using the conventional spot film tunnel with screen film cassettes, the field size can be varied to the size of the cassette. Most spot film devices use either 8 × 10 inch or 9½ × 9½ inch cassettes. Some newer models use 14 × 14 inch cassettes, producing almost full-size radiographic images from a fluoroscopic spot film tunnel.

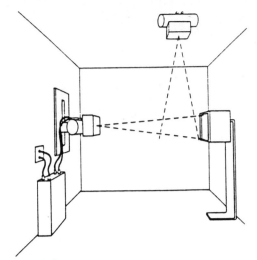

Figure 4-6
**Ceiling-Mounted X-ray Tube for Recumbent
Radiography of the Chest**

*A ceiling-mounted x-ray tube permits the examination
of the chest in the recumbent position. The increased
FFD combined with a low ratio grid results in a radiograph that approximates a conventional chest image.
(Courtesy of Cullinan JE: A perfect chest radiograph—
or a compromise? Radiol Technol 53:2, 1981)*

Chapter 10, Figs. 10-21 and 10-22, for horizontal
beam imaging of the chest in the lateral position.)

If departmental volume does not justify a dedicated chest unit, an existing conventional x-ray
unit can be dedicated to this procedure. Even if a
dedicated chest unit is available, a second radiographic room should be calibrated for chest radiography, since this procedure can account for as
much as 50% of the patient workload in some
facilities.

Daylight Film Loading Systems

Film-handling equipment that loads and unloads
cassettes in normal room light, and that can be directly linked to an automatic processor, has been
available since the late 1960s. Automatic processing of x-ray film is discussed in Chapter 7.

Most of these systems are labeled "daylight-
loading" or "room-light loading" systems. These
units function in normal room light, without the
use of a darkroom, and use wall-mounted film dis-
pensers. Each size of x-ray film requires its own
dispenser and cassettes that cannot be opened
manually. These cassettes can be fed directly into
a central freestanding automatic processor or into

a transportable storage magazine used to carry the
exposed film to an automatic processor. These systems use conventional non-interleaved x-ray film,
without paper covering. Most daylight loading
units require special cassettes; one exception is the
Kodak X-Omatic cassette load system, a freestanding centrally located multiloader that uses the conventional Kodak cassette.

It is possible in some cases, with some units, to
use several different types or speeds of x-ray film.
When only three types of films are needed, these
systems can be relatively small, becoming part of
the processing unit.

Some users claim that the daylight system
eliminates the need for a darkroom. This is not
always true, since many special procedures require specific types of film, film holders, or cassettes. Even with conventional x-ray screens and
films, if a new screen or film is introduced on a
trade-trial basis, it might not be possible to evaluate it in a facility that only has freestanding non-
darkroom processing capability.

The daylight system affords several advantages

The patient does not have to be left unattended,
particularly when only one radiographer is
available.
The image is available to the radiographer immediately, and adjustments to exposure factors,
patient positioning, or additional projections
can be made.
Cassettes do not have to be carried to a central
darkroom.
The option of selecting a faster film is available
for an uncooperative or sick patient.
About half the number of cassettes are needed,
because the cassettes are quickly available for
reuse.
An intensifying screen artifact will quickly become obvious, and the cassette in question can
be removed from the system.

Daylight loading equipment using single emulsion film has been adapted for use with computed tomography, ultrasonography, magnetic
resonance imaging, and nuclear medicine imaging. Daylight film handling equipment increases
productivity, improves work performance, and reduces operating costs.

Automated Film Changers
for Cassetteless Radiography

Dedicated chest radiographic units are designed
with a film transporting mechanism, a pair of in-

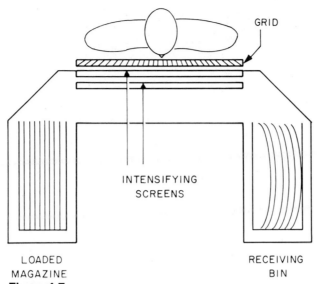

GRID

INTENSIFYING
SCREENS

LOADED
MAGAZINE

RECEIVING
BIN

Figure 4-7
Automatic Film-Changer for Chest Radiography

A film changer, designed for quick and easy evaluation of the chest, holds 100 or more sheets of 14 × 17 inch radiographic film in its loading magazine. The unit is activated by inserting a photoidentification card into a slot on the changer. The film enters the changer, the intensifying screens close, and an exposure can be made. The film is then automatically moved into a receiving magazine for transport to an automatic processor. This unit can also be linked directly to an automatic processor.

tensifying screens, a magazine for housing unexposed film (usually 100 sheets or more), and a receiving cassette for the exposed radiographic film (Fig. 4-7). The x-ray tube moves in synchrony with the film changer; as the height of the changer is adjusted, the tube moves correspondingly. These units can be linked directly to an automatic processor so that a conventional chest radiograph can be made and viewed in less than 2 minutes. A bar can be mounted above the changer to help stabilize the patient in the lateral position.

Cassetteless radiographic tables, linked to an automatic processor, accommodate a variety of x-ray film sizes for routine radiography. The radiographer is able to remain with the patient and the images can be evaluated prior to removing the patient from the table (Fig. 4-8).

Dedicated Head Units

Dedicated head units are used for routine radiography of the skull, sinuses, mastoids, facial bones, and some other small parts of the body. The head unit can also be used in a recumbent position for examination of an immobile patient. Major advantages of the head unit include patient comfort, ease in positioning, and the ability to easily demonstrate air-fluid levels.

Mammographic Equipment

Conventional radiographic equipment should not be used for screen film mammography. Dedicated mammographic units with molybdenum (Mo) anode tubes, a 30-micra Mo filter, and a breast compression platform are essential. Most of these units have an AED as well as a built-in Bucky for high-contrast mammography.

Tungsten (W) target tubes, if used for mammography, should have a beryllium window and minimal aluminum filtration.

Mammography is discussed in Chapter 11, and the xeroradiographic process is discussed in Chapter 13.

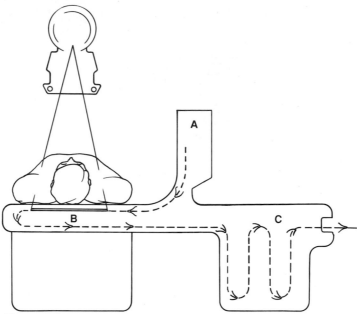

Figure 4-8
Cassetteless Radiographic Table
Supine Bucky tables that can use several sizes or types of x-ray film in an automatic film changer mechanism are available. The Bucky (B) automatically receives x-ray films from a film storage unit (A). An exposure is made and the film is automoatically transported to an x-ray film processor (C).

Radiographic Accessories

The use of radiographic accessories is dependent on the skill and attitude of the radiographer. The following are some of the common radiographic accessories.

1. Compression bands. A compression band made of cloth or nylon (about 10 in wide) can be used on a radiographic table. This band is linked to the table, from side to side, usually across the patient's abdomen. A tightening mechanism can be used to compress the abdomen to an overall even thickness. (See Chapter 5, Fig. 5-3.) An *air-filled rubber bladder* can be used beneath a compression band to compress the ureters during intravenous pyelography. Compression is also important in mammography. (See Chapter 11.)

   Some contraindications for abdominal compression include recent surgery, trauma, acute abdominal pain, known or suspected abdominal mass, and aortic aneurysm. There is a danger of metastasis in patients with an intra-abdominal neoplasm, particularly infants and children; therefore, abdominal compression or prone positioning should be avoided with these patients. Compression should not be used during intravenous urography in patients with a known or suspected ureteral obstruction or suspected ureteral stones.

2. Radiolucent foam rubber positioning aids. Radiolucent foam rubber sponges (circles, squares, rectangles, and wedges of varying angles) help in the positioning of a patient. The angled wedges are used to duplicate comparison positions. Positioning aids also make the patient more comfortable, lessening the chance for lack of sharpness due to motion on the radiograph.

IMPORTANT

Foam rubber sponges can absorb impurities such as barium and iodine, resulting in opaque artifacts on the processed radiograph.

3. Table padding. A study done at the Mayo Clinic found that the table padding can attenuate or absorb 11% to 16% of a 70-kVp three-phase x-ray beam as it exits from a patient-equivalent phantom.* Some low-density materials (referring to the proportion of polyurethane to air, such as ¾-in-thick polyurethane foam) showed a 3% attenuation, whereas high-density (silicone-loaded foam) padding, 1 inch thick, which resembles low-density foam, attenuated 33% of the 70 kVp x-ray beam. Heavy-duty vinyl table pad covers also add 2% to the attenuation factor.
4. Body immobilizers (restraining devices). Pediatric and adult immobilizing devices are used to restrain uncooperative patients.
5. Cassette holders. Cassette holders or tunnels can be placed beneath a patient who cannot be moved to a radiographic table. These tunnels are also used in the operating room during hip pinnings, cholangiography, and so on. Cassette holders, with or without grids, can be used for horizontal beam projection techniques.
6. Radiographic viewboxes. An important radiographic accessory is the x-ray viewbox. Optical density can be influenced by the intensity of the light from the viewbox. The formula for optical density stated as

$$D = \log\frac{\text{incident light}}{\text{transmitted light}} \qquad D = \log\frac{I_o}{I}$$

assumes that the light source incident to the film is calibrated and constant. Often, an image viewed and accepted at the automatic processor may seem either over- or underexposed when viewed on another viewbox, owing to variations in viewbox light output. If the light output of both viewboxes were measured, a significant difference might be found. Viewboxes with different types of fluorescent light will produce "different looks" and may even affect the appearance of the color of the base of the film.

A photographic light meter can be used to evaluate the amount of light being transmitted by individual viewboxes to ensure that all viewbox light emissions are balanced. Periodic cleaning of the glass on the viewboxes should be a part of the quality assurance program.

*Stearns JG, Gray JE: Patient comfort vs. patient exposure. Radiol Technol 53(4):341–342,1980.

(Quality assurance information can be found in Chapter 14.)
7. Emergency equipment. A radiology department is not without its share of emergencies. Radiographers should be familiar with cardiopulmonary resuscitation (CPR) techniques and the location of emergency equipment, including oxygen and suction. Emergency code telephone numbers and departmental emergency guidelines should be posted in a prominent location.
8. Shielding for allied health personnel. Special aprons and apron racks should be provided for employees in the recovery room, intensive care unit, and nursery. Any patient or employee who is pregnant should be removed from or asked to leave an area where an x-ray image is being made. Anyone with reproductive potential who is required to be in the area must be shielded during the making of an exposure. Additionally, the radiographer should notify everyone in the immediate vicinity that an exposure is about to be made.

Mobile Radiographic Equipment

Even though portable x-ray equipment is mobile by nature, all mobile x-ray equipment should not be considered portable. If an x-ray machine can be packed into a small carrying case and transported, it can be called portable. Most transportable x-ray units are lightweight and can be quickly assembled. Mobile imaging services sometimes use this type of equipment to examine patients at home, in a nursing home, or in other remote locations.

In hospital-based radiography departments 15% to 50% of all chest radiographs are made at the bedside. A 30% figure is typical in many hospitals. A third or more of these images may be of poor technical quality owing to limited x-ray output and positioning difficulties (Fig. 4-9).

Rare-earth screen film imaging, combined with 100 mA constant potential mobile equipment, makes it possible to produce images that approach the film blackening of those taken in the radiology department. The use of rare-earth screen film combinations, 600 speed or greater, brings exposure times to acceptable levels with low-output mobile equipment.

Mobile AEDs are available with sensor cassette systems or sensor devices, which are placed behind the conventional x-ray cassette.

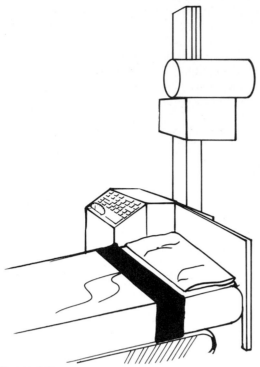

Figure 4-9
Technical Limitations of
Mobile Radiographic Units

A typical high-output mobile radiographic unit; newer mobil units can be either capacitor discharge units or battery operated. With the battery-operated unit, a rotating anode tube is used with a conventional light-beam collimator. Shortened focal film distances are often the norm. Even when the desired FFD is possible, it is difficult to center the x-ray tube to a grid cassette. The weight of the patient or the flexible nature of the mattress often results in cassette rotation and grid cutoff. An automatic exposure device in the form of a paddle, linked by a cable to an AED control panel, helps to produce radiographs of a consistent density. (See Chapter 9, Fig. 9-11.)

Power Supply

An electrical supply is required for both mobile and portable equipment. Lengthy, heavy cables are needed when low-output mobile x-ray units are plugged into an electrical outlet. In older facilities the main current supply may be limited, which will influence the rating of a mobile unit. Even in large facilities, when new equipment and new power lines are available, older sections of a building may have a limited power source. A special "mobile-only" line is helpful in a high-use area such as the emergency room or intensive care unit.

IMPORTANT

A voltage drop or change in an incoming line voltage may cause variations in exposure. Line voltage regulator adjustments can help to overcome variations in current.

A typical portable unit contains the main switch and a rheostat to vary current (mA). The oil-filled, lead-lined head contains an x-ray tube, a step-up transformer, and a step-down transformer. A hand-held mechanical timer is usually used to make an exposure. This type of low-cost timer, also often found on older dental units, will rarely operate accurately below $\frac{1}{10}$th of a second. This limitation is a problem when performing a chest examination because of cardiac motion, and a timer of this nature can rarely be used for the short exposure times needed for pediatric studies.

Milliamperage and kilovoltage output is limited on low-output portable equipment.

Battery-Operated Units

Lengthy trips to the bedside with a battery-operated mobile unit may rob power from the battery. Nickel-cadmium (NiCd) batteries are used for exposure as well as for motor drive assist. The battery source can be recharged from an electrical outlet.

If there is a high volume of work in an area such as the intensive care unit, the mobile unit should be plugged in and left in that area overnight. This policy is also appropriate for the emergency room.

The wet-cell NiCd battery has been an industry standard for many years. However, newer lead-acid batteries are available at about half the initial cost of wet cell batteries and reduce maintenance requirements. Machine up-time is increased.

IMPORTANT

If the battery charge falls off, an inconsistency in generator output may be noticed between exposures. Newer units monitor the condition of their batteries and automatically compensate for power changes, thereby making it possible to obtain more consistent exposures.

Since battery-operated machine output may vary, a repeat radiographic study at the bedside should be made with the same mobile unit, particularly if there is a need for adjustment in technical factors.

Advantages of the battery-powered mobile unit are the availability for triage in remote locations and for use during power outages.

Capacitor Discharge Units

A capacitor (condenser) is a device for accumulating and holding a charge of electricity. Capacitor or condenser discharge mobile units use a conventional electrical source to charge a high-tension capacitor and store a quantity of electricity in the capacitor prior to exposure. Relatively high tube currents can accumulate on capacitors from a standard 110-volt line in a short charging time. When the timer of the capacitor discharge unit is activated, electricity is discharged through the x-ray tube, producing x-radiation. The tube voltage falls off linearly during the exposure.

IMPORTANT

Capacitor units do not maintain a constant kilovoltage value throughout the length of the exposure. For every 1 mAs used during an exposure, these units will drop, in effect, 1 kVp. For example, when a specific mAs value is used, such as 20 mAs at 80 kVp, there is a gradual drop of kilovoltage from 80 kVp to 60 kVp throughout the exposure.

Capacitor discharge units are capable of very short exposure times but are limited if large mAs values are required. According to Thompson, voltage drops off during exposures that are longer than 10 msec.* The capacitor discharge unit is very efficient when low mAs values are used, since only a minor drop in kVp occurs.

A power source should be available in the vicinity of the examining area. Because the charge can leak rapidly from the capacitor, it is not recommended that a unit be charged in one area and used in another area. The unit should be charged immediately prior to use. The use of high-speed, rare-earth imaging, up to 1200 speed, increases the

*Thompson TT: Practical Approach to Modern X-Ray Equipment. *Boston: Little, Brown, 1978.*

film blackening effect of limited output capacitor discharge units.

Battery-operated units have significantly more output than capacitor discharge units and do not drop in kilovoltage during the exposure as mAs is increased.

Field Emission Units

Conventional radiographic tubes use a heated filament to emit electrons; a field emission tube emits electrons from a metal plate. The metal plate is electronegative, with a high-voltage potential between it and its anode. When a sufficiently strong electrical field is applied to this plate, an emission of electrons results.

Field emission mobile units using a microprocessor control can operate at more than 200 kVp. Short exposure times are also possible, reducing radiographic blurring due to patient or organ motion.

Technical Considerations

Most severely injured trauma patients are examined in the emergency area. It is important that experienced personnel handle these patients, because many can quickly develop serious or life-threatening complications that require immediate diagnosis and treatment. The radiographer must learn to work efficiently in this stress-filled environment.

Patients are often examined many times during their hospitalization. Sequential examinations, sometimes several times per day, are common practice. Sequential labeling of the radiographs is important, because in examinations of high quality subtle changes between examinations can be appreciated. A radiograph can never be over-identified (labeled). Positioning angles, technical factors, time of day, and any other pertinent information is a help to the radiologist when interpreting any radiograph, particularly sequential studies.

When using mobile radiographic equipment (see Fig. 4-9), the radiographer must be aware of the potential problems.

1. Poor beam alignment and centering. The central ray can be difficult to align to the center of a grid. Because the mattress and cassette are not always flat, lateral decentering of the grid

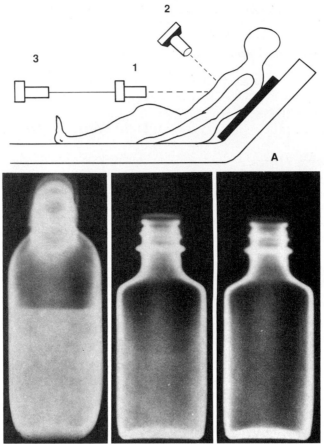

Figure 4-10
Focus Film Distance Variations

(A, top) *An erect bedside examination of the chest is difficult to perform. In the semi-erect position with the tube in a horizontal beam position (1 or 3), a distorted apical lordotic radiograph results. Often it is easier to move the x-ray tube to the foot of the bed (3), producing almost a twofold increase in the FFD.*

Radiographs were made of an 8-oz. bottle half-filled with water (A, bottom). Note the air-fluid level as well as the elongation of the bottle (left) when tube positions 1 or 3 are used (top). When the bottle was imaged with the x-ray tube in position 2, there is no distortion of the bottle but the air-fluid level is not demonstrated (center). (Right) The bottle was placed in the recumbent position and exposed with a perpendicular beam. Because the air-fluid level is parallel to the floor the air-fluid interface cannot be demonstrated. The diffuse gray effect is the result of a perpendicular beam exposure.

If the patient is unable to sit completely erect the x-ray tube can be positioned at an appropriate FFD (2) to ensure proper film blackening. Unfortunately, with this position, an air-fluid interface cannot be demonstrated (bottom, center). See Figure 4-11.

(B) The patient is fully erect as is the bottle in relation to the x-ray tube in position 1. Note the normal representation of the bottle and chest anatomy (bottom, left and right) and the obvious air-fluid interface in both. Once the tube is positioned with the patient partially erect, the cassette can be used as a lever to elevate the patient to the full upright postion. A pillow can be wedged behind the cassette to maintain the erect position.

With the exception of position 2 in A, any of the aforementioned horizontal tube positions can be used to demonstrate an air-fluid level. If air-fluid levels are to be demonstrated, every effort must be made to place the patient in a fully erect position at the appropriate FFD. The central ray must remain parallel to the floor.

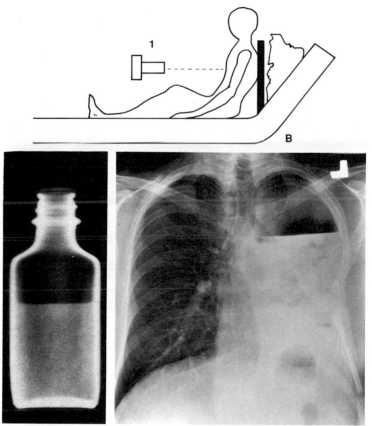

Figure 4-10 *Continued*

can occur. Variations in focal film distance may conflict with the focal range of the grid. Low-ratio grids are often used at the bedside to minimize these problems.

When a non-grid study is made at the bedside, tight beam collimation is mandatory for scatter control. The principles of scatter control outlined in Chapter 5 also apply at the bedside.

2. Positioning difficulties, particularly with decubitus or erect positions. A patient's condition will often dictate positioning limitations. The patient in the intensive care unit may not be able to be elevated to the upright position for a chest study or to inspire fully for maximal ventilation of the lungs. Occasionally, an angled projection with less than optimal inspiration must be taken (Fig. 4-10).

IMPORTANT

A horizontal beam technique is required to demonstrate an air-fluid level in the chest, abdomen, or sinus cavities (Fig. 4-11).

Sometimes horizontal beam radiography cannot be achieved because of the condition of the patient. Unless the patient can be put into the true upright position and a horizontal beam used, an optimal chest radiograph is not produced. It might be advisable to make a supine radiograph for better control of positioning and inspiration. This modification in positioning may produce an image with less motion, since the patient is not in an uncomfortable position.

3. Shortened or increased FFD. A patient in traction with the bed up on blocks may require a shortened FFD, sometimes as low as 20 inches. The location of a bed against a wall may force the use of an increased FFD for a horizontal beam image. Adjustments to techniques must be made to compensate for these variations.

Intensive and Cardiac Care Radiography

Repeat chest radiographs made at the bedside are usually made to monitor postsurgical compli-

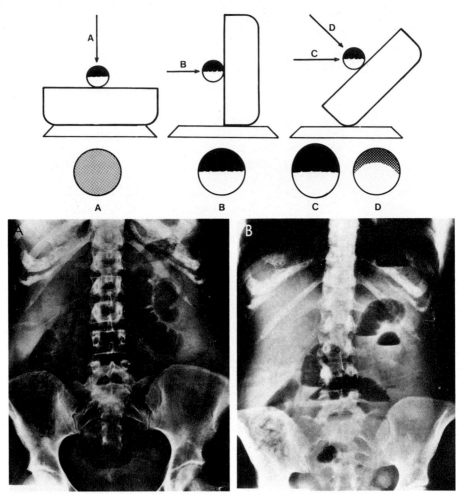

Figure 4-11
Air-Fluid Level Demonstration

For an air-fluid level to be seen on a radiographic image, the central ray must be parallel to the floor (horizontal beam technique). In this illustration, a conventional supine projection is shown (A, top and bottom). Note the air-fluid level in the circular object on the radiographic table. Air is represented by the black superior portion of the circle, fluid by the white inferior portion of the circle. In the full upright position (B, top), there is no change in the air-fluid relation, but the horizontal beam central ray is able to demonstrate the air-fluid interface without distortion. When the table is in the semi-erect position (C, D, top) the air-fluid level will still remain parallel to the floor. When the central ray (C) is used, a distorted elongated image is seen; since a horizontal beam was used, an air-fluid level is demonstrated. Any attempt to avoid this distortion by directing the x-ray beam at an angle to the air-fluid interface (D) will fail to demonstrate this important diagnostic sign. When it is impossible to place a patient in the fully erect position, a lateral decubitus radiograph can be taken to demonstrate an air-fluid interface.

A supine radiograph made to evaluate a mechanical obstruction in the small intestine shows a distended small bowel (A, bottom). The upright horizontal beam radiograph of the same abdomen shows dynamic air-fluid levels (B, bottom). (Abdominal radiographs courtesy of Keats TE: Emergency Radiology. *Chicago: Year Book Medical Publishers, 1984)*

cations or patient progress. Conditions such as pneumothorax, hemothorax, and pneumomediastinum are often followed radiographically.

Placement of airway tubes and catheters must be established; however, tubes, bottles, or other equipment should not be removed or unplugged at the bedside. Do not remove any accessory of any type to obtain a power source. Oxygen and traction devices should not be removed or adjusted without nursing staff approval and help.

Some bedside mobile units have timers that are not accurate at very short exposure times. The increased film blackening of a high-speed, rare-earth screen film accentuates timer limitations when evaluating the neonatal chest in the nursery.

The bassinet of the newborn is often at waist height of the radiographer (see Chapter 9, Fig. 9-7). This fixed FFD, sometimes as close as 20 inches, combined with a high-speed screen film system can cause a fourfold or more increase in film blackening. Newer mobile units allow increases in FFD because of improvements in tube-arm design.

In the lower kilovoltage range the absorption of the x-ray beam by the material used in the cassette front may affect radiographic density.

IMPORTANT

It should be noted that when rare-earth screen film combinations are used, the kVp dependency inherent in most rare-earth intensifying screens causes the system speed to fall off. If 40 kVp or less is used, some rare-earth systems may function at half speed or less. Information on recording media is presented in Chapter 6.

Use of the Mobile Unit in the Operating Room

Whenever possible, a mobile unit should be isolated from routine hospital work and restricted to the operating room to prevent the tracking of contaminated matter into the operating room. This unit must be kept as clean as possible, since the x-ray tube head is often positioned over the sterile field. Debris may fall from the tube head, contaminating the surgical field. The unit should be wiped down before it is used and cleaned again immediately after an operating room procedure. It should be properly covered between examinations.

IMPORTANT

Specific instructions regarding the use of approved cleaning solutions and cleaning methods should be obtained from operating room personnel.

Mobile Radiographic/Fluoroscopic Units

Mobile radiographic/fluoroscopic units can be used in the operating room, critical care unit, coronary care unit, emergency room, or fracture reduction rooms. Fracture reduction, needle biopsy, catheter placement, cardiac pacemaker implant, foreign body localization, and hip pinning procedures are often performed with mobile radiographic fluoroscopic equipment. These units have a C-arm or U-arm configuration and can be linked with videotape, videodisc, or other image storage systems. Images can be digitally stored and displayed. Electronic image subtraction is also possible.

A multiformat camera or laser printer can be used to record fluoroscopic images equal in quality to the original fluoroscopic display.

The C-arm or U-arm can be rotated in many directions around a fixed axis to avoid moving the patient (Fig. 4-12). An image intensifier enables the physician to see a fluoroscopic image in "real" time, which can serve as a baseline for follow-up studies. Field size is limited to the size of the input phosphor of the image intensifier. Confirmation radiographs are often made following the fluoroscopic evaluation.

Mobile imaging systems are no longer limited to conventional radiography. Mobile ultrasonographic equipment, as well as gamma cameras for nuclear medicine studies, are used for medical imaging.

Radiation Dosage Considerations

Radiation protection factors must be considered when performing a mobile examination. These include

1. The exposure control switch should be connected to a long cord (up to 12 feet) to help avoid radiation exposure to the radiographer.
2. A lead apron should be worn by anyone attending these procedures.

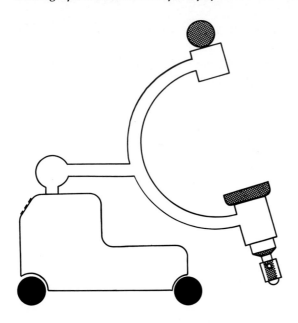

Figure 4-12
C- or U-Arm Mounted Image Intensifier

A mobile image intensifier is available with a C- or U-arm configuration. The C-arm shown is designed with an intensifier and television camera on one end and the x-ray tube on the opposing end. The unit can be rotated around a fixed axis in many directions to avoid moving the patient. As the C-arm is rotated, the relation between the central ray and the input phosphor is maintained. Note that the image intensifier is positioned so that the x-ray beam is always perpendicular to the input phospor.

3. Gonadal shielding should be used on all patients with reproductive potential. Concern regarding the possibility of pregnancy of the patient, other patients in the area, and hospital personnel reflects a professional attitude.

4. Mobile units should not be overlooked when quality assurance tests are being made. Many of the tests used for permanent installations can be used for mobile equipment. The electrical source cables as well as the tube cables of the mobile unit should be evaluated regularly for signs of wear or damage. (Quality control tests are described in Chapter 14.)

I M P O R T A N T

Extension cords or adapter plugs should not be used unless approved by hospital safety officials.

5. Additional radiographs should not be made for the purpose of avoiding a return trip for a possible repeat examination.

Chapter 5

The Production and Control of Scatter Radiation

On a processed radiograph, scatter radiation is seen as a supplemental density that produces a foglike image. More oblique in nature than primary radiation, scatter diffuses in all directions and often travels through longer paths in the body than does primary radiation (Fig. 5-1).

All foglike densities that appear on a radiograph should not be attributed to scatter radiation. Some of these densities may be caused by careless handling or improper storage of x-ray film, use of incorrect safelights, or other film processing difficulties.

The effects of controlling scatter are twofold (1) reduction of dosage to patient and operators, and (2) improvement of image quality.

Production of Scatter Radiation

The production of a radiographic image is influenced by the interactions of x-ray photons with matter. The x-rays may be absorbed totally or partially or may interact with the subject and create characteristic or secondary radiation. As patient thickness and tissue density increase, x-rays interact with more tissue, resulting in an increase in scatter radiation.

In addition to patient thickness and tissue density, the size of the area being exposed to x-radiation has a considerable effect on the production of scatter radiation. The greater the area being exposed to x-radiation, the more scatter radiation produced (Fig. 5-2). In a full-field (14 × 17 inches) radiographic study of the pelvis, 50% or greater of the total number of x-ray photons exiting from the patient consists of scattered radiation.

The x-ray photons that pass through the subject and expose the image detector and the Compton interactions that produce scatter radiation form the remnant beam, which produces the radiographic image.

Angeline M. Cullinan and John E. Cullinan:
PRODUCING QUALITY RADIOGRAPHS, 2ND ED.
© 1987, 1994 J. B. Lippincott Company.

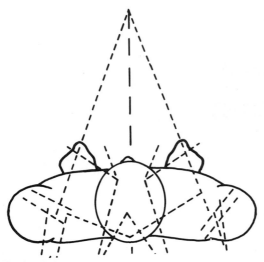

Figure 5-1
Schematic Represenation of Scatter Radiation

Scatter radiation, caused by the interaction of x-rays with matter, is more oblique in nature, can travel through longer paths in the body than primary radiation, and is given off in all directions from the object under study.

As patient thickness increases, scatter radiation also increases. By examining the abdomen in the prone position, patient thickness is decreased; therefore, less scatter is generated. Compression devices can be used with similar results. The use of compression for tissue displacement reduces the area of tissue thickness and therefore the amount of scatter radiation. (See Chapter 4, Radiographic Accessories, for contraindications to compression.) Technical factors can also be reduced when compression is used (Fig. 5-3).

When kilovoltage is increased, the percentage of Compton interaction (scatter) increases and the percentage of photoelectric interactions (absorption) rapidly decreases. Minor increases in kilovoltage provide an increased amount of x-ray photons to the image detector, with a corresponding reduction of absorbed photons. For high-contrast studies, high kVp should be avoided because in general as kVp is increased, scatter radiation is also intensified, resulting in a corresponding decrease in radiographic contrast. As kVp is increased, forward scatter also increases.

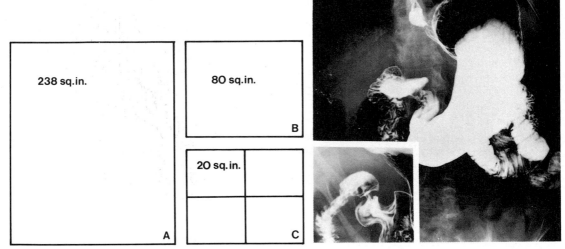

Figure 5-2
The Effect of Collimation of the X-ray Beam

Patient thckness affects the amount of scatter radiation generated in a given examination. The size of the area being examined also has an effect on the production of scatter: the greater the area exposed to x-radiation, the more scatter radiation produced. (A) A 14 × 17 inch field images approximately three times more patient area than an 8 × 10 inch field (B). (C) A typical fluoroscopic spot film (four exposures on one) using a 4 × 5 inch field (one fourth of one 8 × 10 inch film) images 1/12th the field size of the full-frame study (A). (Right) A full-field image of a barium-filled stomach is compared with a tightly collimated fluoroscopic spot film inset. (Radiograph reprinted courtesy Eastman Kodak Company)

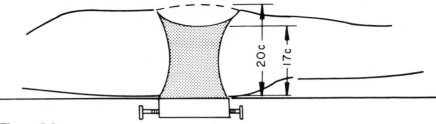

Figure 5-3
Compression Device
The use of a compression device can reduce tissue volume by displacing abdominal tissue to the lateral aspects of the body. Since the x-ray beam is interacting with less tissue, there is a reduction in scatter radiation. Compression is also useful in minimizing patient motion.

Another supplemental density, backscatter—arising from the back of the cassette, the tabletop, or adjoining wall when a wall-mounted upright cassette holder or Bucky is used—can be lessened by the use of lead foil backing in the cassette.

Scattered radiation produced by the object under study or from backscatter contributes to the overall density of the image while diminishing radiographic contrast.

Control of Scatter Radiation

Beam Limiting Devices

The best way to control scatter radiation is to reduce its production. One way to accomplish this is to limit the area being exposed to the primary beam.

Over the years, a variety of beam restricting devices have been developed (Fig. 5-4):

Primary source aperture diaphragms

Conventional cones

Telescopic cones

External lead apertures, including keyhole diaphragms

Variable aperture beam limiting devices, commonly known as light beam collimators, including positive beam limiting (PBL) devices

These beam limiting accessories restrict the area under study to a predetermined field size.

Restriction of the primary ray as close to the source as possible is important. A single diaphragm at source can be more effective than an extension cone or cylinder with its diaphragm some distance from the source (Fig 5-4*A*).

Collimators

Radiographic collimators, variable aperture beam limiting devices, simultaneously adjust several pairs of lead shutters, working synchronously with a beam defining light, to restrict the primary beam. A high-intensity light source, coupled with a reflection mirror, projects the light field, which matches the x-ray field size, onto the part under study. The mirror is part of the inherent filtration of the x-ray tube (Figs. 5-4 and 5-5). The alignment of the light field to the x-ray field (Figs. 5-6 and 5-7) should be checked regularly by quality assurance personnel.

With a PBL, shutter patterns are automatically determined by the size of the cassette being used. Changes in the FFD automatically adjust the beam configuration to the cassette size. In pediatric examinations or serial angiographic studies, the part under study may be smaller than the film size in use, making it necessary to override the PBL feature of the collimator.

Extension Cones and Diaphragms

When extension cones or diaphragms are used in the external tracks of a collimator, the position of the internal collimator shutters is critical. It is easy to add an accessory such as a cone, diaphragm, or keyhole diaphragm and produce an acceptable light beam pattern on the part under study, even when the internal shutters of the collimator are open to the maximum. In this situation, the light beam and not the x-ray beam is being restricted in size (see Fig. 5-4); scatter control is not maximized.

Control of Image Undercutting

If the primary beam does not correspond to the shape of the part under study, scatter from the ta-
(Text continues on page 72)

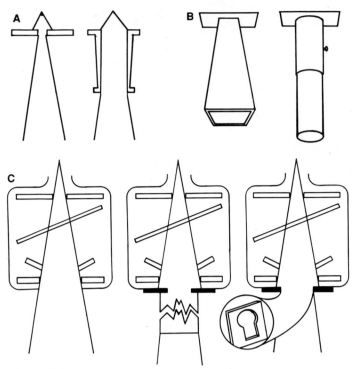

Figure 5-4
Primary Ray Restricting Devices

(A, left) *A primary source aperture diaphragm restricts the x-ray beam as close to the source of x-radiation as possible. An aperture diaphragm of this type can be more effective than a conventional cone or extension cone that does not restrict the primary beam at source (A, right). (B) Conventional radiographic cones can be either square, rectangular, or circular in shape. A specific cone usually used to match a specific cassette size. The rectangular cone is preferred to the round cone because it more closely matches cassette configuration; only the patient area being examined is exposed to radiation. An extension cone can be used for tight primary ray restriction. (C) A light beam collimator uses multiple sets of lead diaphragms mounted at several levels within its housing. A mirror coupled with a light source is used to outline the shutter pattern on the part being examined (see Fig. 5-6). The mirror is considered part of inherent filtration. An extension cone (center) or a keyhold aperture diaphragm (right) can be added to the collimator. Note the position of the internal shutters in relation to the primary x-ray beam. Both of these devices are installed incorrectly in this illustration, since the primary diaphragm of the extension cone or the keyhole aperture is smaller in size than the exit beam formed by the internal collimator shutters. The internal shutters should be reduced in size to conform to the openings in the external aperture. If a keyhole is used and the internal shutters are left completely open, an acceptable light pattern will appear on the object to be examined. Although the light beam has been restricted, the x-ray beam has not been collimated. The effect of collimation has been minimized. (See Chapter 11, Fig. 11-17.)*

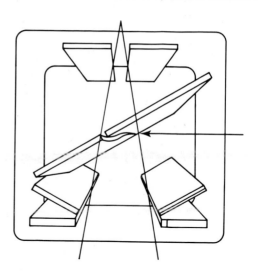

Figure 5-5
The Collimator Mirror as Part of the Filtration System

An exaggerated crack in the colimator mirror is shown. Since the mirror is part of total filtration, the outline of the fracture in the mirror will be seen on lighter areas of the radiograph. A less obvious crack in the mirror can produce an artifact that may simulate a fracture in a large area of bone, such as the skull or pelvis. For a simple test to detect a defect in the mirror, see Chapter 14, Figure 14-8.

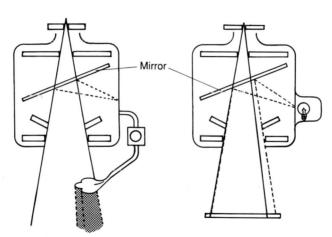

Mirror

Figure 5-6
Gonadal Shielding Collimator Attachment:
Primary Beam/Light Beam Alignment

(Left) A gonadal shield can be externally attached to a radiographic collimator. The shield shown is positioned within the light beam. The shaded area *represents a reduction in primary radiation; therefore, when the shield is properly positioned, a lower gonadal dosage occurs. (Right) A light source is shown in position on the outside of the collimator. Image cutoff can occur if one of the internal shutters of the collimator is out of alignment. The first set of shutters within the collimator is shown out of alignment. The x-ray beam, as a result, is smaller than the projected light beam (dashed lines). This can be a problem particularly with tight field collimation (see Fig. 5-7). For a simple test to detect this problem, see Chapter 14, Figure 14-8.*

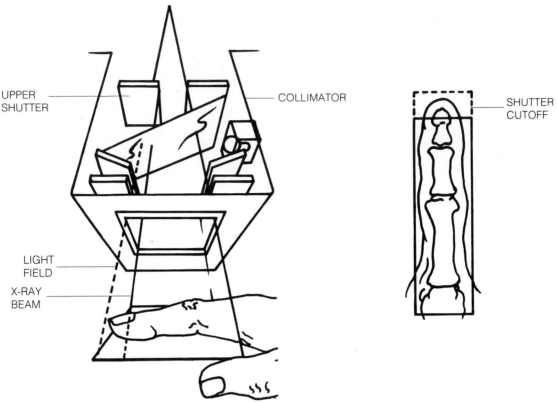

Figure 5-7
Collimator/Shutter Misalignment

Premature closure of a shutter superior to the collimator mirror can result in a cutoff of the image, particulary with a tightly collimated image of a distal extremity. Although the light pattern on the cassette appears adequate, the x-ray beam is reduced in size. For a simple test to demonstrate this problem, see Chapter 14, Figure 14-8. (Reprinted by courtesy Eastman Kodak Company)

bletop may cause "undercutting" of the image, greatly reducing image quality. This is a problem particularly in cerebral angiography or skull radiography as well as in full-field intravenous urography (Figs. 5-8 and 5-9).

Lead rubber-masking or bags of sand, cornmeal, water, rice, or flour placed on the tabletop rather than on the cassette or serial film changer can help to eliminate the undercutting effect generated by a primary beam leak (Fig. 5-10).

Control of Extrafocal Radiation

Ill-defined radiographic details extending beyond the collimated field are often the result of extrafocal (off-focus) radiation, which is produced by backscattered electrons that are re-attracted by the anode in areas other than the actual focal spot

(Figs. 5-11 and 5-12). Extrafocal radiation increases with increases in kVp, mAs, and field size.

The supplemental image formed by the extrafocal radiation, which may represent up to 25% of the "on-focus" radiation, can be partially controlled by lead shutters or a lead iris extending from the top of the collimator and placed as close to the source of the x-ray as possible. Since extrafocal radiation exits at a variety of angles from the x-ray tube, it is important that primary beam collimation begins as close to the source of x-radiation as possible (see Fig. 5-11).

A new x-ray tube was designed to reduce extrafocal radiation. The center of the glass envelope has been replaced with a grounded metal section to collect the electrons that rebound from the target.

The increase in radiographic density on the

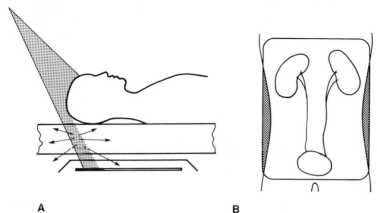

A   B

Figure 5-8
Primary Beam Leak

(A) When an unattenuated primary beam strikes the tabletop, scatter radiation is produced. Scatter is given off in all directions causing an undercutting of the radiographic image. (B) A similar effect occurs with intravenous urography or other abdominal studies where the body configuration does not match the shutter pattern.

image due to extrafocal radiation may be even greater that that seen outside of the collimated field. In the area being examined, particularly in the center of the field where the grid lines are parallel to the central ray, there may be significant density added to the image from extrafocal radiation that is also parallel to the lines of the grid. Because of the oblique nature of extrafocal radiation at the peripheral aspects of the field, this radiation may be absorbed by the canted grid lines, minimizing the significance of the added density on the radiograph (see Fig. 5-11).

Radiographic contrast is also affected by this overall supplemental density.

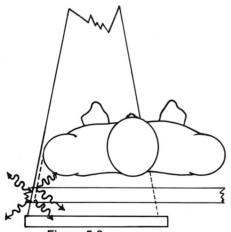

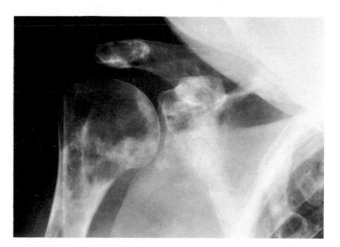

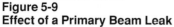

Figure 5-9
Effect of a Primary Beam Leak

(Left) Scatter from the tabletop due to a primary beam leak will undercut the radiographic image. (Right) In a representative radiograph, note the increase in density of the soft tissue structures of the shoulder due to a primary beam leak. The primary beam should be restricted to the part under study.

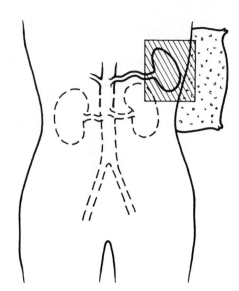

Figure 5-10
Control of Image Undercutting

The use of an underpart filter on the tabletop rather than on the cassette or film changer will minimize undercutting of the radiographic image by attenuating a portion of the primary beam. Bags of sand, cornmeal, water, rice, or flour or lead rubber masking can be placed on the tabletop to absorb the primary ray and minimize the undercutting effect.

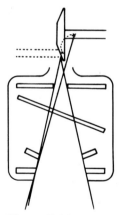
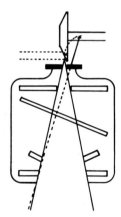
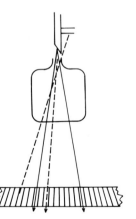

Figure 5-11
Extrafocal Radiation

An additional source of radiation occurs when electrons rebound from the target and strike metallic areas other than the actual focal spot. Extrafocal or off-focus radiation arises from areas of the anode other than the actual focal spot. (Left) For the purposes of this illustration, off-focus radiation is shown emanating from the stem of the anode. Note radiation emanating as a solid line from the stem of the anode. (Center) The placement of a lead diaphragm as close to the source of x-radiation as possible restricts a considerable portion of the off-focus radiation.

Soft tissue details, due to the extrafocal radiation, seen outside of the collimator pattern are considerably lighter than the radiographic image (see Figure 5-12, right). This is probably the result of absorption of the extrafocal radiation by the lateral aspects of the focused grid (right). Although densities seen outside of the x-ray field do not interfere with diagnosis, the extrafocal radiation that overlies the x-ray field can contribute to image blur and increased radiographic density.

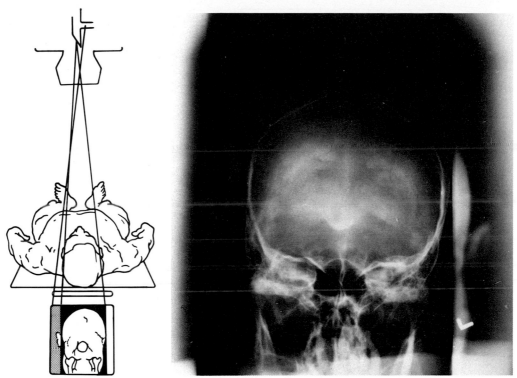

Figure 5-12
Clinical Example of Extrafocal Radiation
On an anteroposterior skull projection, poorly defined soft tissue structures are seen outside the restricted shutter pattern of the collimator as the result of extrafocal radiation. Since extrafocal radiation extends outside of the collimated field, the eyes, thyroid gland, and gonads may receive additional radiation exposure.

Grids

The grid and the Potter-Bucky diaphragm are radiographic accessories designed to minimize the effect of scatter radiation. The use of a stationary or moving grid is recommended for the cleanup of scatter radiation generated by large or dense body parts. A general rule is that a grid or Bucky should be used for any part that is 10 cm or more in thickness. The major exception to this rule is the adult chest, although most modern chest images are made with high kVp/high grid ratio techniques.

Basic Grid Design

Gustav Bucky, M.D., developed a cross-hatch stationary grid in 1913 to assist in the cleanup of scatter radiation. In 1920, Hollis Potter, M.D, redesigned Bucky's grid so that all the grid lines were aligned in the same direction. Potter was then able to move this linear grid back and forth during the x-ray exposure to blur out grid lines. Although the term *Bucky* is used to represent the Potter-Bucky diaphragm or moving grid, in actuality the stationary, cross-hatch grid was invented by Bucky; the moving linear grid was designed by Potter.

Grid design has not changed significantly since its modification from cross-hatch to linear by Potter. Most grids are manufactured with lead lines aligned in the same direction (linear) and separated by organic or inorganic interspacing materials. The radiolucent materials that separate the lead lines permit the passage of the x-ray beam (Fig. 5-13). The interspacing material may be organic (paper, cardboard, fiber), or inorganic (aluminum).

The benefit of aluminum interspacing compared with organic material is that aluminum does not absorb moisture. Aluminum is nonhygroscopic and will not warp. Inorganic material

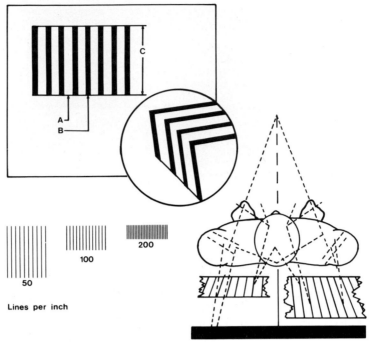

Figure 5-13
Basic Grid Design

Linear grids are designed with their lead lines aligned in the same direction but separated by a radiolucent interspacing material to permit the passage of the primary beam. The lead lines absorb most of the scatter radiation. The interspacing material (A) separates the lead lines (B). Grid ratio is determined by the height of the lead lines (C) compared with the distance between each lead strip (A, also seen in the inset). A low-ratio grid does not absorb as much scatter radiation as a higher ratio grid.

Most grids are manufactured with 100 or more lead lines per inch. When grids are made with an increased number of lines per inch (up to 200), the lead strips must be made narrower. If the grid ratio is to be maintained, the grid lines must be decreased in height, which results in a thinner grid. These extrafine grid lines are virtually invisible on the radiograph, eliminating the need to move the grid to obliterate the grid pattern.

absorbs more x-radiation at lower kilovoltage than do organic materials.

Lines per Inch

Most grids are manufactured with 100 or more lead lines per inch, although many older grids made with 60 or 80 lines per inch are still in use.

The lead strips are relatively thin (0.05 mm), whereas the radiolucent interspaces are relatively thick (0.33 mm). Recent improvements in grid design (up to 200 lines/in) alter this relation. When grids are made with an increased number of lines per inch (up to 200 lines), the lead strips are made

narrower. If grid ratio is to be maintained, there must be a decrease in the height of the lead lines. With these fine-line grids the grid lines are virtually invisible even when the grid is used in the stationary mode. No movement is required to obliterate the fine lead-line pattern (see Fig. 5-13).

Grid Ratio

Grid ratio is defined as the height of the lead lines compared with the distance between each lead strip. As grid ratio increases, the height of the lead lines increases, but the distance between the lead strips remains the same for a given number

Table 5-1. Technical Compensation for Grid Conversions

Type	Ratio	Focal Range (in)	Maximum kVp	+ mAs	+ kVp
Non-grid				1×	
Linear	5:1	28–72	85	2×	+8
Linear	6:1	28–72	85	3×	+8
Linear	8:1	34–44	95	3×–4×	+15
Linear	12:1	36–40	110	5×	+20–+25
Linear	16:1	40	125	6×	+20–+25
Cross-hatch	12:1	28–72	>110	5×	+20–+25
Cross-hatch	16:1	34–44	>125	6×	+20–+25

of lead lines per inch (see Fig. 5-13). The higher the ratio of the grid, the more restrictive its focal range (Table 5-1).

IMPORTANT

The ratio of the grid as well as the amount of lead in the grid are good indicators of the contrast improvement capability of the grid, that is, its ability to remove scatter radiation. A fine-line grid of a given ratio is not as effective in scatter cleanup as the same ratio grid made with lead lines of conventional thickness. For example, a 12:1 ratio fine-line (200 lines/inch) grid may have the cleanup effect of only an 8:1 or 10:1 ratio (100 lines/inch) grid (Table 5-2).

The kVp values selected for a specific examination should be considered in terms of the

part under study and the ratio of the grid used. Kilovoltage must be adequate to produce x-rays capable of penetrating the part. X-rays of insufficient penetrating ability result in increased absorption of the rays by the patient.

IMPORTANT

Lowering the kVp to lessen scatter while raising the mAs is not an acceptable substitute for beam restriction and a proper ratio grid.

Types of Grids

Grids may be either linear or cross-hatch in design (Fig.5-14), as follows:.

LINEAR GRIDS. Most grids are designed with their lead lines arranged in linear fashion, that is, aligned in the same direction. Linear grids can be either parallel or focused.

Parallel grids have lead strips positioned vertically across the entire width of a linear grid. Parallel grids, usually low-ratio, are useful when positioning is difficult owing to limitations imposed by focal film distances and large field sizes. Geometric cutoff can result on both sides of the image when using a parallel grid, particularly at a shortened FFD. The parallel grid is acceptable with smaller size cassettes, since the central portion of the x-ray beam is parallel to the parallel grid lines. With larger field sizes, the divergent beam will bilaterally intercept the parallel grid lines, and bilateral grid cutoff will occur (see Fig. 5-14 and Table 5-1).

Focused grids have the lead strips aligned and tilted bilaterally toward an imaginary predetermined centering point in space. Grid focus or radius is determined when an imaginary line is

Table 5-2. Grid Type Comparisons

Actual Grid Ratio	Lines per Inch	Effective Grid Ratio
12:1 linear 6:1 linear 6:1 linear	100 (Al interspaced)	12:1
12:1 12:1 linear	100 (Al interspaced) 200 (fiber interspaced)	14:1 8:1 to 10:1

Grid ratio comparison must include the lead content, number of lines per inch, the height of the lines, and the type of interspacing materials.

When compared with a conventional 12:1 ratio (100 lines/in) grid, a cross-hatch grid combination cleans up more scatter. The extra layers of aluminum covering on each grid have a cleanup (filter) effect.

The 200-lines-per-inch grid is not as thick as the 100-line grid, and its lead lines can be easily penetrated at high kVp values. See Figure 5-13.

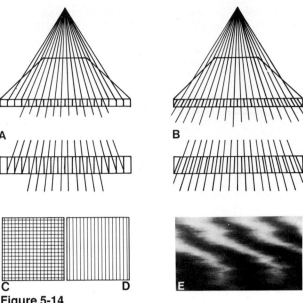

Figure 5-14
Types of Grids

Linear grids can be designed with their lead lines aligned either parallel (A) or focused (B). The lead strips of a parallel grid are positioned vertically across the width of the entire grid. Geometric cutoff can result on both sides of the image with a parallel grid (A). The lead lines of the focused grid (B) are tilted uniformly and bilaterally to a predetermined focal range in a manufacturing process known as canting.

(D) A linear grid is seen from above. Note: Tube angle techniques are possible only if the tube is angled so that the central ray is projected in the direction of the linear lead pattern. (C) When two linear grids are placed at right angles to each other (cross-hatched), maximal scatter cleanup occurs. Tube angle techniques are not possible with cross-hatch grids, since their grid lines run in opposite directions. (E) If two grids are inadvertently positioned with their lead lines running in the same direction, a "moire" artifact is produced.

drawn from the outer aspects of the width of the grid and intersects at this imaginary point. The manufacturing process of inclining the grid lines uniformly and bilaterally is known as *canting*.

IMPORTANT

A focused grid, if positioned correctly, is preferable to a parallel grid over a wider range of focal film distances and for full-field radiography if one wishes to minimize bilateral grid cut-off (see Fig. 5-14).

Moving grids (Potter-Bucky diaphragm) are used during an x-ray exposure to blur out grid lines as well as impurities in grid design. A grid can be made to move continuously during the x-ray exposure. Moving grids can be designed to move in one direction (single-stroke), or they can be driven back and forth, 1-cm to 3-cm (reciprocating). Some grids move forward faster and slower on return (catapult) or can move in a slow, almost imperceptible, circular motion (oscillating). Regardless of the type of movement used, the intent is to blur out lead strips while moving the grid in synchrony with the pulses of the x-ray generator. When the grid moves back and forth, a form of "lateral decentering" occurs, with a loss of as much as 20% of the primary beam.

CROSS-HATCH GRIDS. Two linear grids (parallel or focused) superimposed at right angles to each

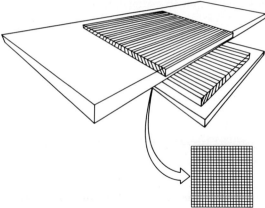

Figure 5-15
A Cross-hatch Grid to Supplement
a Low-Ratio Bucky Grid

When a high-ratio grid is needed to examine a large patient, a cross-hatch grid can be improvised by placing a grid cassette transverse in the Bucky tray with the grid lines of the grid cassette at right angles to the lines of the Bucky grid. Although the lines of the Bucky grid will be blurred by the motion of the grid, the lines of the grid cassette may be seen on the image. An increase in kVp rather than mA or time within the ratings of the x-ray tube in use compensates for the increase in ratio of the combined grids. (Reprinted courtesy Eastman Kodak Company).

other for maximal scatter cleanup form a cross-hatch grid. A higher grid ratio can be achieved if two low-ratio grids are used in a cross-hatch configuration (Figs. 5-14 and 5-15). A cross-hatch grid exhibits a slightly greater improvement in contrast than a comparable ratio linear grid. The combination of two linear grids (cross-hatch) is more efficient in scatter cleanup than a linear grid of a similar ratio.

IMPORTANT

The higher the ratio of the grid, the more restrictive is its focal range. The highest ratio grid used in a cross-hatch combination determines the focal range of the cross-hatch grid (see Table 5-1). A cross-hatch grid must be carefully aligned to the central ray (Fig. 5-16). Tube angle techniques are prohibited.

Related Grid Terminology

The following terms are relevant to this discussion of grids:

Lead content. The amount of lead in a grid, as well as its design, determines the ability of a grid to clean up scatter and improve radiographic contrast.

Selectivity (Σ). The percentage of primary radiation that passes through the grid is known as *primary transmission.* In an ideal situation, a grid would transmit 100% of the primary radiation generated for the procedure. Unfortunately, some primary as well as scatter is absorbed by the grid. The ratio of transmitted primary radiation to transmitted scatter radiation is called *grid selectivity.* Selectivity is determined not only by grid ratio but also by the lead content of the grid.

Contrast improvement factor (CIF). The ratio of radiographic contrast measured in a study using a grid as compared with the contrast in a non-

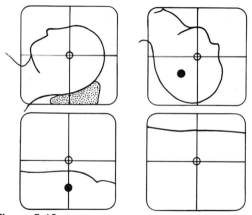

Figure 5-16
The Use of a Cross-hatch Grid

The central ray must be centered to the exact center of a cross-hatch grid to avoid grid cutoff. An open circle is used to represent the center of both grids. A patient is shown positioned for a lateral skull radiograph with the central ray bisecting the intersection of the centers of both grids. Both grids will therefore be in focus (top left). (Top right) A patient is shown in the base position for a lateral study. The central ray (closed circle) is positioned to the area of interest. The central ray is off-center to both the horizontal and vertical grids, which results in grid cutoff on the image. (Bottom left) A cross-hatch grid is shown for an abdominal study. A small patient is positioned with the x-ray beam (closed circle) centered to the abdomen but approximately 4 inches off-center to the horizontal grid. (Bottom right) A larger patient, who in theory should be more difficult to examine, is positioned correctly, with the central ray bisecting both grids in the cross-hatch configuration.

grid procedure, all other factors being equal, is known as the contrast improvement factor.

Grid cassette. When a grid technique is needed for a special projection such as a horizontal beam study (e.g., lateral hip, decubitus chest or abdomen, bedside or operating room radiography), cassettes can be purchased with a built-in grid substituted for the cassette front. When a grid cassette is not available, most radiographers tape a stationary grid to the front of a conventional cassette for these procedures. Grid frames can also be temporarily attached to most existing cassettes. This can be particularly helpful at the bedside when a considerable number of cassettes are in use. A single grid can be used with several cassettes of the same size.

Grid Artifacts

Damage to a grid can produce uneven density patterns on a radiograph (Fig. 5-17). Grid covers or frames are available to minimize grid damage.

IMPORTANT

When an aluminum interspaced grid is purchased, it should be evaluated radiographically for uneven density patterns whether it is intended to be used as a fixed or moving grid. A low exposure (1–5 mAs; 40–50 kVp, depending on the screen film combination used) will produce an acceptable density of approximately 1.0 needed to evaluate an aluminum interspaced grid. If the radiograph is overexposed, grid imperfections may not be obvious.

Grid line artifacts on a radiograph may be caused by the following:

Improper centering of the x-ray tube to the grid. The higher the grid ratio, the more critical the problem (Figs. 5-18 and 5-19)

An increase or decrease in focal film distance. This can produce a widening of the grid lines on the lateral aspects of the radiograph, causing a bilateral decrease in radiographic density (see Fig. 5-18).

Capture of the grid in motion. When a high mA setting is used in conjunction with high-speed, rare-earth screen film combinations, a short exposure can "capture" the grid in motion, accentuating grid imperfections. A widening or banding of the grid lines may be seen. Some types of grid defects never fully "erase" at short exposure times when a Potter-Bucky diaphragm is used (see Fig. 5-17). This is a particularly troublesome problem with the

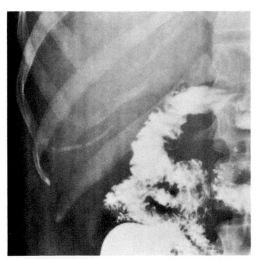
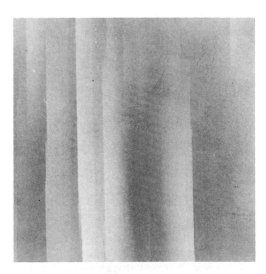

Figure 5-17
Grid Artifacts

A Bucky must be in motion before and after the x-ray exposure. A moving grid can be "captured" in motion by the use of short exposure times. (Left) a widening or banding of the grid lines is seen in this image. This corduroy pattern represents not only widening of the grid lines but also accentuated grid defects. (Right) A damaged aluminum interspaced stationary grid can exhibit low-density banding patterns throughout the grid. Defects of this nature are generally caused by careless handling of the grid. These uneven density bands can be detrimental to image quality.

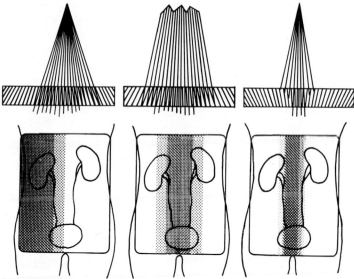

Figure 5-18
Grid Cutoff

(Left) *If the x-ray tube is positioned off-center in relation to the focused grid, severe differences in radiographic density can be noted from one side to the other on the radiograph (see Fig. 5-19). (Center) When an improper focal film range is used, for example, a 72-inch FFD with a grid focused at 40 inch FFD, there is a loss of density bilaterally. One- to 2-inch segments on both lateral aspects of the radiograph can appear underexposed. (Right) When a grid is used in the reverse position, only x-rays parallel to the center of the grid reach the detector. The higher the grid ratio, the more pronounced these defects will be.*

short exposure times used with pediatric techniques.

Poor synchronization of the moving grid to the x-ray exposure. The grid must be in motion before and after the exposure (see Fig. 5-17).

Shifting of the radiographic tube for a stereo technique across the grid lines rather than length-wise with the grid lines (see Fig. 5-18, *left*). Stereoscopic technique is discussed in Chapter 11.

Misalignment of a cross-hatch grid. A "moiré" artifact may occur when a linear grid is placed on top of a second linear grid or grid cassette with the grid lines overlapping rather

Figure 5-19
Tube Off-Center in Relationship to Bucky

This radiograph was made using a 16:1 Bucky with the radiographic tube positioned approximately 1½ inches off-center to the left side of the patient. The right side of the radiograph seems adequatley exposed; the left side is significantly less dense.

As the central ray strikes the slanged lead lines of the grid, which act as an almost solid lead barrier (left side of patient), the focused lines on the opposite side of the grid permit the passage of a higher percentage of the beam, as seen on the right lateral aspect of the image. High-ratio grids are more subject to this type of cutoff than are low-ratio grids.

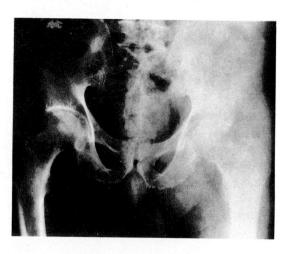

than positioned at right angles to each other (Fig. 5-14*E*).

Pressure on the grid. The weight of the patient can cause the grid in a Bucky to rub against the front of the cassette. If a thick lead identification marker or a marker covered with layers of adhesive tape is used to fasten the marker to the cassette, it can catch onto the moving grid, also producing grid striping artifacts (see Fig. 5-17). The tape may also cause the cassette to move during the exposure (Fig. 5-20).

Grid Cutoff

Grid cutoff occurs when the lead lines of the grid are not focused to the primary beam. Lead strips can be projected radiographically as wider images with a significant absorption of the primary beam (see Fig. 5-18).

The following are common causes of grid cutoff:

Lateral decentering of the grid. If the x-ray tube is positioned off-center to a focused grid, significant differences in radiographic density will occur from one side of the image to the other (see Figs. 5-18 and 5-19). For horizontal beam imaging, the x-ray beam is usually centered to the cassette with the grid lines in a horizontal position (parallel to the floor). With the grid lines in this position, the part being examined must be centered to the grid cassette, regardless of the size of the patient. Positioning the grid cassette with its grid lines perpendicular to the floor will increase positioning latitude. Grid cutoff is avoided unless the tube is shifted off-center, right or left (Figs. 5-21 and 5-22).

Grid-focus-distance centering. The FFD must correspond to the focal range of the grid. A common error is the use of a 72-inch FFD for chest radiography with a grid focused at a 40-inch FFD, causing a bilateral decrease in radiographic density on the image.

With fluoroscopic spot film procedures, although the radiographic tube is usually in a fixed position, the fluoroscopic spot film tunnel changes position with the part being examined. During fluoroscopic procedures, the size of the part under study affects the focal film distance. For example, there is a significant difference in the size of an infant in the supine position compared with an adult in the lateral position.

Lower ratio grids are usually used in fluoroscopic spot film tunnels to avoid grid cutoff

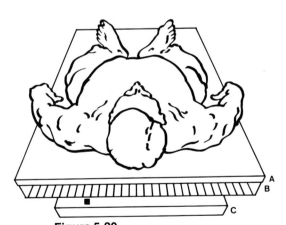
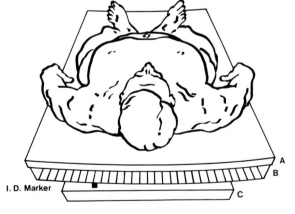

Figure 5-20
Common Causes of Moving Grid Artifacts

Occasionally, an overweight patient, particularly when placed in the lateral position, can cause the tabletop (A) to bend. The pressure of the tabletop against the grid (B) may cause the grid to move erratically, producing a grid artifact. If thick adhesive tape or masking tape is used to fasten a lead marker to a cassette (C); it can interfere in the movement of the grid (right). The taped lead marker can rub against the moving grid and result in a corduroy stripping effect. (see Fig. 5-17). This contact of the grid with the taped marker can also cause the cassette to move within the Bucky tray. (Right) The combination of a large patient and the use of a thick adhesive marker is shown. (Left) A normal table/grid ID marker is also shown.

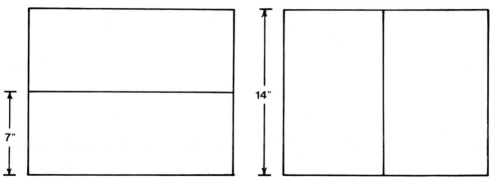

Figure 5-21
Use of a Grid with a Horizontal Beam Technique

(Left) *When a stationary grid is used for horizontal beam radiography with the grid lines parallel to the floor, the center of the patient does not always correspond to the center of the grid. The middle of the cassette and grid may be pefrectly aligned to a larger patient, but a smaller patient may require off-centering of the beam toward the inferior portion of the cassette. (Right) If the grid lines are positioned with the lead lines perpendicular to the floor, then regardless of the size of the patient, tight beam collimation is possible without concern for grid cutoff.*

A problem may occur when using a 14 × 17 inch field for lateral decubitus imaging of the chest or abdomen or air-contrast studies of the colon. When the grid is placed with the lead lines running parallel to the tabletop, it is often assumed that to avoid grid focus difficluties the center of every patient must be exactly 7 inches from the tabletop. This is rarely true. Rather, by placing the grid with the lead lines in the short dimension (14 in) of the cassette, centering is possible anywhere from the table top itself to 14 inches from the tabletop and produces a radiograph without grid cutoff.

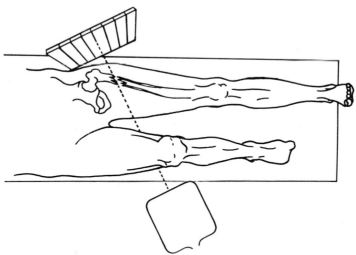

Figure 5-22
Lateral Projection of the Hip: Grid Line Placement

The use of a grid for the lateral projection of the hip often results in grid cutoff. Since patients vary in size, it is unlikely that the center of a 10 × 12 inch grid with its grid lines positioned parallel to the table would be aligned to every patient to be examined. By positioning the grid or grid cassette with the grid lines perpendicular to the tabletop or floor, the central ray can be raised or lowered for large or small patients. A similar positioning approach can be used with cross-table myelography.

(see Table 5-1); however, higher kVp is often needed for studies such as barium procedures for adequate penetration of the contrast medium. The use of a cross-hatch grid in the fluoroscopic tunnel (two 6:1 or two 8:1 linear grids) provides the cleanup needed for higher kVp techniques while permitting significant variations in the focal ranges (see Table 5-1). The development of high-speed, rare-earth intensifying screen film combinations makes the use of higher ratio grids possible for fluoroscopic spot films.

A steep angle target x-ray tube combined with a cross-hatch grid and small focal spot (0.6 mm or less) can result in Bucky-like radiographs (Fig. 5-23 and Table 5-1).

A combination of lateral decentering and a grid-focus-distance problem

The use of a focused grid upside down (see Fig. 5-18). This is a rare occurrence but may be seen with radiographs made at the bedside or any location where mobile radiographic equipment is used.

Grid Identification Markings

Most grids are appropriately labeled as to focal range distance recommendations and grid ratio. If the decal listing this information is unreadable or is missing from a grid, the grid ratio, focal range, and serial number can usually be found

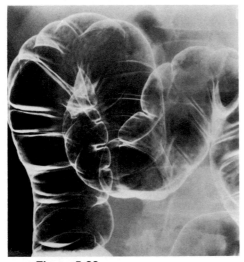 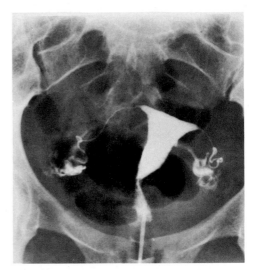

Figure 5-23
Use of a Grid in the Spot Film Tunnel: Small Focal Spot Combined with Cross-hatch Grid

Because of the variability of the focal object distance, grid focal range must be considered when using a fluoroscopic spot film tunnel. A low-ratio grid with an extended focal range is usually installed in a fluoroscopic spot film tunnel. If a higher grid ratio is required, two linear grids can be used in a cross-hatch configuration to overcome the focal range limitations of higher ratio linear grids (see Table 5-1). The second linear grid can be brought into position at a right angle to the first grid for improved scatter cleanup during spot film radiography. For pediatric fluoroscopy of an infant or small child, the fluoroscopic grid can be removed from the fluoro field.

Unsharpness associated with fluoroscopic spot filming due to the shortened FOD can be minimized with the use of a small focal spot. When the small focal spot is used with a cross-hatch grid, fluoroscopic spot films resemble conventional Bucky radiographs. An erect spot film of the hepatic flexure (a double-contrast study; left) and a supine salpingogram (right) are shown. Both radiographs are fluoroscopic spot films but resembel Bucky quality radiographs. The increased film blackening gained by the use of a high-speed rare-earth screen film combination permits the use of a low or moderate mA and a small focal spot. (Reprinted courtesy Eastman Kodak Company).

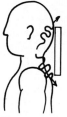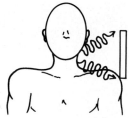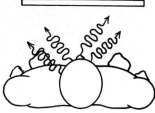

Figure 5-24
Use of an "Air-Gap" to Reduce Scatter Radiation

(Left) *In the anteroposterior position of the cervical spine a grid is required, since the cassette is in close contact with the part being examined. When the patient is separated from the cassette, the effect of scatter radiation on the image is minimized.* (Center) *When the lateral projection is made, an air-gap is formed because the cassette is placed approximately 10 inches from the cervical spine. Much of the scatter from the patient is given off at acute angles to the primary beam and misses the detector. Some of the scatter is reduced in intensity owing to the effect of the Inverse Square Law. Because of the increased OFD an extended FFD (72 in) is required to overcome magnification of the part* (Right) *Another use for the air-gap technique is chest radiography. The patient is positioned 10 to 12 inches from the cassette with the tube positioned 10 to 12 feet from the cassette to overcome cardiac enlargement.*

embossed on an edge of the front or back of the metal covering.

The "Air-Gap" Technique

The scatter emanating from the patient is at acute angles to the primary beam. At only a few inches from its source, scatter is reduced markedly owing to the air-gap effect.

Since the patient is the major source of scatter radiation and since scatter is disseminated in all directions, some of the scatter reaching the detector is reduced in intensity because of the Inverse Square Law principle. If the patient is moved away from the cassette, less scatter radiation will reach the film. This approach is known as the *air-gap technique* (Fig. 5-24). Air-gap techniques are often used as a substitute for a grid or Bucky for lateral cervical spine, chest, and direct roentgen enlargement studies. (Direct roentgen enlargement is presented in Chapter 11.)

Inverted Kodak X-Omatic Cassette as a Grid Substitute

Richard J. Sweeney described the difficulties encountered with proper centering and distance re-

lations between the x-ray source and the grid.* He suggested the use of a Kodak X-Omatic cassette in the inverted position, tube side down, as a grid substitute (Fig. 5-25). This cassette has a thin sheet of lead foil mounted behind the posterior intensifying screen to absorb backscatter. When used as an improvised grid, below 80 kVp, the lead foil backing requires an approximate 30% increase in mAs over a conventional non-grid technique. Sweeney believes that the inverted cassette functions in a manner similar to a 5:1 ratio grid without grid focus concerns. In the higher kilovoltage ranges (up to 120 kVp), he used a low ratio stationary grid with the inverted cassette, taking advantage of the increased technical latitude of higher kilovoltage. He stated that no change in exposure is required over the normal grid technique.

Patient identification problems can occur when using an inverted cassette. The patient identification area of the Kodak cassette is in a predetermined position when the cassette is properly positioned (tube side up). For example, when the cassette is used in the anteroposterior position to radiograph the right femur (lead blocker, superior), the patient identification appears on the medial aspect of the right femur; for a radiograph of the left femur (lead blocker, superior), the patient identification appears on the lateral aspect of the

*Sweeney RJ: The use of an inverted Kodak X-Omatic cassette as an improvised grid. Radiol Technol 49:257–261, 1977.)

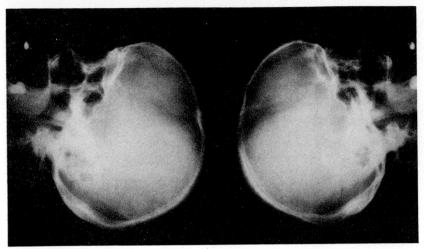

Figure 5-25
Inverted X-Omatic Cassette Compared with a Stationary Grid

The grid exposure of the skull (left) is compared to the exposure obtained with inverted X-Omatic cassette (right) without a grid. (Courtesy of Sweeney RJ: The use of an inverted Kodak X-Omatic cassette as an improvised grid. Radiol Technol 49:257–261, 1977.)

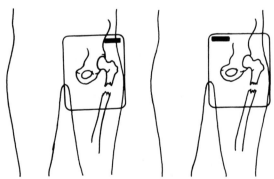

Figure 5-26
Photoidentification When Using an Inverted Kodak X-Omatic Cassette

When a Kodak X-Omatic cassette is used in the inverted position as a substitute for a low-ratio grid, the proper use of identifying right and left lead markers is important. When the cassette is inverted, the relationship of the lead blocker to the anatomic area is reversed. If the correct lead markers are not used, it is easy to confuse the right and left sides of the patient.

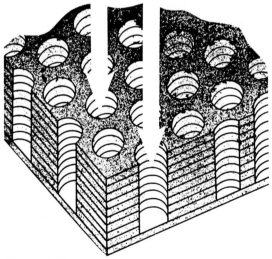

Figure 5-27
New Grid Concept

A new type of grid uses multiple lyaers of thin lead sheeting with 120 holes per inch. At 120 holes per inch, there are almost 1700 openings in the 14-inch dimention and more than 2000 holes in the 17-inch dimension. Each sheet of lead has a total of almost 3½ million openings, with more than 27 million openings in the eight-sheet total. The holes in the lead are aligned using laser technology. Increased positioning latitude is achieved with this new technology, making this grid useful for bedside radiography. (Redrawn, courtesy Eastman Kodak Company.)

left femur. If the cassette is properly placed, tube side up, even when an identifying right or left lead marker is not visible, the radiologist can determine which femur has been examined by the location of the identification blocker. These relationships reverse when the cassette is inverted with the tube side down. The identification marker appears on the lateral aspect of the right femur and the medial aspect of the left femur (Fig. 5-26).

IMPORTANT

When the cassette is used in the reverse position as a substitute for a low-ratio grid, the right- and left-side identification markers must be seen.

New Grid Concept

A new grid has been developed by the Eastman Kodak Company to control scatter radiation. Instead of the conventional lead lines separated by radiolucent interspacing material, this grid uses multiple layers of thin lead sheeting with 120 holes per inch. Eight layers of lead are laminated into a flexible grid. The holes in the lead are aligned using laser technology. The cleanup capability of this grid is approximately equal to a conventional 6:1 ratio grid with an increase in the focal range. It was first developed to overcome technical problems encountered at the bedside (Fig. 5-27).

Chapter 6

Conventional Recording Media

The most common recording media for medical radiography is x-ray film, used either in direct exposure techniques or in conjunction with fluorescing intensifying screens. These screens are mounted in light-proof containers—cassettes—to protect the film from light. Cassettes and intensifying screens, used to enhance the film blackening effect of x-radiation, are described in this chapter. Special image recording media are discussed in Chapter 13.

IMPORTANT

Regardless of how carefully the image is produced, if attention is not given to the processing and handling of the recording media, a poor radiographic image will result. The processing of radiographs is discussed in Chapter 7.

X-ray Film

X-ray film consists of three major components:

1. An emulsion
2. A flexible film base
3. A protective coating

The emulsion is a gelatin mixture containing silver halide compounds (Fig. 6-1). Within the film emulsion are very fine crystals or tablets of silver halide compounds (silver and bromide, chlorine, or iodine) suspended in a pure gelatin base. These compounds are sensitive to both light and x-ray. When silver halide crystals absorb light or x-ray energy, a physical change occurs, which becomes apparent when the film is developed. When the proper level of energy strikes the bromide ions in the silver halide crystals, they emit electrons. These electrons move to a sensitivity center in the halide crystal. The negatively charged electrons attract the positively charged silver ions, and the electron and sensitivity speck interaction causes the silver halide crystal to be converted into atoms of metallic silver.

The degree of absorption of light or x-ray energy by

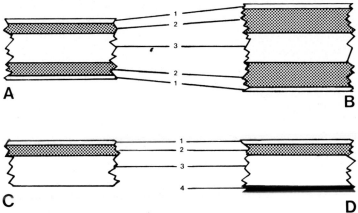

Figure 6-1
Cross-section of Types of Radiographic Films

Most radiographic film emulsions are coated on a blue-tinted base (3). Dual-emulsion medical radiographic film (A and B) has emulsion (2) coated on both sides of the base. A protective coating (1) covers the emulsion to minimize damage from handling.

(A) Medical screen dual-emulsion x-ray film, used with two intensifying screens, is designed to respond primarily to the light emitted by the intensifying screen. (B) Nonscreen radiographic film emulsions respond primarily to the direct effect of x-ray and are considerably thicker than the emulsions used for screen-type radiographic film. (C, D) Single-emulsion radiographic films are generally used with a single high-detail intensifying screen for extremity radiography and mammography or in multiformat cameras for cathode ray tube (CRT) imaging and laser printers. These films, similar to photographic film, are usually designed with an antihalation backing (4).

the crystals produces a latent image, which is converted into a visible image seen as black metallic silver on the film as the result of chemical processing.

By design, radiographic films are more sensitive to one part of the light spectrum than to another. Films are often described as either being panchromatic (sensitive to all colors of the light spectrum) or orthochromatic (sensitive to all colors of the light spectrum except red). Orthochromatic emulsions are sensitive to wavelengths less than 620 nm, whereas the panchromatic emulsions are sensitive to the whole visible spectrum, including the shorter wavelengths (Fig. 6-2). Before

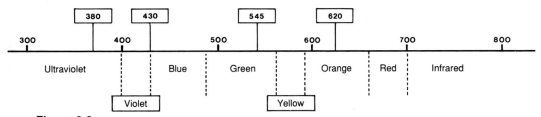

Figure 6-2
Electromagnetic Spectrum

The electromagnetic spectrum is illustrated from 300 nm to 800 nm. Ultraviolet, blue, and green sensitivity ranges are shown. Film is designed to respond to the specific emissivity ranges of the phosphors of intensifying screens.

the early 1970s, x-ray films were primarily blue-light sensitive. With the development of green light–emitting rare-earth intensifying screens, orthochromatic films came into common use.

Most radiographic films have emulsion on both sides of the film base and are used with a pair of intensifying screens so that the least amount of x-radiation can be used to produce a satisfactory radiographic density, thus minimizing patient dosage (see Intensifying Screens).

Silver halide crystals appear as pebble-like grains in conventional emulsions. With new silver halide technology known as *T-grain* (tabular grain), the crystals appear flat and tablet shaped. The tabular grains can be dispersed more evenly throughout the emulsion, resulting in better silver coverage with less tendency to form film grain (Fig. 6-3).

Gelatin is a very good vehicle for the silver compounds because, in a solution, it will swell (become soft and flexible) without dissolving. Gelatin also rehardens quickly during the fixing process. The silver halide particles are dispersed as evenly as possible throughout the gelatin binder. The emulsion, 5µ to 10µ thick, is bound to the film base, approximately 180µ thick, by an adhesive material known as the *substratum.*

The film base used to support the emulsion is made of transparent, nonflammable polyester or cellulose acetate. It must be strong, rigid, and flexible enough to be transported through all cycles of the automatic processor. Polyester shrinks less when immersed in liquid, retains less moisture, and is thinner than a cellulose acetate base. As a rule, radiographic film base is tinted blue to minimize the effect of ambient light passing through large unexposed areas of the radiograph. Some single-emulsion medical imaging films used for procedures such as nuclear medicine imaging are coated on a clear base (see Fig. 6-1*C, D*).

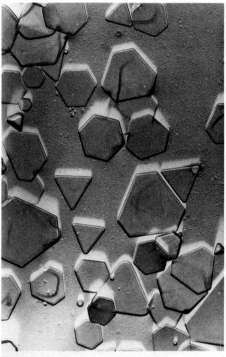 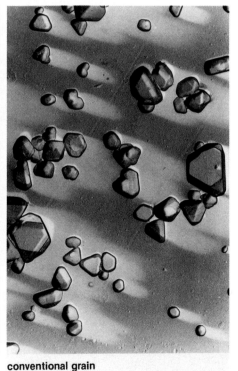

T-grain **conventional grain**

Figure 6-3
T-Grain Emulsion

(Right) Silver halide crystals in conventional radiographic film emulsions can be described as pebble-like grains. (Left) T-grain crystals found in newer film emulsion technology are tabular shaped. These flat grains can be dispersed more evenly throughout the emulsion for better silver coverage. In T-grain technology, a dye is used in the film emulsion to minimize light crossover within the cassette during an x-ray exposure (see Fig. 6-9), resulting in a significant improvement in image resolution. (Reprinted courtesy Eastman Kodak Company)

A protective coating is used over the emulsion to minimize damage resulting from handling.

IMPORTANT

Care must be used to select the proper safelight filter in the darkroom to match the spectral sensitivity of the radiographic film in use.

Characteristics of X-ray Film

Medical x-ray film must possess the following characteristics:

1. Speed (sensitivity). The emulsion must possess the ability to respond to both light and x-ray. Radiographic film is often referred to as being of standard, medium, or fast speed. This type of rating is no longer appropriate with new intensifying screen film combinations. In the past, film could be rated independently of the intensifying screens. If 100-speed intensifying screens were matched to 100-speed radiographic film, the system would be rated at 100 speed. With many rare-earth screen film combinations, faster screens are often used with a slower film. Rather than labeling a screen or a film individually as to speed, screen film combination speed should be considered.
2. Latitude. Latitude can be described in two ways:
   a. Film latitude: The emulsion's ability to record a relatively long range of densities, from the blackest black (gas or air) to the whitest white (dense osseous structures or barium-filled organs), with all shades of gray in between
   b. Exposure latitude: The margin for exposure error with any given technique
3. Contrast. The film must be able to record differences in density. Film contrast is directly related to latitude. A film possessing long-scale contrast will exhibit increased exposure latitude; a film possessing short-scale contrast will exhibit decreased exposure latitude.

Sensitometry

Quantitative measurements, known as sensitometry, can be made of the response of the film to exposure and development.

Variations in Density

A sensitometer is used to expose a stepwedge of photographic densities on an unexposed radio-

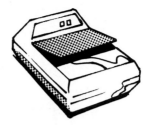

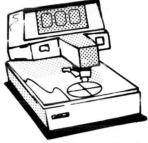

Figure 6-4
Sensitometer and Densitometer

(Top) A sensitometer is used to expose a stepwedge of varying photographic densities on unexposed radiographic film. A high-quality light source with an accurate timer is a prerequisite for this device. The processed image of the stepwedge exhibits sharply demarcated density variations, from clear (white) to black. (Bottom) The stepwedge image is evaluated using a densitometer, which measures the various degress of density on the processed radiograph. These variations are transferred to graph paper to form a sensitometric or characteristic curve that illustrates the properties of the film under study. When the densitometer is properly calibrated and there is no film under the sensor, the reading should be 0.00.

graphic film. To avoid variations in light intensities, a high-quality light source and timer are incorporated into this unit (Fig. 6-4, *left*). The film, exposed to a predetermined level, produces a stepwedge of densities from clear (white) to black after processing. The sharply demarcated density variations are then evaluated with a densitometer, an instrument used to measure degrees of blackening on the processed radiograph (Fig. 6-4, *right*).

Density variations can be displayed on a meter or electronic readout and recorded on graph paper. These readings are used to generate a sensitometric curve, also known as a characteristic curve or an H & D curve after Hurter and Driffield, students of photography in Great Britain who first described the curve in 1890. It is a graphic representation between the exposure received by the film and the densities produced after processing (Fig. 6-5). A typical characteristic curve

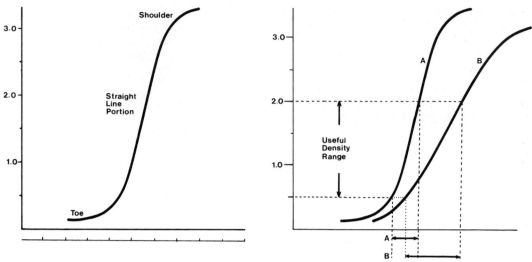

Figure 6-5
Sensitometric Curves

(Left) *A typical sensitometric curve. The vertical axis illustrates increased density; the horizontal axis shows increased exposure. Exposure is expressed logarithmically to confine the graph to a reasonable size. The characteristic or sensitometric curve can be described as follows: toe (the inferior portion), ascending or straight line portion (useful density range), shoulder (top of the curve). (Right) Contrast and latitude parameters of films A and B are compared. Film A in the useful density range (0.25–2.0) exhibits poor exposure latitude, whereas film B, also in the useful density range, exhibits considerably more latitude. Abrupt density differences seen as short-scale contrast will occur with film A. Longer scale contrast seen as more shades of gray will occur with film B.*

Film speed is determined by the position of the sensitometric curve on the graph. Since the horizontal axis documents increased exposure from left to right, film A would require less exposure than film B to achieve a given density of 2.0, as seen on the vertical axis of the graph.

consists of a toe, a straight line portion, and a shoulder. A logarithmic scale is necessary to confine the graph to a reasonable size. A relationship can be expressed between the logarithm of exposure and the radiographic density and is described in Chapter 8.

The toe or lower portion of the curve is measured after an adjustment has been made for base density, which is inherent in every radiographic film, and for base plus fog density. *Base density* is the result of manufacturing parameters and includes the blue tint in the base of the film. *Fog density* is caused by development of unexposed silver halide crystals during processing. Although the base of a single sheet of unexposed processed film may appear transparent to the eye, the superimposition of two or more sheets of clear (after processing) film will demonstrate the presence of a base plus fog density. Some manufacturers use a special dye in the emulsion to minimize the cross-

over of light between intensifying screens (see Intensifying Screens).

At the toe of the curve, the minimal density (D-Min) is the least density recorded on the film after exposure and is usually slightly higher than base plus fog density.

The straight line portion of the curve represents the useful imaging portion of the curve. Average gradient reflects both film contrast and latitude. This is measured on the sensitometric curve from 0.25 density above base fog and 2.0 density above base fog and is defined as the slope of the curve.

The shoulder of the curve represents the area of greatest radiographic density recorded on the film after exposure. Maximal density (D-Max) is read at the shoulder of the curve (see Fig. 6-5).

Variations in density, demonstrated by the characteristic curve, are a function of exposure (photographic effect). As exposure rates are changed, the film changes in density.

Variations in Contrast and Latitude

Contrast and latitude can also be illustrated by the characteristic curve, as follows:

Film contrast: Determined by the manufacturer and influenced by development

Subject contrast: Influenced by tissue absorption differences of the patient

Radiographic contrast: The density differences between adjacent areas of the radiographic image. The combination of subject and film contrast results in radiographic contrast.

Latitude: The range of exposures in the generally accepted medical density range (0.25 to 2.0) (see Fig. 6-5, *right*). As a general rule, an increase in contrast (shorter scale) produces a decrease in latitude and vice versa.

Types of X-ray Film

Three types of x-ray film are used in radiography:

1. Nonscreen radiographic film
2. Medical screen x-ray film
3. Single-emulsion radiographic film

Nonscreen radiographic film responds primarily to the direct effects of x-ray exposure. The emulsion is considerably thicker than the emulsion of screen-type radiographic film and requires significantly more exposure than screen film used in combination with intensifying screens. Because of the thicker emulsion, nonscreen film usually must be manually processed (see Fig. 6-1B). Increased silver content resulting in a thicker emulsion with associated processing limitations and high radiation dosage requirements have discouraged the use of this product. For some special-purpose examinations, such as evaluation for a metallic foreign body, an increase in x-ray exposure may be justified, since a dust artifact on an intensifying screen may mimic or hide a small foreign body.

IMPORTANT

The term *nonscreen technique* is often erroneously substituted for direct exposure technique. Any radiographic exposure using film in a light-proof holder without intensifying screens is a direct exposure. If screen-type film were used in a direct exposure (without screens), it would be three to four times slower than nonscreen film used in a direct exposure. Screen-type film requires the exposure from the fluorescent light emitted by intensifying screens for optimal efficiency.

Medical screen x-ray film, usually dual emulsion, is designed to be used in combination with intensifying screens. The film differs from nonscreen film in that its emulsion layers are considerably thinner (see Fig. 6-1A). It is important that a thin film base be used to support the emulsions. The thinner the base, the sharper the superimposed images and the less image separation caused by the parallax effect associated with tube angle techniques (see Chapter 8).

Medical screen x-ray film responds to the fluorescent light given off by activated intensifying screens. Film blackening or radiographic density is created primarily by this fluorescent light. Radiographic film can be designed to selectively respond to a specific color in the light spectrum. Intensifying screens can likewise be made to emit light (luminesce) in a specific color range (see Fig. 6-2).

IMPORTANT

For optimal results, the color sensitivity of radiographic film should be matched to the light emissivity of the screen. For example, a primarily blue-sensitive film should be used with intensifying screens that are primarily blue emitters.

All radiographic films, whether nonscreen or screen, are also sensitive to the direct action of x-rays.

Single-emulsion radiographic film is used in some radiographic examinations that require highly detailed images, such as mammography or extremity radiography. The film is used for this purpose with a single intensifying screen. Most single-emulsion films have an antihalation backing to minimize light scattering within the cassette, thereby improving image quality (Fig. 6-1D).

IMPORTANT

The emulsion side of the film must be placed against the intensifying screen. If the antihalation backing is placed against the intensifying screen, there will be a significant decrease in radiographic density.

Special recording media are discussed in Chapter 13.

Film Storage and Handling

Heat and moisture hasten the deterioration of radiographic film. High temperatures will produce a foglike density on the processed film. The ideal temperatures for storage of radiographic film vary with unprocessed or processed film.

Fresh, unexposed radiographic film should be stored at 50° to 70°F. After processing, radiographs can tolerate storage temperatures of from 60° to 80°F. Both unexposed and processed film should be stored at a 30% to 50% humidity range.

Radiographic film fog is often caused by out-of-date film, which can lose speed and contrast. The expiration date of the film is listed on every box of film. Unexposed radiographic film must be rotated in storage and the oldest film used first.

Film must be protected from all forms of radiation, including x-rays and light. Radiographic film should be kept in a secure area. These products represent a considerable portion of the departmental operating budget. The potential for theft parallels the need for security.

IMPORTANT

Higher-speed unexposed radiographic films often have a shorter shelf life and increased sensitivity than conventional speed films.

To avoid artifacts from physical pressure, unexposed boxes of film should be stored on their side, not stacked on top of one another. Artifacts such as dark, crescent-shaped marks seen after processing may be caused by bending or pinching of the film before processing. Static electricity is a common cause of film artifacts. Film pulled quickly from its box often builds up an electric charge sufficient to discharge on the radiographic film as treelike static. Smudges occur when electrical discharges follow a path formed by either dust, lint, a rough intensifying screen surface, or a roughened work counter.

Other areas of concern include exposure of radiographic film to chemicals and fumes from gases, formalin, ammonia, and oils.

Intensifying Screens

The emission of light by a material excited by any form of energy is known as *luminescence*. Luminescence, without heat, occurs in both phosphorescence and fluorescence. It should be noted that incandescence is not a form of luminescence.

One of the properties of x-radiation is that it can cause certain substances to fluoresce or phosphoresce. The terms fluorescence and phosphorescence are used to describe the luminescence phenomenon that occurs when x-ray energy is converted into light energy by the interaction of x-rays with certain phosphors (Table 6-1). If the light emission ceases almost simultaneously with the termination of the x-ray energy, the process is known as fluorescence. If the phosphor continues to glow after the activating force (such as x-ray exposure) has been terminated, the process is called phosphorescence.

Properties of Intensifying Screen Phosphors

The purpose of intensifying screens is to "capture" the remnant radiation that has exited from the patient and to convert this energy into light that will expose radiographic film. Almost all intensifying screen phosphors are efficient x-ray absorbers and fluoresce with little or no afterglow. *Afterglow* or *screen lag* describes a persistent light after the x-ray energy has ceased. This is not a desirable feature in intensifying screen design.

Some of the x-ray photons are absorbed by the intensifying screens and are converted into light photons to be used to expose radiographic film. The amount of absorption can vary from one type of screen to another (Fig. 6-6).

Table 6-1. Comparison of Intensifying and Fluoroscopic Screens

Screen Type	Emission	Light Spectrum
Intensifying	Luminescent, fluorescent	Ultraviolet, blue, green
Fluoroscopic	Luminescent, phosphorescent	Yellow-green

Intensifying screens and fluoroscopic screens both possess the property of luminescence. Fluoroscopic screens may phosphoresce or continue to glow after the activating force has ceased. Intensifying screens fluoresce only when activated.

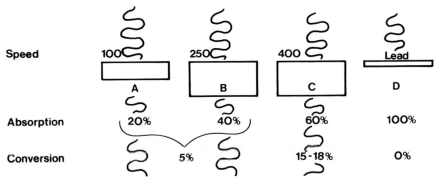

	100	250	400	Lead
Speed	A	B	C	D

Absorption 20% 40% 60% 100%

Conversion 5% 15-18% 0%

Figure 6-6
Absorption/Conversion Ratio of Intensifying Screens

Screen film combinations have been arbitrarily labeled as to speed. Most speed comparisons are made against a conventional-speed blue light-emitting calcium tungstate, medium-speed intensifying screen in combination with a blue-sensitive conventional-speed x-ray film. This combination is labeled speed 100 (A). Before x-radiation can be converted to light, it must be absorbed by the phosphor. An increase in layer thickness will result in an increased absorption of the x-ray photons (B). Rare-earth phosphors (C) inherently absorb more x-ray than conventional calcium tungstate phosphors of an equal thickness (B). A thin sheet of lead, the type used to divide cassettes for multiple images, will absorb 100% of the x-ray beam (D). Absorption, therefore, is only a part of the function of an intensifying screen. The x-ray photons that are absorbed must be converted into light that can be used to expose radiographic film. Conventional 100-speed (A) and 250-speed (B) calcium tungstate screens absorb 20% and 40% of the x-ray beam, respectively, converting 5% of what they absorb into light. A gadolinium oxysulfide rare-earth intensifying screen (C), of equal thickness to the 250-speed calcium tungstate screen, will absorb 60% of the primary beam and convert 15% to 18% of the absorbed x-ray to light. A rare-earth screen absorbs more x-ray per equal thickness and converts more of the absorbed energy to light.

Screen Emissivity

The amount of radiant energy, emitted in the form of light from the screen, is dependent on several factors:

1. The type of phosphor used
2. The design of the screen
3. The crystal size and layer thickness of the phosphor
4. The use of light-restricting dyes
5. The kilovoltage range of the exposure
6. Total x-ray energy used
7. The absorption/conversion ratio of the phosphor
8. Absence or presence of a reflective layer
9. Absence or presence of a light-absorbing layer

TYPE OF PHOSPHOR USED. Calcium tungstate phosphors emit light at approximately 420 nm (4200 Å), primarily in the blue spectrum. Some rare-earth screens, by design, emit light primarily in the green spectrum, approximately 545 nm (5450 Å) (see Fig. 6-3). In reality, all green-emitting screens give off some blue and ultraviolet light as well as green light. Blue intensifying screens, conventional or rare-earth, also emit some green and ultraviolet light.

Screens can be manufactured to emit light that is primarily blue, green, or ultraviolet. Most screens emit a combination of these colors with one spectrum dominating. For maximal efficiency, the films used with the screen must be responsive to the color of light that is primarily emitted (see Fig. 6-2). In general, when green-emitting screens are used with blue-sensitive x-ray film or blue-emitting screens are used with green-sensitive film, system speed is reduced by 50%.

DESIGN OF THE SCREEN. Photon absorption is affected not only by the type of phosphor used but also by the thickness and packing density of the phosphor layer of the intensifying screen (Figs. 6-7 and 6-8). When intensifying screens

Overcoat

Phosphor

Undercoat

Support

Backing

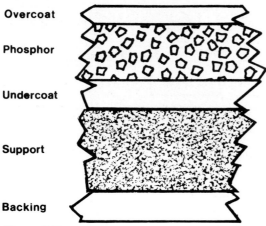

Figure 6-7
Intensifying Screens

A paper or plastic support is used as a base for an intensifying screen. A backing is applied to the support to prevent curling of the screen. An undercoat is used to hold the phosphor layer to the support. The undercoating can be reflective or absorptive (see Fig. 6-9). The phosphor layer is covered with an overcoat to minimize abrasions from handling.

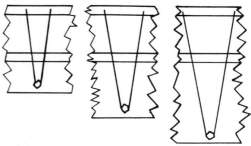

Figure 6-8
Intensifying Screen Design

Intensifying screen crystal size can influence speed. In general, the larger the phosphor crystal, the more light it emits when exposed to x-radiation. Larger crystals cause more image blur than smaller crystals. In actual practice, the crystals vary in size. Layer thickness of the crystals is the primary influence on the speed of the intensifying screen; the thicker the layer, the faster the screen.

A single crystal situated posteriorly in each of the phosphor layers illustrates the effect of layer thickness on sharpness. The thicker screen produces more light spreading in the film emulsion than the thinner screen, resulting in increased image blur. Note: *Crossover of light to the opposite emulsion further increases the spreading of light (see Fig. 6-9).*

were made with phosphors that were low x-ray absorbers, screens of equal thickness were in common use. Rare-earth intensifying screens absorb considerably more x-ray than do conventional calcium tungstate screens (see Fig. 6-6). The anterior intensifying screen in a rare-earth system can absorb a disproportionate amount of x-ray energy, leaving less available for the posterior screen. In order to equally blacken both emulsions of the radiographic film, rare-earth intensifying screens are sometimes asymmetric, with the anterior screen thinner in order to absorb less x-ray.

It would be helpful if the light emitted by the intensifying screen exposed only the emulsion adjacent to the screen. However, light from an intensifying screen passes from emulsion to emulsion through the film base. This effect is called *crossover of light*. As each individual phosphor gives off a cone of light, significant crossover of light with lateral spreading occurs from emulsion to emulsion, resulting in a decrease in image sharpness (Fig. 6-9).

Most radiographic film screen combinations permit a 30% or greater crossover of light. New design parameters cut crossover of light approximately in half. Effective crossover control was first achieved with screens that emitted primarily ul-

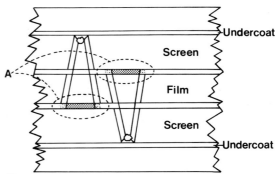

Figure 6-9
Reflection and Crossover of Light

When an x-ray photon penetrates a cassette containing two intensifying screens, the phosphors in the screens give off light in all directions. Some of this light can be reflected forward from the posterior undercoating of the screens to the x-ray emulsion. This light continues to widen (halo effect, A) as it crosses over to the opposite emulsion, producing image blur. About one third of the density of a non-crossover controlled image is the result of "print-through" of the light from the opposite screen.

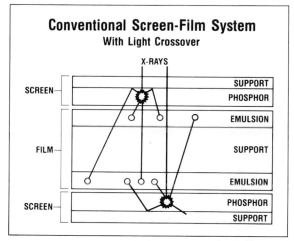

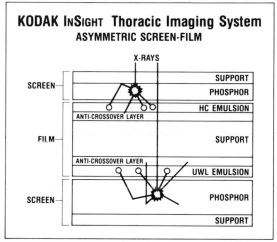

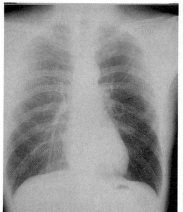
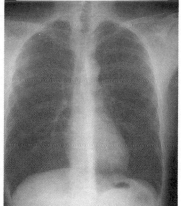
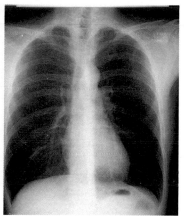

Figure 6-10
Dual Receptor/Zero-Crossover Technology

(Top left) With a conventional screen film system, approximately one third of the light emitted by each intensifying screen crosses over from its adjacent emulsion to the opposite emulsion of the film. This effect increases radiographic density as well as image blur. (Top right) With dual receptor asymmetric screen film imaging, an orange anti-crossover layer on the film support completely prevents the crossover of light from emulsion to emulsion. This anti-crossover dye washes off in the developer. (Bottom right) Two completely isolated screen film receptors of different speeds result in two images recorded on a single sheet of film. The system uses asymmetric screens that differ in speed and spatial resolution. (Bottom left) The high-contrast (HC) emulsion adjacent to the front, thinner screen shows the vascular details of the lungs. (Bottom center) The ultra-wide latitude (UWL) emulsion adjacent to the posterior, thicker intensifying screen adds additional density to the image to record mediastinal information. The posterior combination is about six times faster than the anterior combination. (Reprinted courtesy Eastman Kodak Company)

traviolet light, because the silver halide emulsion absorbs a high percentage of the ultraviolet light.

Some film manufacturers use special dyes added to the film base prior to the coating of the emulsions to minimize crossover. T-grain (tabular grain) technology uses a dye in the film emulsion to minimize crossover, with an improvement in image sharpness (see Fig. 6-3).

In the future, crossover control will become an industry standard, with zero crossover as a goal. This technology is currently available for chest radiography (Fig. 6-10).

When a light-absorbing dye is added to an intensifying screen, the shortest path for light to travel from the fluorescing crystals to the radiographic film is a perpendicular line. As light spreads laterally, considerably more dye must be penetrated, absorbing some of the "halo" effect of the fluorescing crystals. Assuming that each individual crystal gives off light in the shape of a circle, the thickness of the screen, the presence or absence of light-absorbing dye, and the size of the crystal influence the size of this circle of light. The circle continues to widen as the light spreads from emulsion to emulsion. If a light-absorbing dye is used in the screen binder or on the film base, smaller circles of light are produced (Fig. 6-11). The result is an increase in image resolution.

An undercoat is added to the intensifying screens and can be either light reflective or light absorptive. When the undercoat is reflective, unused light is directed toward the film, with an increase in system speed. Unfortunately, this can also cause some loss of image sharpness (see Fig.

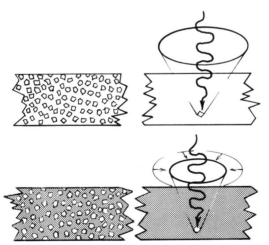

Figure 6-11
**Use of Light-Restricting Dyes
in Intensifying Screens**

(Top right) A typical intensifying screen is shown with a single phosphor as the light source. The x-ray photon strikes the phosphor and a halo of light is produced. Light is given off in all directions from the activated phosphor. Some of the light bounces posteriorly and it's redirected laterally or forward from the posterior reflective layer (see Fig. 6-9). (Bottom, right) If during manufacturing the intensifying screen is impregnated with a dye, the size of the halo of light can be reduced. Much of the light that is reflected or spread laterally is absorbed by the dye, restricting the halo of light from individual crystals. Image blur is reduced.

6-9). An overcoat is added to protect the screen from damage (see Fig. 6-7).

CRYSTAL SIZE AND LAYER THICKNESS OF THE PHOSPHOR. In general, the faster the speed of the intensifying screen (of the same phosphor type), the less detail on the radiograph. This is generally due to the increase in the phosphor layer thickness (see Fig. 6-8). For any given phosphor and crystal size, the greater the number of crystals in the path of the x-ray photons, the greater the absorption. Therefore, increasing the screen thickness increases x-ray absorption if packing density of the phosphors remains constant.

The size of the phosphor crystal is a theoretical concept, since most screens are made with more than a single-size phosphor.

THE USE OF LIGHT-RESTRICTING DYES. For many years, calcium tungstate screens used for detail techniques were deliberately "stained" with a yellow, tan, or pink dye. This produced very slow screens, speed 5 to speed 50 (see Fig. 6-11). For improved sharpness, some mammographic and extremity screens use this principle.

A major exception is the Kodak Lanex medium screen impregnated with a yellow dye to minimize screen blur. This dye absorbs most of the blue light emitted by the screens so that the radiographic film is exposed predominantly by green light. In general, when radiographic films are mismatched to intensifying screens, the system will function at approximately half speed. If a blue-sensitive film is used inadvertently with a Lanex medium screen, a further decrease in film blackening occurs. Instead of a half-speed film density, there is a film blackening of approximately one fifth or less.

IMPORTANT

When screens are accidentally stained or discolored by age or contaminants such as coffee or carbonated beverages, no sharpness benefit occurs. This discoloration is a localized surface phenomenon rather than a dye impregnation of the entire screen.

THE KILOVOLTAGE RANGE USED FOR THE EXPOSURE. Rare-earth intensifying screens are more kVp dependent than most other phosphors. Screen speed differences can occur, particularly in the low kilovoltage range. When a technique chart using a rare-earth film screen combination is formulated and low kilovoltages are required (e.g., for pediatric or extremity radiography), an adjustment often must be made in the mAs factors.

TOTAL X-RAY ENERGY USED. When using a direct exposure film technique, any combination of mA and time produces the same film blackening effect as long as the product of mA and time equals the same mAs. This is known as the reciprocity law.

When film blackening is produced by light photons from an intensifying screen, reciprocity law failure can occur with very short or very long exposures, such as those used in the PA chest exposure (10 msec or less) or with pluridirectional tomographic studies (6–9 sec).

THE ABSORPTION/CONVERSION RATIO OF THE PHOSPHOR. For many years, intensifying screens were made of calcium tungstate ($CaWo_4$) or barium lead sulfate ($BaPbSO_4$). Rare-earth materials such as terbium-activated gadolinium oxysulfide ($Gd_2O_2S:Tb$), terbium-activated lanthanum oxysulfide ($La_2O_2S:Tb$), and lanthanum oxybromide (LaOBr) now dominate screen design. Many of the rare-earth elements used in the manufacture of intensifying screens are more available than the term rare earth implies; however, rare-earth phosphors are expensive and difficult to refine from their natural ores. The phosphors must be as pure as possible in order to control spectral light emissivity. After the phosphor is refined, an activator is added to shift the spectral emission to the predominantly desired light output.

For an equal thickness, screens manufactured with rare-earth phosphors not only absorb more radiation but also have a higher light conversion ratio; that is, they convert more of the absorbed x-radiation to image-forming light (see Fig. 6-6).

ABSENCE OR PRESENCE OF A REFLECTIVE LAYER. See Figure 6-9.

ABSENCE OR PRESENCE OF A LIGHT-ABSORBING LAYER. A light-absorbing layer, as opposed to a reflective layer, may be added between the phosphor and the screen support (see Fig. 6-7).

Screen Speed and Resolution

Intensifying screen film combinations are classified according to their speed and resolution. Generally speaking, slower intensifying screens exhibit improved radiographic resolution (Fig. 6-12).

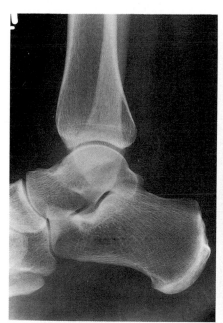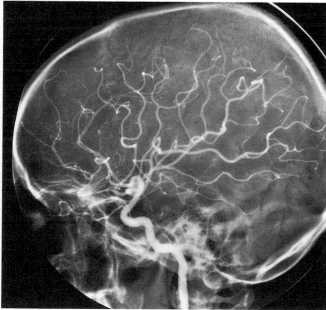

Figure 6-12
Speed 20 versus Speed 1200 Radiographs
For decades all screen film systems were rated at speed 100. Newer rare-earth technology has resulted in system speeds from 20 to 1200. (Left) The radiograph of an ankle was made using a single-emulsion film (see Fig. 6-1D) with a single-detail intensifying screen for a system speed of 20. (Right) The lateral cerebral angiogram was made using fast dual-screen/high-speed dual emulsion film technology for a speed of 1200. The 20-speed system produces excellent osseous and soft tissue detail. The 1200-speed system permits the use of a 0.3-mm focal spot with a frame rate of 2 per second. (Reprinted courtesy Eastman Kodak Company)

Most radiographers compare screen system speeds only, for example, speed-250 calcium tungstate to speed-250 rare-earth gadolinium oxysulfide. Although both of the screens in the given example are the same system speed, the rare-earth screen with its higher absorption/conversion ratio (see Fig. 6-6) produces a considerably sharper radiographic image. Speed-400 gadolinium oxysulfide intensifying screens produce a radiographic image with approximately the same resolution as speed-250 calcium tungstate intensifying screens. T-grain film's crossover control, when used with rare-earth screens, further improves resolution.

Another factor that may affect the speed of intensifying screens is temperature (a theoretical consideration). When room temperature is above 100°F, an intensifying screen will respond slower to x-radiation. When room temperature is below 30°F, the screen will respond faster. The opposite effect occurs with radiographic film. In reality, these effects are probably canceled out, one by the other. Extreme temperature ranges (30° to 100°F) are rarely encountered in radiographic departments.

Advantages of Intensifying Screens

Intensifying screens offer several advantages over direct exposure techniques:

Shorter exposure times

Reduced patient and operator dosage

Less motion, resulting in decreased image blur

Contrast improvement (shorter scale) when lower kilovoltage values are indicated

Extended x-ray tube life

Smaller focal spots

Additional benefits result with the use of rare-earth film screen technology in place of conventional phosphors:

The ability to use the small focal spots when examining larger patients; fractional focal spots (0.3 mm or smaller) may be used for direct roentgen enlargement techniques.

Reduced mAs delivers adequate film blackening with less instantaneous x-ray tube loading, and greater film blackening effect with lower-output generators, such as bedside units (Table 6-2).

Fewer heat units are generated (lower anode thermal loading).

Table 6-2. Film Blackening Effect of Intensifying Screens

		Speed		
mA	100	400 4×	800 8×	1200 12×
50	50	200	400	600
150	150	600	1200	1800
300	300	1200	2400	3600
1000	1000	4000	8000	12,000
1500	1500	6000	12,000	18,000

Disadvantages of Intensifying Screens

Two disadvantages of intensifying screens are radiographic mottle and image blur.

Occasionally unwanted fluctuations in optical densities can be seen on a processed radiograph. This can be described as *radiographic mottle* or noise. Radiographic mottle can be composed of either film graininess, structure mottle from the intensifying screen, or quantum mottle. Radiographic mottle, which is caused by film graininess due to the random distribution of developed silver halide grains, is rarely seen. Structure mottle from variations in intensifying screen crystal sizes is even rarer than film graininess.

Quantum mottle, a variation in optical density resulting from the random distribution of x-ray quanta absorbed by the x-ray receptor, is a more common problem. One can generally categorize the density fluctuations seen on a radiograph as quantum mottle. Quantum mottle exists to some degree in all screen film radiographs. The faster the system speed or the higher the kilovoltage used, the more likely the appearance of quantum mottle (Fig. 6-13). If increased film blackening is achieved with increased mAs, a more homogeneous image is produced and quantum mottle is less likely to be seen.

In addition to the loss of resolution inherent in intensifying screens, image blur can be increased by poor screen film contact. Additional information on image blur can be found in Chapter 8.

Gradient Intensifying Screens

Gradient intensifying screens are often used for full-length vascular studies of the leg or for radio-

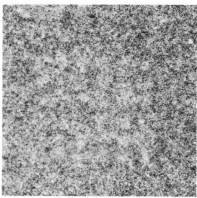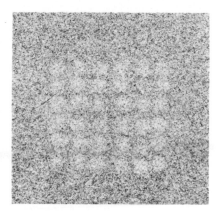

Figure 6-13
Quantum Mottle

Quantum mottle exists to some degree in all screen film radiographs. It can be a problem in studies in which minute radiographic details might be obscured. This mottled appearance is not due to film graininess; it is significantly coarser than film grain and is due to non-uniform light emission from an intensifying screen. (Left) An image made with a relatively fast x-ray system, requiring a minimum amount of x-radiation for exposure; therefore, the mottled pattern is more pronounced. (Right) A slow screen film system was used, which required increased exposure (increased mAs), producing a more homogenous image. Quantum mottle is less pronounced in this image. See Chapter 11, Figure 11-42 for a clinical example of the effect of quantum mottle on an image. Note: *Detail of the plastic bead test object was improved with the slower system. (Reprinted courtesy Eastman Kodak Company)*

graphs of the entire spine. These screens can be up to 51 inches in length, with speeds varying from one end of the screen to the other. For example, a gradient screen may be rated 400 speed at one end and diminish in speed to 100 at the opposite end. The thicker body part is placed over the faster portion of the gradient screen. For a scoliosis study, the faster portion of the intensifying screen is positioned beneath the lumbar region; the slower portions are positioned in the cervicothoracic area. With gradient screens, all regions of the body that are in the x-ray field receive an equal amount of radiation.

IMPORTANT

Compensatory filters should be used instead of gradient screens, whenever possible, to equalize differences in patient density. See Chapter 3 for more information on compensatory filtration.

Screen Maintenance

Screens should be cleaned regularly using manufacturers' recommendations. Cleaning eliminates surface marks, which may result in artifacts on the radiograph. This is particularly important if a screen film combination is used to localize small opaque foreign bodies. Artifacts shield the film from the fluorescent light of the intensifying screen, and a minus density (white) is produced. Dirt or dust particles can mimic or hide small radiopaque foreign bodies.

Intensifying screen cleaner should never be sprayed directly on an intensifying screen. Excessive spraying or improper drying of the screen can cause screen damage.

Cassettes

Cassette Design

The cassette, a container for exposed and unexposed radiographic film, is used to protect the film from light. Most cassettes have fronts made of either bakelite or magnesium. Low x-ray–absorbing materials that lessen the absorption of the primary x-ray beam are available for cassette fronts and radiographic tabletops. The designers and manufacturers of these products claim a 35% or greater improvement in film blackening when compared with conventional cassette front or tabletop materials.

IMPORTANT

Although an improvement in film blackening due to the low absorption front material seems impressive, rare-earth film screen combinations produce up to a 1200% increase in film blackening when compared with a medium-speed calcium tungstate system (speed 100) (see Table 6-2).

Intensifying screens are mounted within the cassette. A thin sheet of lead foil is often mounted underneath the back intensifying screen to absorb backscatter (Fig. 6-14).

Film screen contact must be maintained to minimize blurring of radiographic details caused by lateral spreading of light from the activated phosphors in the screen (Fig. 6-15). Often, poor screen film contact seen as segmental blurring of the radiographic image is mistaken for motion blur. Bending or warping of the cassette can cause

poor screen contact. Sometimes the weight of a patient placed directly on a cassette can produce a temporary contact problem. (See Chapter 14 for a film screen contact testing procedure.)

When conventional cassettes are used for high-detail extremity radiography or mammography, a single intensifying screen is often used with a single-emulsion antihalation-backed radiographic film.

Direct exposure film holders are sometimes used for extremity radiography. These holders protect the film from light and may also contain a lead foil backing to minimize backscatter.

Specialty Cassettes

Special cassettes have been designed for mammography, tomography, and unusual positioning techniques.

Curved cassettes, available in 8 × 10 inch and 10 × 12 inch sizes, are used for the following:

1. To evaluate the head of the femur in the lateral position when a conventional radiograph cannot be made

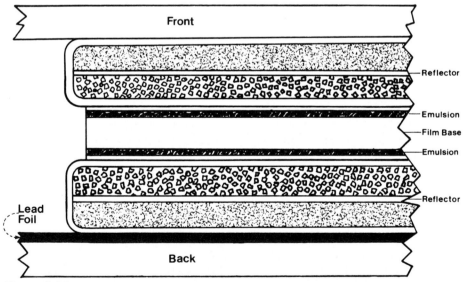

Figure 6-14
Cross-section of Cassette, Screens, and Radiographic Film

The cassette is a container for both exposed and unexposed film. A pair of intensifying screens in intimate contact with a dual-emulsion x-ray film is shown in a light-proof cassette. The cassette front is usually made of bakelite, magnesium, or some type of low radiation–absorbing material. A thin sheet of lead foil is often mounted underneath the posterior intensifying screen to absorb backscatter.

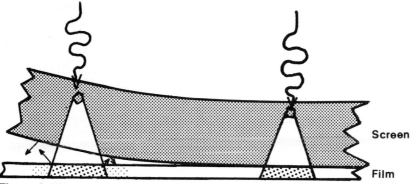

Figure 6-15
Screen Film Contact

Screen film contact is essential to minimize blurring of the radiographic image. Bending or warping of the cassette can cause poor screen contact. As the screen is pulled away from the film emulsion, the halo of light widens. If the screen is not in contact with the film, light from the screen can reflect in many directions, producing segmental blurring of the image. See Chapter 14, Figure 14-20, for screen film contact test information.

2. To examine the knee in the anteroposterior position when the knee is flexed and cannot be extended

3. For an axillary image of the shoulder

Multiscreen (book) cassettes can be used for simultaneous multilevel tomographic studies. These cassettes hold from three to seven pairs of intensifying screens to produce three to seven tomographic sections at ½-cm or 1-cm increments, with only one exposure. An increase of approximately 2½ times the mAs over the original exposure value of the single section is needed with a book cassette. Because the beam must penetrate through multilevels of intensifying screens, low kilovoltage levels are not acceptable. Generally, 70 to 75 kVp is the minimal kilovoltage recommended with a book cassette. Special intensifying screens arranged in order of increasing speed, from front to back, are required. For example, in a five-screen-pair book, the first screen pair may be 50 speed, the second may be 100 speed, and so on. This progressive increase in screen speed works fairly well with calcium tungstate screens because of their low absorption properties. It is difficult to design a book cassette using rare-earth intensifying screens because of the high absorption nature of rare-earth phosphors. The first screen pair would absorb most of the beam, leaving little or no radiation for the remaining pairs of intensifying screens. The images are often of marginal quality, and this technique has not been well accepted.

A special type of book cassette with closely matched intensifying screens (1.0 mm apart), known as a *plesiocassette*, holds four pairs of intensifying screens for use in a Bucky tray. The exact 1.0-mm spacing of the pairs of intensifying screens in the plesiocassette produces four equidistant radiographic images with one exposure. For example, when a tomographic fulcrum is set at a specific level such as 10 cm, the first pair of screens in the plesiocassette will image the anatomy at that focal range (10 cm). The second, third, and fourth will image, in descending order, 9.9 cm, 9.8 cm, and 9.7 cm of body tissue.

A *reduced exposure mammographic cassette* is available, with a polycarbonate and polystyrene front for minimal absorption of the primary beam. The low absorption front is important for screen film mammography because of the low kilovoltage required for this study. Very thin cassette edges permit placement of the cassette in close contact with the chest wall.

Vacuum cassettes have also been used with mammographic techniques. There are two types of vacuum cassettes. A flexible reusable polyvinyl chloride cassette is available, with a built-in vacuum valve and an internal envelope, which can be removed for easy film loading. When reloaded, the end of the vacuum bag can be resealed with a plastic spacer. The air is evacuated from the bag by means of the vacuum valve, which is attached to either a hand pump or a motor-driven suction unit. A second type of thin polyethylene bag can be loaded, evacuated, and heat sealed in the dark-room with special equipment designed for this task. This bag absorbs significantly less radiation than does the reusable polyvinyl chloride bag.

Automated Film Handling

Daylight or room-light handling systems use spe-cial cassettes that can be loaded and unloaded in an illuminated room. These room-light systems are useful in the emergency ward, neonatal unit, and pediatric and orthopedic areas.

Radiographic tables that hold boxes of film with a single pair of intensifying screens can also be used to expedite workflow. The automated ta-bles are often linked to a freestanding automatic film processor. (See Chapter 4, Fig. 4-8.)

The dedicated chest unit has been available since the mid-1960s and is considered an indis-pensable part of large radiographic departments. The unit is loaded with a box of radiographic film, and one hundred or more radiographs can be made before additional loading is required. (See Chapter 4, Fig. 4-7.)

Film Identification

Most cassettes have a lead insert in a predeter-mined corner of the cassette to shield the film from x-ray exposure during the making of the radio-graph. In a given product line, this lead blocker is in the same area of every cassette. The shielded (unexposed) portion of the film is used for the photographic transfer of patient information.

Some identification printers can be used only in the darkroom. When the exposed film is removed from the cassette and placed in a given position on a printer, patient information can be photo-graphed (contact printed) from an identification card to the unexposed portion of the film.

Other types of identification cameras permit in-formation to be transferred to the radiographic film under room-light conditions while the film is still in the cassette (Fig. 6-16).

Fluoroscopic Screens

Intensifying screens are used for static imaging. A fluoroscopic screen is required for dynamic evaluation of organs and structures. For fluoro-scopic examinations, an x-ray tube is mounted beneath a radiographic table. Radiation passes

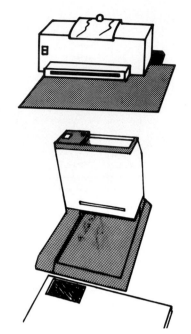

Figure 6-16
Radiographic Film Identification Systems
(Top) Most cassettes have lead inserts in a predeter-mined location to shield a small area of the radiographic film from x-radiation. After an exposure is made, this unexposed portion of the film is exposed in the dark-room with an identification printer. Patient informa-tion, typed on an identification card, is photographi-cally transferred to the film by means of contact printing prior to processing. (Bottom) Another type of identification camera, used with specially designed cassettes, records patient information on the unexposed film, in normal room light. See Chapter 5, Fig. 5-26, for potential medicolegal problems with cassette identifica-tion systems.

through the patient to the fluoroscopic screen to produce a visual image on the screen. The basic phosphor used in the manufacture of fluoroscopic screens is zinc cadmium sulfide (ZnCdS). The property of phosphorescence known as lag or af-terglow is characteristic of fluoroscopic screen phosphors. The crystals absorb x-ray energy and convert it to visible light, similar to the crystals in intensifying screens (see Table 6-1). Fluoroscopic crystals are considerably larger than intensifying screen crystals. A fluoroscopic screen can tolerate the lack of sharpness produced by the larger crys-tals because the fluoroscope is primarily used as a positioning device or for organ motion evaluation. Fluoroscopic screens give off a yellow-green light. This luminescent effect, although in the range that the human eye can see, is not diagnostically useful unless the eyes are adapted to darkness. The brightness of a conventional fluoroscopic screen is a fraction of that of a radiograph as seen on a viewbox. Red adaptation goggles, almost an historical curiosity with the advent of the image intensifier, must be used for up to 20 minutes to prepare the eyes for a dimly illuminated conventional fluoroscopic screen. The image-intensified fluoroscope described in Chapter 12 produces brighter images than a conventional fluoroscope and is helpful in reducing patient dosage.

Chapter 7

Radiographic Processing

Latent image is the invisible change in a radiographic film that is caused either by a controlled exposure to x-radiation or the light from a fluorescing intensifying screen. The latent image is made visible by the process of development.

Processing Considerations

Safelight Filter Selection

Care must be made in the selection of safelight filters. Special filters are required to match the spectral sensitivity of the film in use.

For years, the Eastman Kodak Wratten Series 6B Safelight Filter was in common use. This filter was designed to be used with blue-sensitive medical x-ray films. With the introduction of orthochromatic-sensitive medical x-ray film, a filter had to be designed that could be used with blue- and green-sensitive film products. This filter is the Kodak safelight filter type GBX-2.

IMPORTANT

The use of a safelight designed for blue-sensitive film with orthochromatic x-ray film (primarily green sensitive) results in fogging of the film. Light bulb wattage level information and a simple safelight test kit are available from most film sales representatives.

A dark green filter is available for photofluorographic and cinefluorographic panchromatic films. These films should be handled in total darkness until at least one half the development time has expired.

Potential Hazards of Processing Chemicals

Sore throats, sinusitis, skin rashes, constant headaches, nausea, aching joints, fatigue, confusion, and heart irregularities have been linked to sensitivity to processing chemicals.

Angeline M. Cullinan and John E. Cullinan:
PRODUCING QUALITY RADIOGRAPHS, 2ND ED.
© 1987, 1994 J. B. Lippincott Company.

A comprehensive report entitled *Radiographic Film Processing Procedures Guidance Notes for the Provision of a Safe Work Environment and Safe Work Practice for Radiographers and Darkroom Technicians, 1990*, includes information on the responsibility for a safe working environment, the potential hazards in x-ray film processing, the assessment of hazards, the effects on health, safe work practices, and emergency procedures.*

Manual Processing

Before the design of the automatic processor, all x-ray films were manually developed. Hand processing is still practiced in some low-volume facilities, whereby, under safelight conditions, exposed film is attached to four corners of a metal hanger, placed in the developer, and hand agitated so that uniform development can be obtained.

Developer reduces the exposed silver compounds in the film emulsion to black metallic silver. After a predetermined period of development, usually 3 to 5 minutes, development is halted by placing the film in the fixer. The unexposed silver compounds are removed and the gelatin containing the black metallic silver is hardened. Normally, the developed radiograph is briefly agitated in a water bath, then moved to the fixing tank. A stop bath of a diluted acetic solution, recommended to neutralize the alkaline developer, is sometimes used. The manual fixing process requires approximately 10 minutes, or twice the time of the development process. After clearing and hardening of the emulsion in the fixer, room lights can be turned on. The film is then moved to the wash tank, where 20 or more minutes of washing is required to remove residual fixer. The radiographs are either air dried or placed in dryer cabinets equipped to circulate heated air. As much as 90 minutes may be required before a dry radiograph is available for interpretation. It may be difficult to make an accurate diagnosis from a wet radiograph, and a final decision is usually withheld until the dry image can be reviewed. If an immediate diagnosis is required, the radiograph can be interpreted while wet.

*This booklet (ISBN 0-477-04616-9) can be obtained by writing to MA Gordon, Wi Tako Street, Manakau, RD 31, Levin, New Zealand.

IMPORTANT

Care must be taken to avoid crowding the radiographs in the dryer. If radiographs are placed too close to each other during the drying process they may stick together.

For many years, despite its limitations, manual processing satisfactorily served the needs of radiology departments. As the workload increased, however, hand processing techniques took too much time, making it difficult to complete processing tasks in a reasonable period of time or to maintain quality control. Space to accommodate the drying of large numbers of radiographs presented an additional problem.

Automatic Processing

In the 1940s, automated film processors were designed that moved the films on hangers from tank to tank. There was less manual labor involved but very little saving in time. In the late 1950s, the first roller transport processor was made commercially available by the Eastman Kodak Company. The 1-hour, or longer, dry-to-dry processing previously required was reduced to 6 minutes (Fig. 7-1). With automatic processors, time of processing is exact because of the constant speed of the motor-drive system.

The purpose of an automatic processor is to transport film through the processing cycles in a controlled manner and to deliver a dry radiograph at the end of the drying cycle. To accomplish this goal, the solutions must be constantly agitated, temperature controlled, and replenished.

With hand processing, time, temperature, agitation, and replenishment were difficult to control because of the human factor. Radiographers could, and did, allow films to remain in the developer longer than recommended to make up for underexposure and prematurely removed films from the developer to compensate for overexposure. This arbitrary approach to development, although not encouraged, was frequently practiced. Safelight viewing of radiographs often resulted in the contamination of the solutions as depleted developer drained back into the developer tank, hastening the exhaustion of the solution. If a small amount of fixer were splashed into the developing solution, it would contaminate the developer, making it ineffective.

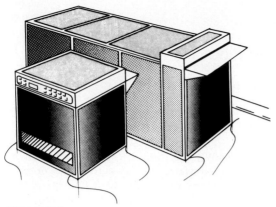

Figure 7-1
Evolution of the Automatic Roller
Transport X-ray Film Processor

The first commercially manufactured roller transport processor (Eastman Kodak Company) had a 6-minute, dry-to-dry processing cycle. The roller racks of the early processor were so cumbersome that a ceiling-mounted crane was required to remove the racks from the solution tanks for repair or cleaning. A typical present-day automatic processing cycle requires 90 seconds to process a film dry-to-dry. Newer rapid processing units require considerably less floor space and can process a radiographic film in 30 seconds.

Two other essentials, agitation and replenishment, have also been considered in the design of the automatic processor. Improper agitation can result in streaks and uneven densities on the radiograph. The rollers of the transport system and the recirculation pumps continually agitate the solutions. Replenishment solutions are added as each sheet of film is fed into the automatic processor. The system is designed so that a precise amount of developer and fixer replenisher is fed into the tanks for every centimeter of film that passes over the entrance roller. There are specific recommendations for the proper feeding of sheet or roll films into the automatic processor (Fig. 7-2).

Processors can be modified to transport films according to the specific needs of the user. Most modern radiography departments use a rapid transport system of approximately 90 seconds or less for medical x-ray films. New rapid processing units can deliver a radiographic film, dry-to dry, in 30 seconds. This rapid process requires special processing chemicals with special x-ray films.

Other uses require a longer processing cycle. For example, an extended cycle process is sometimes desired for mammograms. Film speed and film contrast are increased by extended cycle pro-

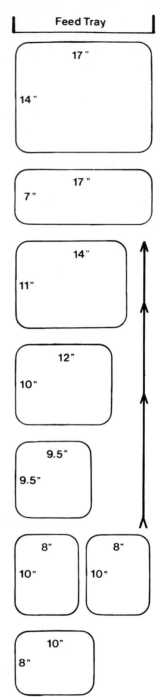

Figure 7-2
Automatic Processor Film
Alignment Feeding Patterns

Processor manufacturers recommend specific film alignment feeding patterns to maintain proper replenishment rates. The feeding patterns shown ensure the recommended amounts of replenishment solutions per square foot of film processed. A change in feeding patterns could result in over- or under-replenishment of the solutions.

cessing, and reduced exposure factors can be used. Ideally this automatic processor should be dedicated to single-emulsion mammographic film, and the use of proper chemicals and replenishment rates is critical.

The Need for Special Solutions

The solutions used in the automatic processor have a longer solution life and differ from the solutions used for manual processing techniques.

With manual processing techniques, when the film is placed into the developer, its emulsion gets soft and swells. In the stop bath and fixer solutions, the emulsion contracts and begins to harden. As the film is passed from one solution to another, it varies in thickness and stickiness. This is not a problem as long as films do not come in contact with one another.

In an automatic processor, film is always in contact with the rollers in the transport systems, therefore the degree of swelling and stickiness of the film must be controlled. A film that is too thick slows down the transport system and causes a jam as the next film catches up to it. A film that is too thin can slip into or between the rollers and could also cause a jam. If the film becomes too sticky, it could adhere to or wrap around a roller.

Because of the unique requirements of the automatic processor, special chemicals were formulated that contain hardeners in the developer and the fixing solution; these hold the thickness and stickiness of the film within the tolerances needed for automatic processing. These special chemicals, along with controlled replenishment and recirculation, reduce processing and transport time.

The Developer

Developer chemistry (an alkaline solution) used for automatic processing usually contains the following:

Sulfite (sodium or potassium) as a preservative
Carbonate (sodium or potassium) as a buffer and a source of alkali
Hydroquinone (a developing agent) to provide upper scale density (black)
Metol or phenidone (a developing agent) to provide intermediate or lower scale densities (shades of gray to white)
Hydroxide (sodium or potassium) as the activator in the developer (a source of alkali)

Gluteraldehyde as a hardening agent (not found in manual processing developer solutions)
Potassium bromide as an antifoggant and restrainer (used to minimize fog and maintain chemical balance between fresh and seasoned chemicals; a suppressor of the phenidone activity on unexposed silver crystals, thereby helping to maintain low base fog levels)
Water to aid in the swelling of the emulsion; the solvent for the developer chemicals

The Fixer

The automatic processor fixer contains well-buffered acidic solutions; therefore, a stop bath is not required. The fixer contains the following:

Sodium thiosulfate or ammonia thiosulfate (hypo) as a silver solvent to remove unexposed silver crystals from the film
Sodium sulfite as a preservative for the ammonia thiosulfate
Acetic acid (a source of hydrogen ions) as a buffer
Aluminum sulfate (a hardening agent) to help reduce drying time
Water as the solvent for the fixer chemicals

IMPORTANT

Never substitute manual processing chemicals for automatic film processor chemicals.

Components of the Automatic Processor

All manufacturers have specific processor design parameters, which vary from unit to unit. In this book, only the factors common to all processors will be discussed. The details of installation and servicing can be found in the service manuals provided with each model.

The automatic processor consists of three major parts (Fig. 7-3):

1. A film loading area (Fig. 7-3*A*). The film is fed into the processor in the darkroom. An audible or visual signal is emitted when the film completely passes over the entrance roller. This indicates to the darkroom personnel that the unit is ready to accept another film. If a second film is prematurely fed into the processor, overlapping of the films and possible jamming could occur. Even if a jam does not occur, the

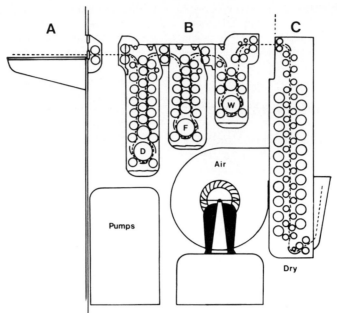

Figure 7-3
Automatic Roller Transport Processing

Three major sections constitute the automatic processor. In the dark-room, film is fed into the processor by means of a film feeding tray (A). The remainder of the processor (B and C) is usually in-stalled outside the darkroom. Developer, fixer, and wash tanks with their roller transport components make up a major section of the sec-ond portion (B) of the processor. Temperature controls and recircu-lation and replenishment pumps are vital components of section B. Section C is the dryer portion of the roller transport system, consist-ing of the air blower, heaters, and the dryer roller transport system. A receptacle for processed dry radiographs completes the final seg-ment of the processor.

Most automatic processors are linked to a darkroom. Freestanding processors with special feeding mechanisms can be used with room-light cassettes. These cassettes can be automatically loaded under room-light conditions and placed in a special feed mechanism on the freestanding processor, eliminating the need for a darkened film feed area.

overlapped radiographs would be improperly developed or fixed and often not of diagnostic quality.

2. The film solution processing tanks, roller transport system, temperature controls, and recirculation and replenishment pumps (Fig. 7-3B)

3. Heaters and air blowers to facilitate drying of the radiographs, a roller transport system in the dryer, and a receptacle for the processed, dried radiographs (Fig. 7-3C)

Processor Systems and Cycles

The major purposes and functions of the various components of the automatic processor are out-lined in Table 7-1.

THE ROLLER TRANSPORT SYSTEM. The roller transport system consists of a series of gears and chains connected to rollers that are used to trans-port the films through the processor while provid-ing constant, vigorous agitation of the solutions against the film surfaces.

Table 7-1. Automatic Processor System Functions

Roller Transport System

Transport film
Control processing time
Control replenishment time
Help prevent film overlap
Agitation
Squeegee action

Recirculation System (Developer)

Develop film
Maintain solution activity and concentration
Control temperature
Agitation
Constant filtration
Control recirculation

Recirculation System (Fixer)

Stop development
Clear film
Harden emulsion
Maintain solution activity and concentration
Agitation
Control recirculation

Recirculation System (Water)

Wash film
Control water flow
Agitation
Keep developer overflow clean
Temperature control

Air Circulation System

Dry film
Control temperature
Control air recirculation

Replenishment System

Replenish solutions
Control replenishment rates
Maintain solution activity and concentration
Prevent and control backflow of replenisher

The roller transport system includes

An entrance roller assembly
Crossover racks (not in all processors)
Turnaround racks located between roller
     assemblies
A squeegee assembly to remove excess moisture
     from the film surfaces
Dryer rollers to transport the film through the
     dryer section.

THE RECIRCULATION SYSTEMS. The recirculation systems keep solutions evenly mixed and provide chemical agitation to ensure uniform solution coverage of the film while it is transported through the solutions. Overflow solution is carried over the top of the tanks into a well, known as a *weir*, to a drain.

This system also includes heaters, thermostats, heat exchangers, and filters. In some systems, the temperature of the solutions may be controlled by contact with the common walls of the solution tanks and the temperature of the wash water.

THE WASH SYSTEM. An adequate supply of water is necessary to remove residual fixer from the processed radiograph. Adequate washing helps to preserve the radiograph while in storage, thereby improving its archival properties. The wash system is not part of the recirculation system. Water is passed through the processor at a constant rate and flows over a weir into a drain.

THE DRYER. As the film is transported through the dryer section, heated filtered air is directed over both sides of the film by a wind box, commonly called a *phlenum*. Humidity and temperature are carefully controlled. Proper venting must be provided for dryer heat as well as for chemical fumes.

Automatic standby controls, used to reduce energy costs and water consumption, de-energize the processor when film is not being processed.

CHEMICAL REPLENISHMENT SYSTEM. Over-replenishment of the developer may result in lower radiographic contrast. Severe developer under-replenishment may cause film to stick in the dryer.

Over-replenishment of the fixer does not greatly affect image quality but is expensive and wasteful. Under-replenishment of the fixer results in poor clearing and insufficient hardening of the emulsion, with possible failure of the film to transport properly. The archival quality of the film can be affected by under-replenishment of the fixer.

Replenishment keeps the solutions at proper strength and level in the processing tanks while extending solution life. As radiographic films pass through the processor, they change the balance of developer alkalinity and fixer acidity. The automatic replenishment system works accordingly to keep these chemistries in balance.

Developer and fixer are automatically added to the automatic processor to compensate for the volume of work. As the film passes into the developer, a microswitch in the entrance roller closes, activating the replenishment pumps. Replenisher solutions flow into the proper tanks. The rate of replenishment is determined by the film size (see Fig. 7-2). After the film passes over the entrance roller, the switch opens and replenishment ceases. The new solutions are blended into the tanks by the recirculating system.

The replenishment system includes a strainer, a device to control backflow, and instrumentation to measure replenishment rates.

It is difficult to maintain the developer solution at a stable processing level in an automatic processor used for a low volume of film. *Flooded replenishment* is a method in which developer replenishment containing starter solution is introduced into the processor at timed intervals. Replenishment is independent of the number of films processed. Flooded replenishment is particularly helpful with a medium to low volume of single-emulsion films, such as is used for nuclear medicine scans, computed tomography, and ultrasound imaging.*

Automatic Mixer and Replenishment Systems

In some large radiology departments that are serviced by an in-house central replenishment facility, bulk chemistry is often mixed at a remote location and pumped to several automatic processors. In departments without a central replenishment facility, developer and fixer replenishment tanks holding up to 50 gallons of each solution are usually located close to the automatic processor.

Automatic mixer and replenishment systems contain concentrated developer and fixer replenishment, which are automatically mixed with water as required, in 5-, 10-, or 15-gallon mixing and holding containers. The dispenser compartments are color- and letter-coded, and their openings are shaped to accept correspondingly shaped bottles (Fig. 7-4). Electronic probes sense the chemistry level and mix the precise amount of concentrated solution and water. One automixer can be used for one or two processors. This equipment is simple to operate and can be cleaned and maintained with hot water.

Cine or Strip Film Processing

Seventy-millimeter or 105-mm fluoro spot films and 14-inch-wide roll film used for serial angiography can be taped to a leader of x-ray film and

*Specific information on this process can be found in Frank ED, Gray JE, Wilken DA: Flood replenishment: A new method of processor control. Radiol Technol 52(3):272–275, 1980.

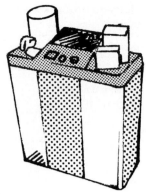

Figure 7-4
Automatic Mixer and Replenishment Units
Processing consistency is ensured with automatically mixed replenishment solutions. Concentrated developer and fixer replenishers can be automatically mixed with water as required. Electronic probes within the automixer sense chemistry levels in the replenishment tanks and add the precise amount of concentrated solutions and water. The developer and fixer replenishment bottles are of different shapes and colors and are letter-coded.

processed in a conventional automatic processor. The leader piece of film should be 7 inches or longer and as wide or wider than the roll film to ensure proper transport through the automatic processor. Scotch Brand electrical tape No. 850 (1 inch wide) can be used to butt-splice the roll film to the leader film.

IMPORTANT

The adhesive side of the tape must not come in contact with the roller transport system.

Professional cine processors that can accommodate 8-mm to 70-mm films are available. They are similar to medical x-ray film processors in that they control time, temperature, agitation, replenishment, and wash water flow rates. Special drive transport systems ensure proper film tension and help to eliminate film breakage during transport.

Silver Recovery

The residual silver halide in the fixing solution of the processor can be collected by either a metallic replacement cartridge or an electrolytic plating cell. These reclamation procedures can be carried out "in house." To collect the silver from the fixing solution, a drain is connected to the fixing tank. Instead of emptying the exhausted fixer solution into the main drain, it is allowed to flow into a collecting receptacle or directly into a silver recovery unit. If solution is being passed into an electrolytic silver recovery unit, a broken connection (an air space) in the tube is needed so that no electrolytic action can follow the solution back into the processor and cause corrosion or plating of silver. Recovered silver can be sold to provide an additional source of revenue for the radiology department or hospital.

Chemical precipitation of used fixer is generally performed in commercial facilities or in departments with centralized collecting systems.

Another form of silver recovery is the removal of the black metallic silver on processed radiographs or the unprocessed emulsion of unexposed film. The film is usually purchased by reclaimers who are equipped to remove the silver in an efficient, cost-effective manner, either by burning or by chemical methods.

Radiographic Quality

Image quality describes those qualities that are always present, in varying degrees, in all radiographic images. The quality of the radiograph determines the diagnostic information available for interpretation.

All radiographic images exhibit certain characteristics: *photographic and optical density* (overall blackness), *radiographic contrast* (differences between two or more densities), *definition* (sharpness of the structure being imaged), and *distortion* (size or shape of the image relative to the true size and shape of the object being examined). Density, contrast, definition (often referred to as recorded detail), and distortion can be controlled and affected by technical factors and radiographic accessories. If these imaging qualities are optimum, they will be easy to discern on the processed radiograph. The physical parameters that control or affect image quality can be adjusted by the radiographer to accommodate the preferences of the interpreter.

Radiographic images are transparencies and, therefore, their light-absorbing properties are measured as transmission densities. When a reflective support is used to record the image, such as in the Polaroid technique or xeroradiography, reflection densities are measured.

A proper blend of technical factors affects the appearance of the radiographic image. Some of the factors used in the production of a radiograph are standard, whereas others must be changed depending on patient condition, size, ability to cooperate, and equipment limitations. Image quality will be discussed in terms of how radiographic principles affect the radiographic image and the relation of controlling factors to each other.

There are four primary exposure factors that are used to change the photographic effect of the image. They are kilovoltage (kVp), milliamperage (mA), time (expressed in seconds), and distance (D). The photographic effect can be expressed as:

$$PE = \frac{mA \times T \cdot kV^2}{D^2}$$

Angeline M. Cullinan and John E. Cullinan:
PRODUCING QUALITY RADIOGRAPHS, 2ND ED.
© 1987, 1994 J. B. Lippincott Company.

Additional formulas that are needed to accomplish technical changes are presented in Appendix II. The purpose of grouping all formulas together is to provide easy access when they are needed as a reference for conversion of technical factors. Chapter 10 is devoted to the application and evaluation of the imaging principles presented in this book.

Radiographic Density

Density as applied to mass per unit volume should not be confused with photographic or optical density. Photographic density is defined as the log of the intensity of the incident light falling on the image to the intensity of the light transmitted through the image. Radiographic density is usually described in terms of the overall blackening of a processed film.

The radiologist refers to density as an anatomic or pathologic change that absorbs x-radiation (Fig. 8-1), for example, a solid mass within the lung that stops x-rays from reaching the detector, decreasing film blackening in that area. X-ray absorption is dependent on the atomic number as well as the thickness of the part doing the absorbing, whether it is a solid tumor, an osseous change, or fluid.

The radiographer thinks of density as it refers to overall film blackening, which is an optical or photographic property. A radiolucent area created by decreased absorption will produce an increase in film blackening.

The image as viewed by transmitted light, usually on a viewbox, consists of variations in the amount of black metallic silver remaining on the film after chemical processing (Fig. 8-2). The exposed silver emulsion is converted into black metallic silver by the process of development. The degree of blackness on a radiograph is determined by the amount of exposure reaching the emulsion of the film.

The overall blackness and relation of the intensity of the incident light from the viewbox to the light transmitted through the film can be measured and the density on the film expressed as

$$D = \log \frac{\text{incident light}}{\text{transmitted light}}$$

Differences in density represent the contrast within the image. Images with only a few density

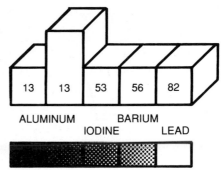

Figure 8-1
Effect of Absorption on Radiographic Density
Physical density (mass per unit volume) should not be confused with photographic or optical density. A step-wedge of densities of four different materials and their atomic numbers are shown. The four materials, aluminum, iodine, barium, and lead, are displayed as equal-sized objects. Equal thickness of dissimilar materials are used to demonstrate subject contrast. A rectangular structure of aluminum (the second step) represents a twofold increase in thickness compared to the other objects. Note the difference in absorption in the simulated stepwedge. The x-ray beam produces a blackened step for the first thickness of aluminum, since most of the radiation would pass through this substance. The double thickness of aluminum absorbs more x-ray and therefore attenuates the x-ray beam to a greater degree. Iodine (atomic number 53) and barium (atomic number 56) absorb a similar amount of radiation. Lead, on the other hand, absorbs all of the x-radiation in this example. An object having increased mass determined by the atomic number or tissue thickness will absorb more x-radiation, with decreased film blackening. The differences in adjacent densities represent contrasts. When multiple density changes are seen, long-scale contrast is present. Abrupt density differences indicate short-scale contrast.

variations are said to exhibit short-scale contrast. Greater density variations result in longer-scale contrast.

To graphically portray the response of x-ray film to known amounts of exposure, density may be measured by a densitometer and plotted on a graph. The resultant curve drawn from the graph is called an H & D curve, sensitometric curve, or characteristic curve (see Chapter 6).

Most radiographic film has a blue tint in its base, which adds to overall density. An increase in density can also be caused by chemical fog from development of unexposed silver halide crystals.

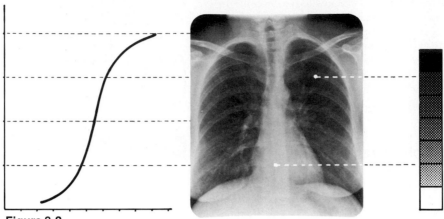

Figure 8-2
Optical Density

A densitometer is used to measure the response of x-ray film to known amounts of exposure. Overall blackness (optical density) and the relationship of the intensity of the light transmitted through the radiographic film to the amount of light incident to the image from the viewbox can be measured. These measurements can be plotted on a graph known as a characteristic curve (left). Radiographic density increases as exposure is increased. Exposure factors are represented logarithmically at the bottom of the graph (see Fig. 8-5). A chest radiograph as viewed by transmitted light is keyed to a stepwedge of the differences between densities (contrast) (right). Dotted lines from the sensitometric curve pass through representative areas of density on the chest radiograph and are aligned to comparable densities on the stepwedge.

Control of Radiographic Density by mAs

Radiographic density, as a result of x-ray exposure, is primarily controlled by mAs.

The energy spectrum of the x-ray beam is not changed by a change in the mA value. As mA is raised, the quantity of x-ray production is increased, but the energy of the photons is not affected. The combination of mA and time of exposure (T) determines the total number (quantity) of x-rays produced. Since mAs is the product of mA × T, as expressed in seconds, an increase or decrease in either factor results in a change in density on the radiograph.

Milliamperage is used to control the number of electrons made available for interaction with the target and time is used to control the length of exposure. Milliamperage and time are inversely proportional to each other; therefore, it is easy to maintain a given density when either variable must be changed. Increasing mA or time will cause a corresponding increase in radiographic density.

IMPORTANT

A 30% to 40% increase im mAs is required to detect a visible change in density on a radiograph.

Milliamperage and time, expressed in seconds or fractions of seconds, can be varied to maintain a preselected mAs with no change in radiographic density or may be changed in combination with kVp to maintain or vary radiographic density and contrast. A high mA combined with a short exposure time is sometimes needed to stop motion. However, several problems can occur with extremely short exposure times and high ma values. These include:

"Blooming" of the focal spot
"Capture" of the grid in motion
Minimal response time difficulties that may occur if an automatic exposure device is used

The Effect of Distance

Variations in focal film distance (FFD) are rarely deliberately used to affect image quality. A minor

Table 8-1. Geometric Designators

Original Terminology

FFD—Focal film distance	TFD—Target film distance
FOD—Focal object distance	TOD—Target object distance
OFD—Object film distance	OFD—Object film distance

Optional Terminology

FRD—Focal receptor distance	SID—Source image receptor distance
FOD—Focal object distance	SOD—Source object distance
ORD—Object receptor distance	OID—Object image receptor distance
	SSD—Source skin distance

A variety of geometric designators are listed. The designators FFD, FOD, OFD were selected for use in this book since they are in most frequent use.

increase in FFD may require a major change in technical factors (Tables 8-1 and 8-2). A change in FFD not only affects radiographic density but can influence radiographic detail (see Recorded Detail).

In practice, it may be necessary to adjust mAs because of distance restrictions imposed by the patient's condition or the use of a grid, or by x-ray equipment limitations. Because less radiation reaches the film as the FFD is increased, mAs must be changed to compensate for changes in distance (Fig. 8-3). The intensity of the x-ray beam varies inversely with the square of the distance, when I = beam intensity and D = focal film distance:

$$\frac{I_1}{I_2} = \frac{D_2^2}{D_1^2}$$

IMPORTANT

Doubling of the distance would result in a reduction of radiographic density by a factor of four, necessitating an increase of four times the mAs required to maintain the given density (see Table 8-2).

If distance is changed with a grid technique, the radiographer must remember that grid focal ranges are predetermined by the manufacturer to coincide with the grid ratio. (See Chapter 5, Table 5-1.)

The Effect of Kilovoltage

The kVp range determines the penetrating ability and quality of the x-ray beam. More higher energy

Table 8-2. Distance (D) Relations

	Field Size: Directly Proportional to D	Area Coverage: Directly Proportional to D²	Density: Inversely Proportional to D²	Beam Intensity: Inversely Proportional to D²	Exposure Value: Directly Proportional to D²
1/2 (D)	2 × 2.5 in	5 sq in	4.0	4 (R)	1/4 (mAs)
(D) Value	4 × 5 in	20 sq in	Unit of density	R (given)	mAs (given)
2 (D)	8 × 10 in	80 sq in	1/4	1/4 (R)	4 (mAs)

Representative distance changes are shown, with D indicating the distance for a normal study. Field sizes change in a linear fashion, whereas area coverage is directly proportional to the distance squared. For example, doubling of the distance produces a twofold linear, fourfold area field coverage. Density and beam intensity vary inversely to the distance squared. See Appendix II for related formulas.

The density and beam intensity changes in this table are accomplished with adjustments in distance only. In practice, when distance is changed, technical factors are adjusted to maintain the desired radiographic density.

The Exposure Value column shows adjustments needed in the mAs values to overcome changes in distance. The exposure changes are directly proportional to distance squared. Variations in Kilovoltage are not shown as part of this table, since kVp is not linear. It is difficult to recommend changes in kVp over the wide range of focal film distances shown.

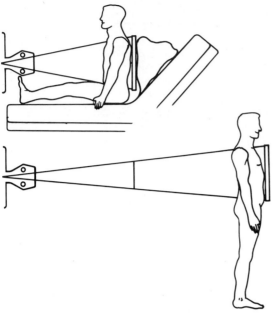

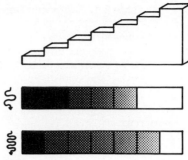

Figure 8-4
Penetrating Ability of Kilovoltage

This representation of an aluminum stepwedge includes two simulated x-ray beams to show the effect of different x-ray wavelengths on penetration. The longer wavelength (low KVP) results in short-scale contrast, which produces sharp demarcations between structures. Kilovoltage must be adequate to penetrate the part under study to show radiographic details within the structural borders. The shorter wavelength (high kVp), which is more penetrating, produces multiple density changes from black to white with intermediate shades of gray, demonstrating a wider range of structures (latitude).

Figure 8-3
Effect of Focal Film Distance on Density

*The intensity of the x-ray beam varies inversely with the square of the distance. If the exposure factors used for a bedside chest study (*top*) at 36-inch FFD resulted in a proper radiographic density, a fourfold increase in exposure factors would be required to duplicate this image at a 72-inch FFD (*bottom*). See Table 8-2 for representative distances.*

photons will penetrate the part under study; therefore, a greater effect is evident on the radiographic image. Increased kVp results in the production of radiation with a shorter wavelength, increased penetration, and greater Compton effect (scatter). When a longer x-ray wavelength achieved with a lower kVp technique is used, more of the low-energy photons are absorbed by the body (Fig. 8-4).

IMPORTANT

Kilovoltage must be sufficient to penetrate the object. No reasonable amount of mAs can compensate for inadequate kVp.

However, the relation of kVp to radiographic density is not linear. The amount of kilovoltage needed to double or halve the density on a radiograph varies according to the kilovoltage level

used. At lower kVp levels, an increase of less than 10 kVp is sufficient to double the density on a radiograph. At higher kVp levels, much more kilovoltage is needed for a doubling effect, if all other factors remain constant. A 15% change in kVp is required to double or halve density. Compare this change with the linear relation associated with the adjustment of mAs to control density (Fig. 8-5).

The scatter generated by an increase in kVp is also reflected in the density on the radiograph, since scatter radiation produces a supplemental density. It is difficult to measure the effect of scatter in each given situation.

The Effect of Tissue Thickness

The density (mass per unit volume) of the patient or of the part under study can affect radiographic density. Thicker body parts absorb more radiation. This factor is generally thought of in terms of differential absorption, which is related to radiographic contrast, since kVp is often used to compensate for thicker body parts (Fig. 8-6).

The use of compression devices will reduce overall tissue thickness by displacing tissues bilaterally, thereby influencing radiographic density.

EXPOSURE CONTROL & SENSITOMETRY

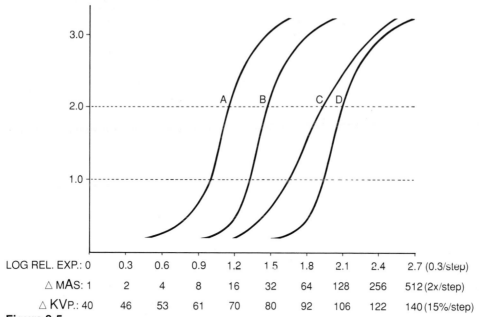

LOG REL. EXP.: 0	0.3	0.6	0.9	1.2	1.5	1.8	2.1	2.4	2.7 (0.3/step)
△ MAS: 1	2	4	8	16	32	64	128	256	512 (2x/step)
△ KVP.: 40	46	53	61	70	80	92	106	122	140 (15%/step)

Figure 8-5
Relationship of Exposure Factors to Radiographic Density

Typical sensitometric curves are labeled A, B, C, and D. Relative exposure values are used to logarithmically indicate the doubling of radiographic exposure values (twofold increase in exposure per 0.3 step). Logarithms are necessary to confine this scale to a reasonable size.

The doubling of density by a change in mAs is conceptually easier to grasp than a logarithmic change, since mAs changes are linear. Kilovoltage is not linear and requires an approximate 15% change to double radiographic density. The doubling or halving of mAs or a 15% incremental change in kVp produces approximately the same effect on radiographic density. These changes are usually expressed as logarithmic increments.

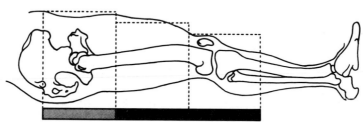

Figure 8-6
Effect of Differential Absorption on Density

Thicker body parts absorb more x-radiation. A body part can vary in thickness as well as mass density. In this illustration of the acetabulum and lower leg, the hip requires more x-radiation than the knee. However, if an adequate exposure were used to image the hip, the femur would be approximately two times overxposed and the knee approximataely four times overexposed. Conversely, proper exposure for the knee would result in an underexposed hip radiograph. Individual exposures of each region should be made for adequate density and contrast. If the entire leg must be visualized for orthopedic measurement, the use of a compensatory filter near source can overcome the gradation differences in tissue density from the hip to the midportion of the lower leg. (See Chapter 3, Fig. 3-12.)

The Effect of Scatter Radiation

Scatter radiation, although detrimental to image detail because it can mask useful information, also adds to radiographic density. Controlling scatter radiation, if all other factors remain the same, reduces radiographic density. Control of scatter radiation is discussed in Chapter 5.

Grids reduce the overall density on a radiograph by preventing scatter from reaching the film and by absorbing some primary as well as most secondary radiation. To maintain a given density, the use of a grid requires an appropriate increase in exposure factors, usually kVp.

Beam restriction by the use of cones, collimators, or diaphragms limits the production of scatter radiation, thus improving radiographic contrast (shorter scale). Overall density is reduced by restricting the supplemental density created by scatter. As compensation, technical factors are adjusted to maintain a given density. Technical factor selection is discussed in Chapter 9.

When the added density created by scatter is reduced by tight beam collimation, for example, an AED will adjust for the change in density by lengthening the exposure time until the predetermined density has been reached. It follows that the degree of collimation affects radiographic density. Undercutting of the image by scatter can cause the AED to prematurely shorten the length of the exposure, resulting in an underexposed radiograph. (AED information can be found in Chapter 2.)

The Heel Effect

The position of the x-ray tube can have an effect on radiographic density. This variation in intensity is known as the *heel effect*. The heel effect is less noticeable when an increased FFD or a small field size is used, because the x-ray beam is more uniform nearest the central ray. Additional information on the heel effect can be found in Chapter 3.

The Effect of Filtration

Any material that attenuates the x-ray beam will reduce density on the radiograph. Depending on the type of filtration, its method of use, and its purpose, this effect may or may not be obvious. Low-energy wavelengths that are filtered out by inherent and added tube filtration do not appreciably affect density. Wedge, trough, and other compensating filters, however, are often used to affect density changes on a given portion of the radiograph. Absorptive tabletops or cassette fronts have a filtration effect on the x-ray beam and can decrease radiographic density.

The Effect of Intensifying Screens

Intensifying screens are designed to increase the efficiency of the x-ray beam and are frequently used to influence radiographic density. High-speed, rare-earth screen film combinations are frequently used to compensate for low-output x-ray equipment. The reduction in the amount of exposure needed to produce an image results in the added benefit of a reduction in dosage to patient and operator.

The Effect of Radiographic Processing

Processing conditions greatly affect radiographic quality. Changes in development time, developer temperature, transport time (in automatic processing), and the degree of concentration or exhaustion of developer can affect radiographic density. Chemical fog due to overdevelopment or chemical imbalance may produce a supplemental density on the radiograph. Cold or weak solutions can result in films that are underdeveloped and lack adequate density. Film storage conditions can also affect radiographic density. Additional information on radiographic processing can be found in Chapter 7.

Radiographic Contrast

Radiographic contrast is an important image quality that takes into consideration subject contrast and film contrast and is defined as the differences between two or more adjacent densities on a radiograph (Fig. 8-7). The radiographer is able to control several factors to affect radiographic contrast (Table 8-3).

Radiographic contrast can be better understood if only the density differences between black and white (short-scale contrast) are considered. Using a sensitometer to evaluate a clear processed film, the reading would begin at D-Min. (See Sensitometry in Chapter 6.) A totally blackened radio-

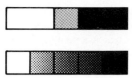

Figure 8-7
Radiographic Contrast
The difference between two or more adjacent densities on a radiograph is defined as radiographic contrast. *Short-scale contrast (top) is usually associated with low kVp, high mAs values. Long-scale contrast (bottom) is associated with high kVp, low mAs techniques. A higher kVp range that produces long-scale contrast can be of advantage when the object being examined contains many subtle densities. In the chest long-scale contrast is preferred; the heart must be penetrated for mediastinal details and the lungs not overexposed. When a low kVp is used for chest radiography, the ribs will appear chalklike, the lungs blackened, and the mediastinal structures underpenetrated.*

graph would be read at D-Max. If the conditions that produced these two radiographs could be reproduced so that the two densities were adjacent to each other on the same radiograph, short-scale contrast (abrupt difference in densities) would be evident (see Fig. 8-7).

As a greater number of density changes are produced, the contrast scale increases. The longer the scale of contrast, the wider the range of structures that can be imaged. This widened range of density differences is referred to as *latitude* (see Figs. 8-4 and 8-7).

Subject Contrast

The ratio of the x-ray intensity transmitted through one segment of the part in a study to that

transmitted through a more absorbing adjacent segment is known as *subject contrast*. The density and atomic number of the part affect subject contrast, as does radiation quality. Kilovoltage settings, total filtration, and the tube target material all influence beam quality. Tungsten and molybdenum tube target material comparisons are described in Chapter 11.

A major influence on subject contrast is the effect of scatter radiation, which can be controlled by collimation or grid and compression techniques. Subject contrast is also affected by the use of contrast media to outline organs or vessels. Specific information about the selection of technical factors for use with radiopaque or radiolucent contrast media can be found in Chapter 9.

Equal thickness of dissimilar materials, that is, materials having different atomic numbers, will radiographically demonstrate subject contrast (see Fig. 8-1). If a single radiograph were taken of two identical objects of equal thickness and material content, no density difference would be evident. If the two objects show no density differences, contrast is not present. One could also choose objects of dissimilar materials of unequal thickness to demonstrate the absence of radiographic contrast as long as the densities are the same.

Film Contrast

Film contrast refers to the contrast inherent in the radiographic film. A radiographer cannot control film contrast, since it is a design parameter. Radiographic film is manufactured to exhibit high (short-scale) or low (long-scale) contrast (Fig. 8-8).

Processing conditions, fog level, and other sources of radiation can affect film contrast.

Table 8-3. Radiographic Contrast (Short-Scale)

Controllable Factors*	Recommendations
Kilovoltage	Sufficient to penetrate the part under study
Scatter control	
Collimation	Restrict field size to cassette size or smaller
Grid or Bucky	Match grid ratio to highest kVp to be used; use recommended grid focal range
Extrafocal radiation	Restrict the x-ray beam as close to source as possible
Compression	Use to flatten tissue to reduce scatter; helpful in mammography; may be contraindicated in some examinations

*Some factors that are controlled by departmental preferences or quality assurance practices include selection of filtration material, film screen products, processor temperatures, and the use of contrast media.

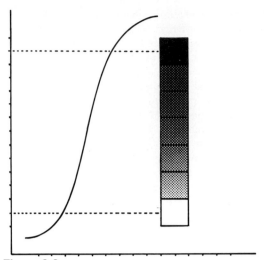

Figure 8-8
Sensitometric Representation
of Radiographic Contrast

A typical sensitometric curve is shown, with dashed lines *representing the useful density range for medical radiography. The lower* dashed line, *just above the toe of the sensitometric curve, is represented by the whitest portion of the stepwedge. The upper* dashed line, *crossing through the highest-density portion of the stepwedge, is represented as black. As the curve ascends from the toe to the shoulder, there is an increase in density. The differences between the seven density steps in this illustration denote radiographic contrast. For additional sensitometric information see Chapter 6.*

Control of Radiographic Contrast by kVp

Kilovoltage is used to control both radiographic contrast and penetration of the part. Kilovoltage determines whether the radiation will be of sufficient strength to penetrate the object and whether the radiation consists of long wavelengths, some of which would be absorbed by the object. In the diagnostic kilovoltage range, two x-ray interactions with matter are significant photoelectric effect (absorption) and Compton effect (scatter). (X-ray interaction with matter is discussed in Chapter 1.)

Scatter radiation does not affect the entire image in a uniform manner. It is detrimental to radiographic contrast, since it affects the whiter areas on the radiograph to a greater degree than the blacker areas. Segments of the image that have reached D-Max cannot get blacker.

As kilovoltage is increased, the number of photons of all energies up to the peak kilovoltage is increased, adding additional high-energy photons to the x-ray beam. Above 80 kVp, the primary interaction is Compton effect, which reduces short-scale contrast.

The Effect of Scatter Radiation

The purpose of a grid or Bucky is to prevent most scatter radiation from reaching the x-ray film.

Beam restriction limits the area of tissue interaction with the primary beam. The smaller the field size, the less scatter radiation generated, and the result is shorter scale contrast (Fig. 8-9).

Compression reduces the amount of tissue available for interaction with x-radiation, thereby reducing the amount of scatter radiation generated. The reduction in scatter radiation improves radiographic contrast. (See Chapter 4, Radiographic Accessories, Compression Bands, for contraindications to compression.)

The Effect of Beam Filtration

Filtration attenuates the low-energy photons in the beam by the photoelectric process. Small increases in aluminum filtration do not appreciably affect contrast, because low-energy photons are not contributing to the image, having already been absorbed by the patient. If the amount of added filtration is sufficient to reduce density on the radiograph, shorter scale contrast results.

The Effect of Intensifying Screens

Radiographic contrast is affected by the use of intensifying screens. The fluorescent effect of the screens on the film results in shorter scale contrast compared with images made by the direct action of x-radiation alone. When sensitometric test radiographs are made and evaluated, the slope of the characteristic curve will change more abruptly on screen film images, indicating a shorter scale of contrast.

The Effect of Radiographic Processing

Processing solutions can affect radiographic contrast. Solutions that are too hot can produce

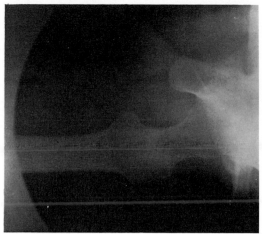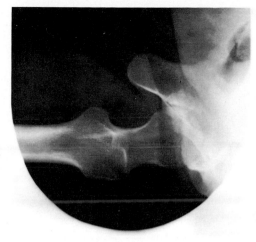

Figure 8-9
Contrast Improvement with Scatter Control

Scatter diminishes radiographic contrast. An attempt was made to demonstrate the relation of the head of the femur to the acetabulum. The nongrid, full-field image (left) demonstrates the effect of scatter on both contrast and detail; the relation of the head of the femur to the acetabulum is barely visible.

A reduction in field size will limit the amount of tissue that can interact with the x-ray beam to produce scatter. The tightly coned grid image (right) exhibits excellent radiographic contrast and recorded detail.

chemical fog. If development time is too long owing to extended immersion in the solutions because of increased transport time in an automatic processor or increased development time in manual processing, the lower-density regions of the radiograph will be affected by the developer chemicals, and shortscale contrast will be decreased. Proper time/temperature processing is required to maintain contrast and density.

Recorded Detail

Recorded detail is a visual quality. Radiographic *sharpness* or *detail* is used to describe the impression of the boundaries or edges of structures on a radiograph. The sharpness of the structural edges of the radiographic image or its definition is usually referred to as detail. Detail in a radiograph can be affected by geometric limitations and by those controllable factors that make the details visible to the observer (Table 8-4).

Four basic categories of image blur may be present on a radiograph and may contribute to a loss of detail

1. Image geometry
2. The effect of the shape of the structure on beam absorption
3. Characteristics of the intensifying screen
4. Motion artifacts

Geometric Blur

The boundary of a structural edge of an image can appear blurred owing to lateral spreading of the image, whether by motion, geometry, or inherent receptor blur. Geometric blur is defined in terms of the umbra (distinct shadow) evident on an image, and it can be affected by several factors.

Table 8-4. Radiographic Detail (Geometric)

Controllable Factors	Recommendations
Focal spot size	As small as possible
Position of object	Perpendicular to central ray to minimize distortion
Focal object distance	As great as possible within grid focal range
Object film distance	As short as possible to minimize enlargement
Plane of the object	Parallel to receptor

Note: Since the x-ray beam widens as it travels from the actual focal spot to the image receptor, there is often unequal distortion of portions of the anatomy. Some degree of magnification occurs with all studies.

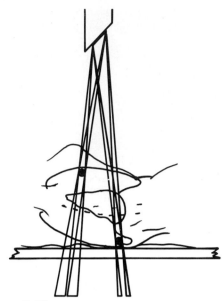

Figure 8-10
Effect of Focal Spot Size on Image Sharpness

Ideally, radiation should originate from a point source for optimal sharpness (recorded detail). Since x-radiation arises from a focal area on the target that is greater than a point source, structural edges may appear unsharp. The widened divergent beam passing over the edges of the structure produces a penumbral effect immediately adjacent to the sharp umbral shadow. The degree of image blur is dependent on the size of the focal spot and the distance that the object is placed from the recording media. As the object is brought closer to the detector, or as the FFD is increased, recorded detail improves. The optimal image is generated by an increased FFD, minimal OFD, and a microfocal spot.

Focal film distance (see Fig. 8-3). FFD is usually standardized, with 40 inches used for most radiographic imaging and 72 inches used for chest or lateral cervical spine imaging.

Focal spot size. Ideally, radiation should originate from a point source; however, x-radiation usually arises from an area on the target called the actual focal spot (Fig. 8-10) and travels in straight lines in a divergent beam. The use of a small focal spot helps to reduce image blur.

Object film distance. The degree of blur is dependent on the distance the beam travels from the source to the object and the location of the object in relation to the detector (Figs. 8-11 and 8-12). Even when the OFD is minimal, nothing can be done to overcome the tabletop/Bucky tray (TT/BT) distance. Many radiographic tables have a TT/BT relation of 6 cm to 13 cm. The part under study, although in intimate

contact with the radiographic table, can be as great as 13 cm from the image detector. For example, when a patient measuring 30 cm thick is placed in the lateral position for a lumbar spine study, the center of the vertebral column is 15 cm from the tabletop, with a 28-cm OFD. Unless a small focal spot of 0.6 mm, or smaller, is used, image blur will increase (see Fig. 8-11). An increase from a 40-inch FFD to a 50-inch FFD reduces image enlargement and decreases image blur. When the patient is examined in the anteroposterior supine position for the orbits, which can be 20 or more cm from the tabletop, there is at least a 30-cm OFD. The part under study can be magnified as much as 50% (see Fig. 8-12). Although a radiographer would not consider making a radiograph of a hand placed 30 cm from a cassette with a large focal spot, a similar effect occurs when the orbits or lumbar spine is evaluated using a 13-cm TT/BT distance. When using a fluoroscopic spot tunnel, the size or position of a patient determines the FFD (Fig. 8-13). Because of the shortened TOD

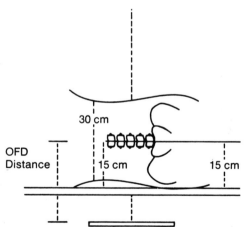

Figure 8-11
Tabletop/Bucky Tray (TT/BT) Relation

Every effort should be made to position the object under study as close to the image receptor as possible for optimal recorded detail. In this illustration, the patient is placed in the lateral position for an examination of the lumbar vertebrae. The patient measures 30 cm through the thickest portion of the abdomen, with the lumbar vertebrae 15 cm from the tabletop. An additional increase in OFD is caused by the TT/BT distance, which can vary from 6 to 13 cm. The vertebrae in this illustration are 28 cm from the cassette. A small focal spot (0.6 mm or smaller) is essential to maintain image sharpness. (Reprinted courtesy of Eastman Kodak Company)

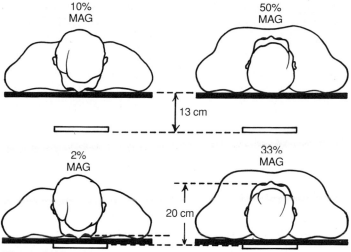

Figure 8-12
Table Bucky Versus Grid Cassette Placement

A patient is positioned prone and supine for orbital evaluation. In the prone position, the orbits are almost in contact with the tabletop. In the supine position, the orbits are approximately 20 cm from the tabletop. (Top) The tabletop/Bucky tray distance increases the OFD. A 40-inch FFD, in the supine position, will create an approximate 50% enlargement of the orbits (right) and an approximate 10% enlargement in the prone position (left) owing to the increased TT/BT distance. (Bottom) If the patient were then examined in the prone and supine positions using a grid cassette, the increased OFD generated by the TT/BT spacing would no longer exist. In the prone position (left) the part is positioned directly on the grid cassette, minimizing the OFD with only a 2% increase in enlargement. In the supine position (right) the magnification is 33%.

of approximately 20 inches, image blur can occur.

The relative plane of the object. Blurring will be influenced by the alignment of the object to the central ray and image receptor and the divergent effect of the x-ray beam (Figs. 8-14 and 8-15). Even with the proper alignment of the central ray, cassette, and body part, an additional view made at right angles is needed to demonstrate any deviation in the position of

Figure 8-13
Fluoroscopic Spot Film Tunnel Geometry

The size or position of the patient, or both, determines the FFD used for fluoroscopic spot films. The relationship of the part to the detector influences image sharpness. (Right) In the left lateral position, anatomic structures on the left side of the patient will be greatly magnified. The structures on the right side of the patient should be somewhat sharper because of the reduced OFD and increased FFD. (Left) When a small focal spot (0.6 mm or smaller) is used with a fluoroscopic spot film tunnel, image blur is reduced. The image blur associated with the shortened FOD (approximately 20 in) is minimized.

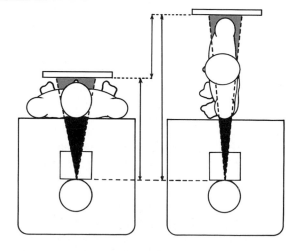

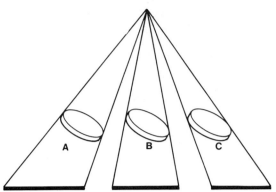

Figure 8-14
Tube Angulation/Part Relationship

A flat disc at an increased OFD is tilted at an angle and radiographed with an angulated beam (A), a beam that is perpendicular to the detector (B), and a reverse angle beam (C). Note the changing shape of the disc, from elongation (A) to foreshortening (C), depending on the position of the x-ray tube.

fracture fragments (Fig. 8-15, *right*) or the anterior or posterior location of a lesion.

An object in the path of the beam may not be imaged as a distinct shadow because of the widened divergent beam passing over the edges of the structure. The recorded image may possess a region of blur described as *penumbra,* immediately adjacent to the umbral shadow.

Blur Resulting from the Heel Effect

In addition to the potential image blur caused by the size of the focal spot and the position of the body part, one must also consider the variation in sharpness along the projected x-ray field. The projected focal spot increases in size from anode to cathode along the axis of the x-ray tube. (See the Heel Effect, Chapter 3.)

Blur Resulting from Extrafocal Radiation

Extrafocal radiation increases image blur. Structures outside the collimated shutter pattern are often seen as indistinct shadows. The extraneous de-

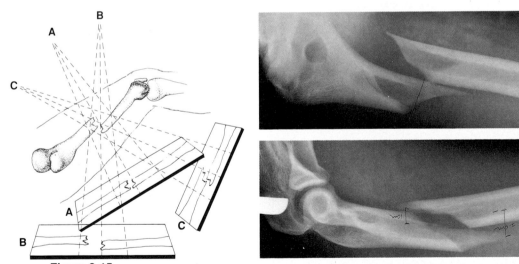

Figure 8-15
Distortion Associated with Tube, Receptor, and Object Alignment

(Left) The x-ray tube and receptor in position A are in proper alignment with the central ray perpendicular to the film. A slight separation of the fragments of the femur is demonstrated. The tube-receptor relation in position B gives the illusion that the fragments are further separated. The tube-receptor angulation technique in position C gives the impression of overlapping fragments. (Right) A fracture of the lower end of the humerus is viewed in both anteroposterior and lateral positions. In the lateral view (bottom) the fragments seem to be in good apposition. In the anteroposterior view (top) there is signifcant displacement of the fragments. Images made at right angles to each other are essential to determine fracture alignment. (Radiographs courtesy Cullinan AM: Optimizing Radiographic Positioning. *Philadelphia: JB Lippincott, 1992)*

tails, while esthetically unattractive, do not affect diagnosis. Unfortunately, a portion of the primary x-ray beam consists of extrafocal radiation and adds to image blur. Extrafocal radiation can be controlled by the placing of the primary shutters of the collimator or an aperture diaphragm as close to source as possible. (See Extrafocal Radiation, Chapter 5.)

Absorption Blur

Absorption blur describes the effect produced when a three-dimensional object is recorded in a two-dimensional plane. The blur seen in the recorded image is caused by variation in the absorption of the beam throughout the structural edges and the location of the object in the path of the beam.

The combination of the penumbral effect and the absorption effect results in the radiographic demonstration of indistinct borders in many internal body structures (Fig. 8-16).

Intensifying Screen Blur

Any unwanted variation in optical density (mottle) on a screen film study can be categorized as radiographic noise and may consist of receptor graininess, structure mottle, or quantum mottle. Although screen or film graininess is rarely seen, quantum mottle can affect image resolution.

Photographic scientists have developed complex objective testing procedures to evaluate resolution. Resolution is measured as line pairs per millimeter (lp/mm), line spread function (LSF), and modulation transfer function (MTF). MTF can be used to measure image detail (resolution) of a radiograph made of a metallic test pattern. With this method, an attempt is made to reproduce the sharp edges of the test pattern with no loss in contrast. This technique helps physicists to determine the limitations of the imaging system.

Performance and evaluation of tests such as MTF and LSF, which measures the ability of a film screen system to accurately measure the bounda-

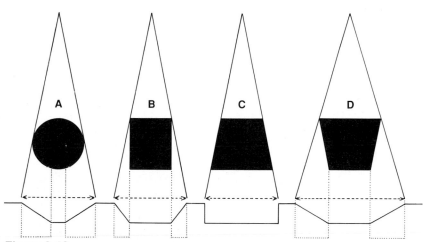

Figure 8-16
Variations in Absorption of Structural Edges
Three different-shaped objects are shown: a sphere (A), a rectangular object (B), and a wedge-shaped structure, approximating the pattern or shape of the divergent x-ray beam (C). All objects are positioned with an increased OFD. Note that objects A, B, and C produce approximately the same size x-ray shadow.

Object A absorbs more x-ray in the center and less x-ray bilaterally to produce an image with unsharp, overexposed edges. B is enlarged, and again the lateral aspects of the beam strike the upper edges of the object resulting in a penumbral effect. Object C, which conforms to the beam shape, appears as the sharpest image in the series, because absorption is equal throughout the entire structure and artificial boundaries or edges are not created by structures proximal to the x-ray source. When C is inverted to make D, image blur is further increased. If object C is used to represent a segment of the anatomy of a patient in the supine position, object D illustrates the increased image blur associated with the same structure in the prone position.

ries of an image, should not be attempted without appropriate training. These tests require specific test tools and must be carried out according to manufacturers' recommendations. Measurement of resolution and perception of sharpness are subjective. A detailed explanation of MTF and LSF is not the intent of this book.

The degree of image blur resulting from the use of intensifying screens is dependent on the following:

Type of phosphor used in the manufacture of the screen

Size and layer thickness of the phosphor

Use of a reflective or absorptive undercoat layer

Use of light restricting dye (if any)

Degree of film screen contact present in the system

Tube angulation techniques, which can result in increased image blur caused by the parallax effect (Fig. 8-17)

The properties of intensifying screens are discussed in Chapter 6.

Motion Blur

Voluntary or involuntary motion will diminish recorded detail. Immobilization of the part and short exposure times can help to minimize this problem.

Motion blur can also occur at the source of the radiation as a result of vibration in the x-ray tube or crane. Defective Bucky lock assemblies can permit motion of the cassette in the Bucky tray, or rotating anodes with damaged bearing assemblies can vibrate; either movement produces blur on the recorded image.

Motion can be deliberately used to advantage in tomography to blur out structures, as described in Chapter 11. Shallow breathing techniques using a low mA setting and long exposure times can be used to blur out the pulmonary markings and ribs for studies of the thoracic spine and sternum.

Visibility of Detail

Recorded detail and contrast are dependent on each other. Visibility of detail is greatly influenced by radiographic contrast. A quality radiograph must possess sufficient contrast to render the structural details visible. Reduction in contrast

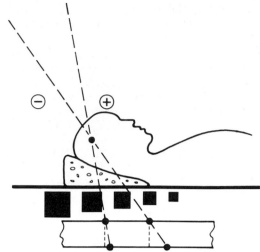

Figure 8-17
Tube Angle Technique Concerns
One concern with tube angulation is the potential for image blur due to the parallax effect. A black dot in the skull in this illustration represents an area of pathologic interest. A shallow tube angle of 10 degrees is shown with the dot projected onto a dual emulsion film. Note the separation of the image from the front to the back emulsions. When a tube is angled 10 degrees or less, the unsharpness attributed to the parallax effect is less than the intrinsic unsharpness of the film screen combination. When the tube angle is increased beyond 10 degrees, image blur increases. At 25 degrees, there is a greater separation on the image (represented by the black dots). If a small focal spot (0.6 mm or smaller) is available, the skull can be elevated on a 15-degree sponge, as shown in this illustration. The 25-degree tube angle can then be lessened to 10 degrees, minimizing the parallax effect. Whenever possible, a perpendicular beam should be used to minimize the parallax effect.

In this illustration, differences in focal spot size related to the line focus effect are shown from cathode to anode. At the anode end of the x-ray tube, the focal spot is smaller than the effective focal spot as measured at the central ray; at the cathode side, the focal spot is larger. There is also a variation in intensity across the long axis of the x-ray tube; therefore, film blackening will not be uniform.

can result from scatter radiation or underpenetration of the object.

Chemical fog generated by processing difficulties and other types of fogging of the image can also reduce the visibility of recorded detail.

Distortion

Distortion is the radiographic difference (misrepresentation) in size or shape compared with the actual object. Radiographic images are larger than the objects being evaluated owing to the divergence of the x-ray beam. Image distortion must be considered when evaluating image detail (Figs. 8-15 to 8-20). Distortion may be categorized into two major types size and shape.

Equal or overall enlargement of the image is known as magnification. With magnification, the shape of the object is accurately reproduced, but the recorded details of the image are enlarged (see Fig. 8-18).

Any angulation of the x-ray beam, the recording plane, or the object in the path of the beam will result in distortion (true distortion) on the recorded image. Depending on the position of the x-ray tube and the patient, the image will demonstrate either elongation or foreshortening (see Figs. 8-15, 8-18, and 8-19).

Distortion can sometimes be used to advantage (see Fig. 8-20). It is sometimes necessary to deliberately distort anatomy when an air–fluid level interface requires a horizontal beam technique to be seen. (See Chapter 4, Figures 4-10 and 4-11.) Distortion can also be used to project superimposed anatomy away from the area of interest.

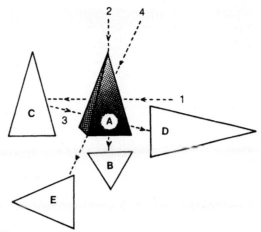

Figure 8-19
Shape Distortion
A three-dimensional pyramid (A) illustrates shape distortion. A central ray (1) is positioned perpendicular to the apex of the pyramid for the projection represented by a two-dimensional triangle (C). When an image is made from position 2 the base of the pyramid is shown without shape distortion (B). An angled projection (3) creates an elongated image (D). An image obtained with the central ray at position 4 will be foreshortened (E). A clinical example of this shape distortion can be seen in Figure 8-20.

The Effect of Distance

The distance of the object to the film plane affects the size of the object. The closer the object is placed to the film, the less magnification is evident on the image (Fig. 8-21). If the object is moved farther away from the recording plane, magnification increases (see Fig. 8-12).

The relation of focal film distance to object film distance also determines image size (see Figs. 8-11 and 8-12). If an object cannot be placed in close proximity to the recording plane, size distortion (magnification) can be reduced by increasing the FFD.

The Effect of Focal Spot Size

The closer the focal spot size approaches a point source, the less penumbral effect and the greater the detail on the magnified image. The degree of penumbra on the image can be determined mathematically using the formula

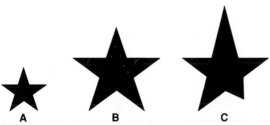

A   B   C
Figure 8-18
Magnification-Distortion Relation
Distortion is the radiographic misrepresentation in size or shape in a radiographic image when compared with the object under study. Star A is a normal-size radiographic image. If the object under study is magnified (B), equal (overall) enlargement occurs, that is, an increase n the size of the object without a change in the shape of any of its parts. When portions or all of the structure under study are distorted (elongated or foreshortened), shape distortion occurs (C). This effect can be due to the angulation of the part, detector, or x-ray tube. Star C exhibits two forms of distortion, an elongated as well as a foreshortened point.

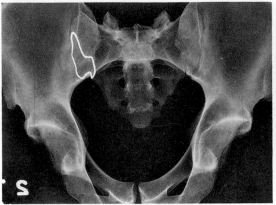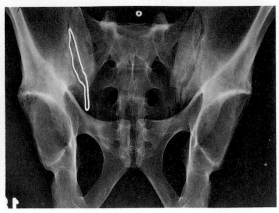

Figure 8-20
Clinical Application of Distortion

On occasion, distortion can be used to clinical advantage. A soft wire was shaped to conform to the sacroiliac joint on the right side of a pelvic specimen. (Left) A conventional anteroposterior projection of the pelvis does not clearly show the relation of the sacroiliac joints to the pelvis. (Right) The x-ray tube was then angled 35 degrees cephalad, elongating the pelvis. Note the elongation of the metallic wire and the sacroiliac joints, which are now well visualized. (Reprinted courtesy Eastman Kodak Company)

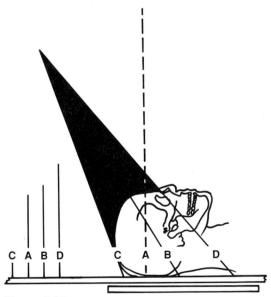

Figure 8-21
Disproportionate Anatomic Enlargement

Segments of anatomy are enlarged depending on their position within the structure being examined. Tube angulation further distorts anatomic segments. Note that the entrance point of the beam at A, B, and D is approximately the same, but different degrees of distortion occur in the image. The posterior portion of the skull (C) is less affected by tube angulation. To reduce image blur, it is sometimes necessary to use an alternative position. (See Fig. 8-12.)

$$\text{Penumbra (P)} = \frac{\text{effective FS} \times \text{OFD}}{\text{FOD}}$$

See Appendix II for additional information.

Total Unsharpness

Unsharpness in all forms detracts from the resolution of the image.

A recording medium should be able to produce well-defined structural outlines. To evaluate total resolution, the product of the components that enter into the resolution of the imaging system must be considered. Some factors that may affect resolution include focal spot size, geometric enlargement and distortion, motion, parallax, and screen film blur (Fig. 8-22).

A more useful approach would be concern for individual components of the imaging chain as a way to avoid compromising image quality. To illustrate, if a radiographer carefully selected the proper technical factors to obtain an optically sharp image; used a high-detail screen film system; carefully positioned the part with concern for OFD, FFD, and central ray alignment; collimated appropriately; and used the proper ratio grid in an attempt to improve radiographic contrast but did not use a small focal spot, the result could be a

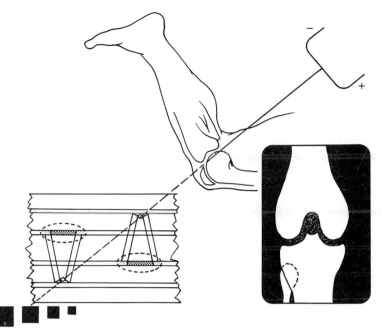

Figure 8-22
Total Unsharpness

Many factors contribute to image blur. This illustration is of a tunnel projection of the knee. The increased angle required for this projection causes the images on both emulsions of the film to separate, owing to the parallax effect (bottom, left). *If a non-crossover control screen film combination is used, approximately one third of the density on the radiograph is the result of crossover of light from opposing intensifying screens, further increasing image blur. The unsharpness associated with the cathode side of the x-ray tube, owing to the line focus effect* (bottom left) *further adds to this problem. Other factors, such as extrafocal radiation, can also contribute to image blur.*

The rectangular collimated x-ray field permits the unattenuated primary beam to strike the tabletop, producing scatter radiation (bottom, right). *The soft tissues of the knee are "undercut"; soft tissue structures may be overexposed.*

poor-quality radiograph. The weak link in this example is the focal spot size, which diminished the total MTF of the system.

Nevertheless, a compromise is often necessary, since image quality and a diagnostic image are not necessarily synonymous. Although a radiograph may seem to possess excellent image quality, it may not be diagnostic. For example, the abrupt black and white of a short-scale contrast image of the lung fields may mask subtle pulmonary vascular details. A short-scale contrast image of an extremity may fail to demonstrate a subtle soft tissue change.

Conversely, a radiograph that is not of optimal radiographic quality may be adequate for diagnostic purposes. For example, a child suspected of ingesting a coin should have his or her entire alimentary tract evaluated. If the first image is made of the abdomen and the coin is not found, cervical and chest radiographs are needed. The coin, if lodged in the esophagus, could migrate to the abdomen while the abdominal radiograph is being processed. If chest and cervical studies are made, a negative study could also result. A large-format (14 × 17 inch) study using high kVp and low mAs helps to avoid this problem while minimizing exposure to the child. An infant can often be placed diagonally on the cassette to image the entire alimentary tract from the nasal cavity to the rectum. If 85 kVp or greater were used without a grid for this study, the overall appearance of the radiograph would be photographically unattractive but diagnostically adequate. Although the technique used for this single exposure is not one that would be recommended for any specific area, the anatomic details would still be visible in relation to the high-contrast metallic foreign body.

As with all technical factor selection, the radiographer must do more than simply select kVp, mA, time, and distance. Radiographic quality can also be affected by the selection of radiographic accessories and processing techniques.

Technical Factor Selection

Selecting technical factors to produce an optimal radiograph can be a complex process. In 1940 Harold G. Petsing wrote, "One of the problems coincident with the art of radiography has been the search for satisfactory and practical methods of selecting and recording desirable techniques for different anatomic regions."* This statement is still appropriate more than a half century later.

Technique charts offer baseline values for specific examinations. An experienced radiographer can predict an expected outcome in a clinical situation and, with a solid knowledge of the principles of exposure, can modify technical factors to arrive at acceptable compromises.

The technical suggestions made in this chapter are based on the presumption that x-ray units are calibrated regularly and that automatic processors are maintained according to manufacturers' recommendations. A fourfold variation in exposure range can be due to processor conditions. Processing conditions of this magnitude can even negate the latitude inherent in some film products.

Technical factor selection should be considered only after adequate calibration of the equipment has been ensured. Minor differences in generator output, grid ratio, screen film selection, and processing criteria can have a cumulative effect on the final image. Although these variations affect radiographic quality, variations in technique by the radiographer occur more frequently.

Many radiographers and radiologists will critique a radiograph and suggest a minor change to improve a study. When this occurs, every effort should be made to use the same room in which the initial study was performed. A minor change in a repeat radiograph may have little or no effect, or an exaggerated effect if the image is made in a different radiographic unit.

A technique chart is not intended to be used interchangeably from x-ray room to x-ray room. Even with identical

---

Petsing HG: Evolution of the technique chart. X-Ray Technician (Radiol Technol) 11(4):125–131, 1940.

Angeline M. Cullinan and John E. Cullinan:
PRODUCING QUALITY RADIOGRAPHS, 2ND ED.
© 1987, 1994 J. B. Lippincott Company.

Table 9-1. Grid Ratio and Technique Comparisons

Grid Ratio	Fixed kVp, Variable mAs	Variable kVp, Fixed mAs
6:1 grid cassette	75 kVp	30 mAs
8:1 upright Bucky	80 kVp*	40 mAs*
12:1 table Bucky	85 kVp	>50 mAs

*With the patient in an erect or decubitus position, an additional increase in kVp or mAs may be needed to compensate for the increase in tissue thickness caused by the dependent portion of the abdomen.

Note: The above examples are presented to demonstrate the variation in x-ray technique that may be necessary when grids of different ratios are found in the same x-ray room.

equipment, a variation in calibration may affect techniques. If the x-ray table, upright cassette holder, and grid cassettes in the same room have grids of a different ratio, separate technique charts will be required (Table 9-1). Every radiographic machine, including mobile units, should have a technique chart.

IMPORTANT

Tube rating charts should be prominently displayed in radiographic rooms. Focal spot size, generator type, and grid ratio should also be posted on or near the x-ray control panel.

When making changes in technique, the radiographer is often influenced by who will interpret the radiograph. Radiographers sometimes believe that a specific radiologist has a preference for a particular technique. These assumptions often arise when a radiologist requests a repeat examination for a specific reason. For example, if a radiograph is exposed at a lower kilovoltage value, a dense osseous structure may not be adequately penetrated and underlying pathology may still be in question. A modification in mAs might be requested with a 10- to 15-kVp increase to image this suspicious area. If this type of request is made with some regularity, a radiographer might assume that the radiologist prefers higher-kilovoltage techniques for all examinations. A professional discussion between the radiographer and the radiologist can help to clarify why a technical adjustment must be made. Radiographers should not feel that a request for a repeat film is a criticism of their work or of the validity of the departmental technique charts.

Although the type of technique used is often based on the preference of the interpreter, the quality of the image is under the control of the radiographer.

Errors in technical judgment or in equipment calibration can negate the effect of a technique chart. Although a major technical error is usually easily recognized, several small technical errors can collectively result in an unacceptable image (Table 9-2).

Technique Charts

Technique charts are guides to the exposure factors needed to produce an image that meets the given standards of a radiology department. They are formulated so that predetermined contrast and density ranges can be consistently produced by all radiographers on all radiographic equipment within the department. In a large facility where many radiographers rotate from room to room, technique charts are not only helpful but also essential to maintain image quality. A technique chart that is too complicated and cannot be easily used, or that is proved to be inaccurate, should be replaced.

Radiographers should not rely on a favorite technique for a given body part. The radiographer, who would not consider increasing a patient's medication, in fact increases radiation dosage to a patient if a repeat x-ray examination is required

Table 9-2. Cumulative Effect of Variations from Standard*

Error	Density Increase
Overmeasurement	up 30%
Processor temperature elevation	up 30%
mA setting, 200 mA; actual mA, 220 mA	up 10%
36-in FFD used instead of 40 in FFD	up 20%
Total	up 90%

*The error in measurement produced a 30% increase in density, which is all that is required to produce a perceivable density change on a radiograph.

The shortened FFD produces an additional increase of approximately 20% in film blackening.

The elevation of the processor temperature and the increased mA output results in an additional 40% error.

The cumulative effect of errors in technique will result in an unacceptable radiograph. It may be difficult to identify the problem if more than one error occurs at the same time.

because of an arbitrary selection of technical factors for the original image.

Primary Exposure Factors

The four primary exposure factors used to change the photographic effect of the x-ray image are the following:

1. Milliamperage. Milliamperage determines the quantity of the x-ray to be used for a specific technique and can be described as the amount of current flowing through the x-ray tube. As mA values are increased, an appropriate reduction in time of exposure is possible. Unfortunately, higher mA settings often necessitate the need for a larger focal spot and an increase in the risk of blooming of the focal spot of the x-ray tube, which increases image blur. The mA stations must be constantly monitored for mA linearity (Table 9-3).

2. Exposure time. The length of the exposure and the mA value are the major controlling factors of radiographic density (Table 9-4). In general, shorter exposure times are recommended to lessen the image blur associated with voluntary or involuntary motion. The time of exposure can be controlled manually or with the use of an automatic exposure control. (A detailed explanation of the use of automatic exposure devices can be found in Chapter 2.)

Table 9-3. Variations in Milliampere Output*

	mA Setting			Actual mA	
mA	*sec*	*mAs*	*mA*	*sec*	*mAs*
100	1	100	85	1	85
200	1/2	100	220	1/2	110

*Any combination of milliamperage and time that results in the same milliampere second value should yield a radiograph of similar density. In the examples shown, the 100 mA station was assigned to a small focal spot, whereas the 200 mA station was assigned to the large focal spot. Although both mAs combinations should result in 100 mAs, a variation in mA output results in about a 30% increase in film blackening at the 200 mA station as opposed to the 100 mA station. The milliampere setting of 100 mA yields an output 15% lower than expected, and the 200 mA setting yields an output approximately 10% higher than expected. If it were necessary to change techniques from the 100 (small) to the 200 (large) mA setting, a 25% difference in the expected density would occur.

Table 9-4. Technical Factor Manipulation to Maintain Density

mA	Second	kVp	S/F Speed
100	1/2	70	200
200	1/4	70	200
400	1/8	70	200
400	1/16	82	200 (may require large focal spot)
200	1/16	82	400
100	1/8	82	400
100	1/4	70	400

Note: Any of these technical factors will produce a similar radiographic density. The higher kVp images would exhibit longer-scale contrast; the shorter exposure times would help to stop motion.

IMPORTANT

When a change in mAs is needed to increase radiographic density while maintaining radiographic contrast, there is a tendency to raise the mA value rather than increase the length of exposure. From a practical standpoint, high mA settings with short exposure times are useful to stop motion for specific studies such as angiography, chest radiography, and some pediatric procedures. Most organs or organ systems are relatively static and do not require short exposure times. Image blur due to organ motion can also be minimized by medications such as glucagon, which is frequently used to stop peristaltic motion during double-contrast gastrointestinal studies.

Physiologic gating of the exposure using sophisticated electrocardiac devices can be used with cineangiographic techniques. Focal spot blooming and tube loading are concerns with falling load techniques, even when exposures are as short as possible. With conventional generators, modest mA settings can be used with longer exposure times to avoid blooming of the focal spot. If longer exposure times are a problem, then high-speed screen film combinations should be considered. With high-speed, rare-earth screen film combinations, the short exposure times required with high mA can "capture" the grid in motion, producing grid mottle.

The use of long exposure times at low mA values help to blur out pulmonary vascular markings when evaluating the sternum or the lateral thoracic spine.

Table 9-5. Typical Kilovoltage Range Selection for Various Body Parts

kVp Range				
55	75	90	120	150
Extremities	Abdomen Skull	Thick body parts	Chest Barium studies Pelvimetry	Chest
		Lateral lumbar spine Air contrast studies		

Note: Grouping of body parts according to kilovoltage ranges is an accepted approach to a fixed kilovoltage technique chart. When formulating a technique chart using a rare-earth screen film combination, very low or very high kilovoltage values should be carefully evaluated for possible falloff in screen response.

3. Kilovoltage. Kilovoltage controls radiographic contrast, determines the quality of the x-ray beam, and influences the amount of scatter generated. As kilovoltage is raised, the relative absorption differences between structures is lessened, and it is possible to "see through" dense structures. Specific kilovoltage ranges are recommended for certain body parts (Table 9-5).

High mAs techniques, frequently used with low kVp to produce short-scale contrast, should not be used as a substitute for scatter control. If low kVp is used, portions of the anatomy may not be adequately penetrated. Images produced with high-frequency generators are similar in contrast to those produced with three-phase equipment. If a change in film density is necessary it should not be at the expense of image contrast, particularly in studies using positive contrast media.

4. Distance. Variations in focal film distances are rarely used to change radiographic density. Small changes in FFD can affect large changes in radiographic density. A significant increase in image blur is caused by an increase in OFD, unless a fractional focal spot is used. In general, the OFD usually remains constant with a given body part. However, if an increase in the FFD is needed to minimize the effect of an increased OFD, an increase in exposure is required for adequate film blackening (Table 9-6). The 40- to 48-inch FFD change requires an approximate 45% increase in mAs to duplicate the original density. With three-phase, constant-potential, or high-frequency generators, a twofold increase in film blackening can occur in the same exposure time frame. This makes it possible to use an increased FFD, such as 48 inches, to minimize image blur.

A detailed discussion of the effect of the four primary exposure factors—mA, exposure time, kVp, and distance—can be found in Chapter 8.

Formulating a Technique Chart

A technique chart should contain all pertinent technical data and should be mounted in an easily accessible area. In addition to the primary exposure factors of mA, time, kVp, and distance, it should indicate the following:

1. Tube warm-up procedures as recommended by the manufacturer as well as the focal spot size to be used
2. Changes in exposure factors related to tissue thickness and body type or the use of a contrast medium
3. Projection of central ray, including tube angulation recommendations
4. Appropriate screen film combination (Table 9-

Table 9-6. FFD Conversion Table

	40 in	48 in	72 in
40 in	—	1.44	3.24
48 in	0.69	—	2.25
72 in	0.24	0.44	—

Note: Minor variations in FFD can produce significant changes in radiographic density. Most FFD conversion tables list many distances, most of which are not in common practice. Distance changes of 40, 48, and 72 inches are shown. If a 72-inch chest study needed to be repeated at 40 or 48 inches, the conversion factor multiplied by the original mAs would indicate the technique conversion needed to maintain the original density. If, for some reason, the original 40-inch study had to be repeated at 72 inches, more than a 300% increase in mAs would be required if kilovoltage remained constant. If a 72-inch study were repeated at 40 inches and kilovoltage remained constant, approximately one fourth the mAs would be required. It is not necessary to memorize this table. The calculations can be made using the formula for mAs/distance/intensity.

Table 9-7. Relative Exposure Levels of Some Image Detectors

Type of Detector	Relative Exposure Level
Detail (rare-earth)	up to 100
Medium (CaWo4)	100
High (CaWo4)	250
Rare-earth (medium speed)	250–300
Rare-earth (high speed)	400–1200

Note: These screen film speeds are not representative of any manufacturer but are commonly accepted approximations. A medium-speed screen film combination (calcium tungstate) is shown with a representative speed of 100. In practice, most radiology departments use higher screen film combinations, with speed 400 (rare-earth) being the industry standard.

7). The screen film combination can influence the amount of radiation received by patient and operator. Minor changes in technique should be made with caution when using ultra-high-speed, rare-earth screen film systems. When using a 1200-speed system, a technical change will have 12 times the film blackening effect of the same change made with a 100-speed system.

5. Location of the grid (table, upright stationary grid or Bucky, or grid cassette)
6. Grid ratios and focal ranges
7. Gonadal or breast shielding or other radiation protection options
8. Generator phase (single-phase, three-phase, and so on; see The Influence of Equipment Generator Phase later in this chapter)

Technique charts cannot always be followed precisely. They should not be thought of as the answer or cure-all for technical problems. Before making an exposure, radiographers should review the patient's clinical history on the examination request. A standardized technique chart does not take into consideration the nature of a patient's pathologic or physical condition. A repeat examination can often be avoided if the radiographer is aware of a suspected pathologic condition that could require a change in technical factors.

Technical Factor Adjustments

Technical factor adjustments should be made after considering the following rules or principles of radiographic exposure:

1. To maintain a given density, (a) increase kilovoltage by 15% and reduce mAs by one half,

or (b) decrease kilovoltage by 15% and double mAs (Fig. 9-1).
2. When kVp is increased, short-scale contrast decreases; a wider latitude, long-scale technique results. When kVp is decreased, short-scale contrast increases.
3. The use of a grid or Bucky improves contrast. A grid will also absorb some primary radiation, as well as scatter radiation, resulting in a decrease in radiographic density. (For factor conversion information when using grids of different ratios, see Chapter 5, Tables 5-1 and 5-2.)
4. When using intensifying screens of the same phosphor type, system speed increases with a possible decrease in radiographic detail. X-ray cassettes should have prominent intensifying screen identification labels so that the screen film combination can be easily determined.
5. A smaller focal spot results in increased detail but may require the use of a lower mA value and an increase in exposure time.
6. An increase in FFD improves recorded detail but decreases radiographic density (see Table 9-6), unless an increase in exposure factors is made.
7. An increase in OFD or a decrease in FFD results in image enlargement, with an increase in image blur.
8. Any increase in scatter radiation diminishes radiographic contrast and visibility of detail.
9. Any type of extraneous fog (e.g., chemical, visible light, safelight) increases overall density, diminishing radiographic contrast and visibility of detail.
10. Angulation of a part, an image receptor, or the x-ray tube (Figs. 9-2 and 9-3) or the divergent effect of the x-ray beam can produce anatomic distortion. Angulation of the x-ray tube also results in an increased FFD.

The Effects of Tissue Density and Pathology

Some radiographers are reluctant to measure the part under study and prefer to substitute a "rule of thumb" for measurement. Failure to measure the part to be examined can be a major cause of exposure error. There must be agreement as to where to measure the part (Fig. 9-4). For example, depending on where measurement of the shoulder is made, part thickness can vary from 10 cm to

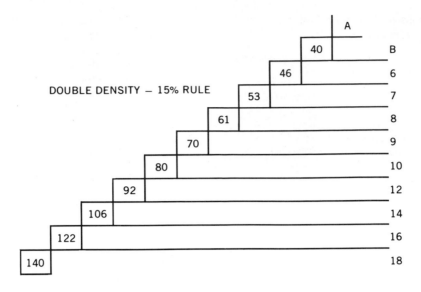

DOUBLE DENSITY — 15% RULE

	A
40	B
46	6
53	7
61	8
70	9
80	10
92	12
106	14
122	16
140	18

A. Original Kilovoltage Value
B. Increase in kVp Needed to Double Density

Figure 9-1
The 15% Rule Versus a "Rule of Thumb" for Density Changes

Kilovoltage values ranging from 40 kVp to 140 kVp are shown (A), with the 15% increase in kilovoltage (B) needed to double radiographic density. A "rule of thumb" adjustment of kVp is sometimes substituted for the 15% kilovoltage change. This rule states that radiographic density can be maintained if an adjustment of ½ mAs is accompanied by an increase of 10 kVp. The reduction of 10 kVp and the doubling of mAs has the same effect on density. In the typical kilovoltage range (60–80 kVp) used for most medical radiographs, this rule of thumb approximates the 15% calculation. As kilovoltage is lowered to the 40 kVp range or elevated to 125 kVp or greater, the 10 kVp adjustment is no longer valid.

Figure 9-2
The Divergent Effect of the X-ray Beam

In this representation of the lateral chest, three black circles are used to represent lesions, with the central ray passing through the most posterior circle. Since these representative lesions are at different distances from the tabletop, they will be enlarged to different degrees. Owing to the divergent effect of the x-ray beam, the circles will also appear distorted (elongated) on the radiograph. The posterior circle (C; 5 cm from the tabletop) is the most accurate representation. The central circle (B; 10 cm from the tabletop) is enlarged and slightly elongated. The anterior circle (A; 15 cm from the tabletop) is also enlarged and more elongated because of its position relative to the central ray. When a patient is being examined for multiple lesions, a positioning compromise must sometimes be made. In the above illustration, the central ray should pass through B to minimize distortion and elongation of the remaining circles.

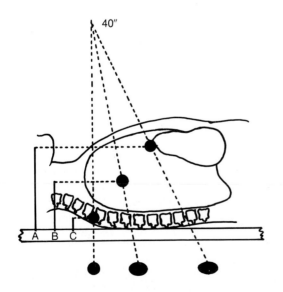

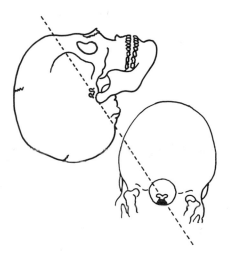

Figure 9-3
The Use of Tube Angulation for Deliberate Anatomic Distortion

Tube angulation, from 25 to 35 degrees caudad, with the patient in the anteroposterior Towne position to project facial structures off of the occiput, is an accepted technique. The central ray passes through the dorsum sellae of the sella turcica, projecting it into the foramen magnum (right). Both posterior clinoid processes can be visualized free of superimposed facial structures.

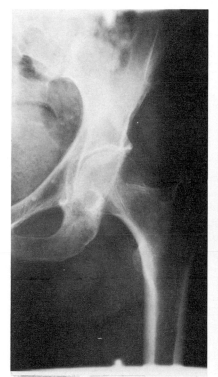
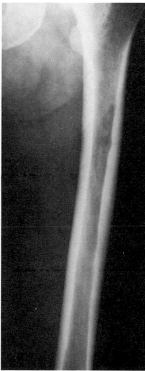
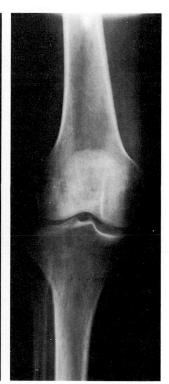

Figure 9-4
Technical Factor Adjustments for Variations in Patient Thickness

These three separate radiographs from the hip to the lower leg used 70 kVp and 12:1 grid. As body thickness or density decrease the mAs was reduced by half; the hip was exposed at 100 mAs, the femur at 50 mAs, and the knee at 25 mAs, using a 100-speed screen film combination. The use of the same exposure factors for all three images of the leg would have resulted in over- and underexposed images. Measurement of each segment of anatomy should be made for proper exposure.

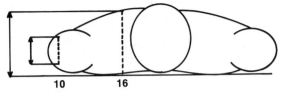

Figure 9-5
Measurement Concepts

The use of a measurement caliper is essential for variable or fixed kilovoltage techniques. There must be agreement as to where to measure the part under study. In this illustration, the measurement over the glenoid fossa was 10 cm. If the patient were measured over the center of the clavicle, a significant increase in the measurement (16 cm) would occur. This difference in measurement could produce more than a 100% density change on the processed radiograph.

20 cm in the same patient (Fig. 9-5). This could represent more than a 100% change in radiographic density.

If a patient is seen only in the recumbent position, covered with street or hospital clothing, plaster or mechanical splints, and so on, reliable categorizing as to body habitus (size, shape, and tissue density) can be difficult. The recumbent position can cause tissue to spread laterally, influencing measurement.

The type of tissue to be examined can influence the selection of technical factors. The use of measurement calipers with a hands-on approach may help to determine whether or not a patient is muscular. A patient may be obese or pregnant; may have fluid in the chest, abdomen, or extremities; or may have osteosclerotic or osteolytic bones. Some diseases or conditions that require an increase in technical factors include ascites, cirrhosis of the liver, osteoarthritis, atelectasis, hydropneumothorax, and cardiomegaly.

An emphysematous patient requires a reduction in technical factors to avoid overexposure of the lungs. Emaciation, an atrophic limb, gaseous distention of hollow viscera, osteoporosis, degenerative arthritis, pneumothorax, and emphysema are types of radiolucent pathologic changes.

Radiographers have often been taught that a significant increase in exposure is necessary for a wet versus a dry plaster of Paris (calcium sulfate) cast. Gratale, Turner, and Burns demonstrated that this is not always a valid rule.* The amount

*Gratale P, Turner GW, Burns CB: Using the same exposure factors for wet and dry casts. Radiol Technol 57(4):325–329, 1986.

of plaster used to reinforce a segment of a cast may also require an increase in exposure factors (Fig. 9-6). Newer, lightweight cast materials are easier to penetrate.

The age and size of the patient must be considered when selecting technical factors. The osseous structures of a newborn child have a low calcium content. With modern neonatal technology, babies weighing 2 lb or less often survive and are categorized as newborns. Whereas an average newborn baby weighs from 6 to 7 lb, many newborn babies weigh 10 lb or more. There is a 500% difference in weight between the 2-lb premature newborn and a large, full-term baby. Pediatric technique charts that have been formulated according

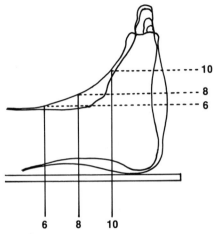

Figure 9-6
Technique Selection for Casted Extremities

Traditionally a wet plaster cast was thought to require considerably more exposure for adequate penetration than a dry plaster cast. According to Gratale and colleagues, if most of the water has been expressed from the plaster prior to its application, the wet or dry cast should require approximately the same exposure factors. The amount of reinforcement plaster used with the cast must also be considered. In this illustration extra plaster was used to reinforce the cast anterior to the ankle mortise in the anteroposterior dimension. Note the configuration of the leg compared with the cast. A measurement taken just above the ankle joint is 6 cm; adjacent to the joint, 8 cm; and below the ankle joint (including the extra plaster), 10 cm. Higher kilovoltage may be necessary to demonstrate the ankle mortise. The use of a grid or Bucky at 80 kVp or greater will result in a high latitude technique with adequate contrast, demonstrating the tibia and fibula as well as the ankle joint. This technique helps to overcome the variations in thickness of plaster used to strengthen casts.

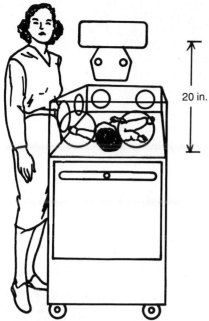

20 in.

Figure 9-7
Technical Complications in Neonatal Imaging
Many bedside x-ray units have restricted tube heights. A 40-inch FFD may not be able to be achieved with the neonate positioned in a basinette. In this illustration, the x-ray tube is restricted to a 20-inch FFD. This shortened FFD requires one fourth of the exposure needed for an image at a 40-inch FFD. Since most mobile units have a fixed mA setting of 100 mA or greater, the shortest possible exposure time, usually 1/120th of a second, must be used. If these factors are used with a 400-speed or 600-speed rare-earth screen film combination in an attempt to minimize radiation dosage to the neonate, the image will be significantly overexposed. Since the mAs cannot be reduced, it is common practice to lower kVp to the 40 to 55 kVp range. With rare-earth technology, the screen emissivity is lessened by the kVp dependency effect. To improve the image, a slower speed screen exposed at 70 kVp or greater should be considered.

only to the age of the patient—for example, newborn, 3 months, 6 months, and so on—can be misleading. The weight of the child should influence the selection of technical factors. Screen film selection and FFD limitations complicate neonatal imaging (Fig. 9-7).

Pediatric technique charts cannot be adapted from adult charts. Infants and children require special technique charts. The late John Hope, M.D., of Philadelphia was fond of reminding radiographers that "infants are not little people."

For example, the infant chest is almost round in shape, measuring approximately the same in the anteroposterior and lateral dimensions, as opposed to the significant difference in the posteroanterior and lateral adult chest measurements.

There is significant variation in weight, height, and muscularity among adolescents. A larger adolescent may require adult techniques.

Special technical consideration must be given to older patients. Atrophic and osteoporotic tissues often require lower kVp to maintain radiographic contrast. Because adequate subject contrast may not be present in severely demineralized structures, radiographic contrast may be difficult to produce in these patients, regardless of technical factor compensation.

Contrast Media

Positive Contrast Agents

The following descriptions are of commonly used positive contrast media.

Barium Sulfate

Barium sulfate is used for opacification of the gastrointestinal tract. Since barium is not absorbed, it does not alter normal physiologic function. It can be used in various suspension weights to image the esophagus, stomach, small bowel, or colon. Barium is also used for mucosal coating studies of the gastrointestinal tract (Fig. 9-8).

Iodinated Contrast Materials

AQUEOUS. Aqueous ionic contrast media are iodinated salts that are intravenously injected in the form of a hypertonic solution and excreted by the kidneys during intravenous pyelography (see Fig. 9-8) or secreted by the liver during intravenous cholangiography. These agents are also used for opacification of blood vessels during angiography. A direct injection of aqueous iodine into the biliary ductal system results in a cholangiographic study (Fig. 9-9).

Aqueous iodine can be used for gastrointestinal studies when barium sulfate is contraindicated, for example, when a bowel obstruction or perforation of a hollow viscus is suspected.

NON-IONIC CONTRAST. Non-ionic contrast media are molecular water solutions. Although adverse affects can occur with any contrast media, non-

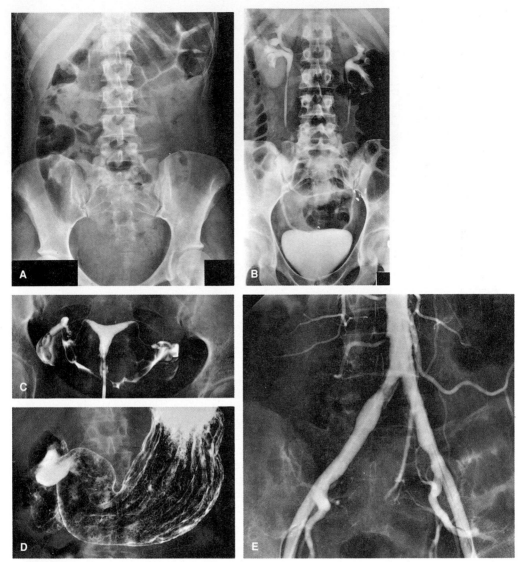

Figure 9-8
Use of Contrast Media in the Abdomen

(A) *A survey radiograph of the abdomen demonstrates the need for positive and negative contrast media to show abdominal structures. Radiolucent gas patterns can be seen throughout the intestines. Radiolucent flank stripes, extending from the lateral rib margins to the iliac crests bilaterally, are also seen. (B) After injection of an iodinated contrast agent, an intravenous urogram demonstrates the renal outlines, renal collecting systems, ureters, and urinary bladder. Newer imaging techniques can also be used to image the kidney. (See Chapter 12, Fig. 12-7.) (C) A retrograde injection of an oil-based or thickened water-based iodinated contrast media is used for salpingography to opacify the female reproductive organs. (D) Barium sulfate (positive contrast) and air or gas (negative contrast) are often combined in a double contrast study to better visualize the mucosal lining of the stomach during an upper gastrointestinal examination. (E) After the retrograde placement of a catheter into the upper abdominal aorta through a femoral artery, an aqueous iodinated contrast medium is injected using a power syringe to opacify the abdominal aorta and associated arteries. The catheter can be manipulated under fluoroscopic guidance for selective and subselective opacification of specific arteries. (F) During myelography, a radiopaque water-soluble contrast agent is introduced into the*

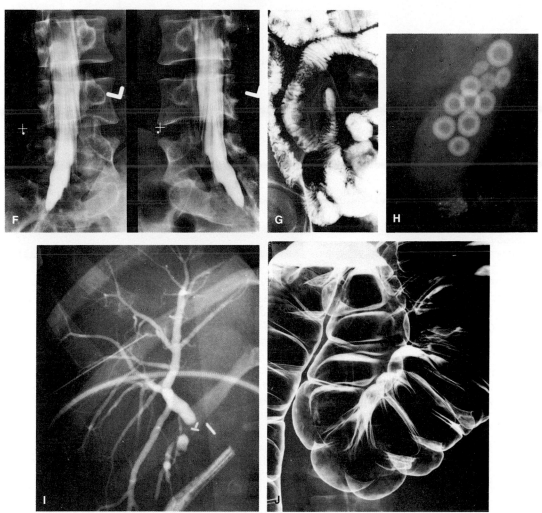

spinal canal by spinal tap to visualize the subarachnoid space of the spine. Oil-based contrast agents were used for many years for this study. Magnetic resonance imaging is currently used to visualize the spinal cord without an injection of contrast material. (G) Following the ingestion of barium sulfate, a series of full-size radiographs may be required over a period of several hours to visualize all segments of the small intestine. A second method uses a small bowel enema with both air and barium. (H) The gallbladder requires iodinated contrast tablets or capsules, taken by mouth, to determine the concentration of bile and the emptying capabilities of the gallbladder. Note the calcific rimmed gallstones. Ultrasound is currently the preferred imaging modality for imaging of the gallbladder. (See Chapter 12, Fig. 12-11.) (I) Following gallbladder surgery, a postoperative cholangiogram may be needed to determine the patency of the biliary ductal system or to check for residual calculi. An aqueous opaque contrast agent is injected directly into the biliary system through a drainage tube inserted into the ductal system at surgery. (J) The lower gastrointestinal tract can be opacified by a barium sulfate enema for a full-column study. Double-contrast enemas require both barium and air or gas to distend the lumen of the colon for visualization of the mucosal lining, small polyps, and intraluminal tumors. The image shown is a fluoroscopic spot film. (Radiographs reprinted courtesy Eastman Kodak Company)

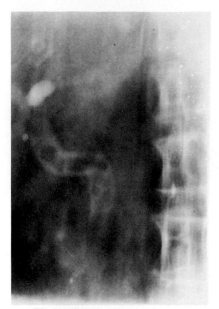 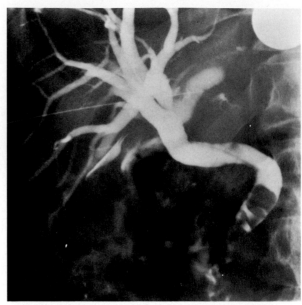

Figure 9-9
The Effect of Kilovoltage on Contrast Media

The kilovoltage range needed to produce adequate radiographic contrast when using a contrast medium depends on whether the medium is injected directly or intravenously. (Left) A tomographic section of an opacified biliary system shows multiple radiolucent filling defects. The iodine (intravenous injection) was diluted by bile. A low kVp, high mAs technique is required to augment a poorly visualized iodinated shadow. (Right) A direct injection of undiluted contrast material is shown in a percutaneous transhepatic cholangiogram. A needle was inserted into the abdomen into the biliary system, bile withdrawn, and undiluted aqueous iodine injected directly in the dilated biliary ducts. Note the radiolucent defects near the end of the distal common duct. A high kilovoltage technique (above 90 kVp) will penetrate dense opacified biliary ducts.

ionic contrast media are associated with a lower risk of adverse affects than ionic materials.

WATER-SOLUBLE IODINATED THICKENED SUSPENSIONS. These solutions are used for hysterosalpingography (see Fig. 9-8), retrograde urethrography, and draining sinus injections, among other procedures.

OIL-BASED IODINE. Oil-based iodine is used for myelography or bronchography. Non-ionic, water-soluble contrast agents are currently used for myelography.

IODINATED PILLS OR CAPSULES. Iodinated pills or capsules are used for oral cholecystography (see Fig. 9-8).

Negative Contrast Agents

Radiolucent or negative contrast agents include gas, air, oxygen, helium, carbon dioxide, and nitrous oxide. Radiolucent contrast agents were initially used for visualization of the ventricles of the brain during pneumoencephalography or ventriculography, and for injection into the abdomen or retroperitoneal space to outline organs. Air is occasionally used as a contrast agent for myelography. Computed tomography, which is discussed in Chapter 12, enhances the differences in contrast between soft tissue structures and has replaced most of these examinations.

The most common use of air as a contrast medium is for chest radiography. Full inspiration fills the lungs with radiolucent contrast medium (air). The diaphragms are moved downward, and the cardiac shadow assumes its true size and configuration. When an expiratory film is made, the diaphragms are elevated, giving the illusion of an enlarged heart. In Figure 9-10 the right side of the chest is shown after expiration and compared with an image made at full inspiration. The same technical factors were used for both exposures. Note the increase in radiographic density on the inspiration image due to aeration and expansion of the lung tissue.

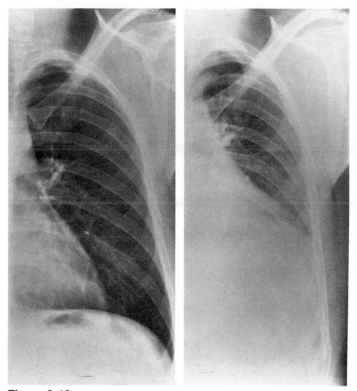

Figure 9-10
Use of Air as a Radiolucent Contrast Media
for Chest Radiography
*The left side of a posteroanterior chest is shown on full inspiration (left)
and expiration (right). The difference in radiographic density is due to
the degree of inspiration. These exposures were made without an automatic exposure device. A fully inspired lung field produces a normal-
appearing left lung. The image made on full expiration appears to be
significantly underexposed, even though the same exposure factors were
used. The elevated diaphragms create the illusion of an enlarged heart.
The base of the lung seems congested in the expiratory film. If this examination were made using an automatic exposure device, the densities
would be matched, since the AED would permit exposure until a preselected density were reached. The study would not be diagnostic; the heart
would be difficult to evaluate. (Modified from Thompson TT:* Primer of
Clinical Radiology, *2nd ed. Boston: Little, Brown, 1980)*

Air or gases are used with barium examinations to perform double-contrast studies of the
stomach and colon. Barium sulfate is used to outline the mucosal pattern of the stomach, which is
then distended by a gaseous substance introduced
orally or by way of a gastric tube. For the double-
contrast barium enema, barium is used to partially
fill the colon, and air is then introduced to dilate
the hollow viscus. Barium coats the walls of the
air-distended colon. Studies that use air as a contrast agent in combination with barium require

low to moderate kilovoltage values to maximize
radiographic contrast (see Fig. 9-8).

Selection of Technical Factors
for Use with Contrast Media

The radiographic perception of an object is influenced by the density of the material surrounding the object. A body part, when surrounded by
a more radiodense material, will appear radio-

lucent; if surrounded by a radiolucent material, it will appear relatively opaque. Air, fat, water (mostly soft tissue), and bone are naturally occurring tissue densities. Fatty tissue sometimes outlines and separates body structures from one another.

When a survey radiograph of the abdomen is made, the osseous structures of the lower ribs, spine, and pelvis can be seen. The liver and spleen, as well as both kidneys, are sometimes represented by faint radiolucent outlines owing to fatty tissue envelopment. Gaseous pockets are often seen throughout the hollow viscera of the gastrointestinal tract. The lateral margins of the psoas muscles can also be seen (see Fig. 9-8).

Pathologic conditions can produce gas, fat, or calcium deposits as well as other increased or decreased tissue densities.

The stomach, small and large intestines, and biliary, urinary, and vascular systems require contrast media in order to be seen radiographically.

The route or method of injection of the contrast medium also affects technical factor selection. Higher kVp values (100 kVp or greater) must be used to penetrate large, dense, barium-filled hollow viscera. The use of shorter exposure times will help to overcome motion blur that results from peristalsis or patient motion.

Some studies, such as the cystogram, require direct injection of large amounts of aqueous contrast by means of a urethral catheter into the urinary bladder. An opaque, dilated bladder is extremely dense and can mask radiolucent or radiopaque calculi or other disease processes. The use of moderate to high kilovoltage (85–100 kVp) to penetrate the distended, opaque bladder produces an image with longer scale contrast.

With the transhepatic cholangiogram, when there is a direct injection of undiluted contrast material, a dense radiopaque shadow is produced. Since non-opaque biliary calculi can be obscured by a dense contrast agent, higher kilovoltage values of 85 kVp or greater are required to penetrate the opaque, often dilated, ductal system (see Fig. 9-9).

A low or moderate kilovoltage of 70 kVp or less should be used for optimal visualization of the contrast-enhanced organs when there is an indirect routing of an aqueous iodine contrast medium, such as with intravenous urography or intravenous cholangiography (see Figs. 9-8 and 9-9). The amount and concentration of the contrast agent delivered by intravenous injection to the urinary or biliary system depends on the function of the kidney or liver, respectively. A low-to-moderate kilovoltage level is needed for adequate radiographic contrast.

A considerable difference in contrast is evident in a common duct made visible by intravenous cholangiography compared with a direct-injection, percutaneous transhepatic cholangiogram (see Fig. 9-9).

The Influence of Equipment Generator Phase

When a technique chart is being developed, generator output must be considered. A single-phase study at 80 kVp, 100 mAs that produces a satisfactory radiographic density can be duplicated at 70 kVp, 100 mAs on a three-phase, 12-pulse unit. There should be no obvious difference in radiographic contrast between these images, since the effective kVp from the three-phase equipment is higher than the effective kVp generated with the single-phase unit. There is, however, a significant reduction in heat units when using three-phase equipment with appropriate technique adjustments (Table 9-8).

Constant-potential and high-frequency generators produce heat units similar to three-phase, 12-pulse generators. Heat units are discussed in Chapter 3.

Table 9-8. kVp and mAs Adjustments and Their Effect on Heat Units

		Heat Units	
kVp	mAs	S∅	3∅
53	400	21,200	29,892
61	200	12,200	17,202
70	100	7,000	9,870
80	50	4,000	5,640
92	25	2,300	3,243

Note: A representative technique, 100 mAs at 70 kVp, is selected as a starting technique (center line). Kilovoltage changes made using the 15% rule are shown with mAs adjustments to maintain a given density. (See Fig. 9-1.) Note the difference in the heat units generated using single-phase equipment, full-wave rectified vs. three-phase, 12-pulse equipment.

An adjustment of 15% in kVp from the original 70 kVp setting (61 kVp or 80 kVp) generates either 17,202 HU or 5640 HU, respectively. This represents more than a 300% increase in heat units at the lower kVp setting.

If a similar kilovoltage value, such as 80 kVp, is used for both exposures, a reduction in mAs of approximately 50% can be made for the three-phase study. This will produce an image in half the time or perhaps permit the use of a smaller focal spot at a lower mA value to reduce image blur. The overall contrast of the three-phase radiograph will be of a longer scale since the effective kVp is greater. When working in the 65- to 85-kVp range, with a single-phase unit, an increase in 10 kVp with one half the original mAs will produce similar radiographic density to that of a three-phase unit. This assumes that the same make and ratio grid, same screen film combination, and same collimator shutter pattern are used.

The difference in the scale of contrast generated with single- or three-phase equipment at the same kVp setting can present a problem when performing examinations such as iodinated contrast studies, chest radiography, conventional tomography, and mammography. When selecting the optimum kilovoltage for an iodinated contrast study, it should be noted that the generator phase has a significant effect on radiographic density and contrast. The proposal to determine an appropriate kVp for interaction with the K-edge of iodine was first made years before three-phase equipment became available. A survey of physicians, physicists, and radiographers about the proper kVp needed to image structures made opaque by iodinated contrast media would reap a variety of opinions, from 55 kVp to 75 kVp. For the purpose of discussion, it is assumed that 70 kVp is appropriate for imaging an iodinated contrast medium, as determined by using single-phase equipment. This implies that images made on a three-phase unit would only require 62 kVp for optimal imaging (see Chapter 2, Fig. 2-6).

Types of Technique Charts

The technical options in this chapter are conceptual and are not meant to be used with a specific x-ray unit. Exposure charts can be formulated to reflect one or more of the following techniques.

Fixed mAs, Variable kVp Technique

The fixed mAs, variable kVp technique combines a predetermined fixed mAs value with a variable kVp, which is determined according to the mea-

Table 9-9. Variable vs. Fixed Kilovoltage Techniques

Variable			
mAs	20	20	20
kVp	62, 64, 66	72, 74, 76	80, 82, 84
cm	17, 18, 19	20, 21, 22	23, 24, 25
Fixed			
kVp	75	76	76
mAs	10	20	25

Note: A representative technique chart for the abdomen is shown with centimeter measurements from 17 to 25. The variable kVp portion (top) shows kilovoltage variations of 2 kVp per centimeter measurement with a fixed mAs. The fixed kVp chart lists 75 kVp for all centimeter measurements, with variations in mAs.

sured thickness of a body part. Differences of 1 to 2 cm in tissue thickness necessitate an adjustment of 2 to 3 kVp (Table 9-9). As tissue mass increases and the required higher kVp is used, scatter radiation increases.

Fixed kVp, Variable mAs Technique

The fixed kVp technique with varying mAs introduced in the 1940s is often labeled the *optimum kilovoltage* technique. With the fixed kilovoltage technique, pioneered by the late Arthur W. Fuchs of the Eastman Kodak Company, body parts fall into an average thickness range. In 1955, Fuchs reported that the average thickness range of most body parts was similar in approximately 75% of patients.[*] Thickness of extremities is average in almost 100% of the patients. With this technique, patients are divided into general categories such as small, medium, large, and extra large, and centimeter measurement groupings are used to determine the mAs settings (Table 9-10).

A fixed kilovoltage was selected to adequately penetrate the part under study, while maintaining adequate contrast. Fuchs used relatively high kilovoltage values, considering the low-ratio grids (6:1 or 8:1) available at that time. The kilovoltage levels, 80 kVp or greater, were probably necessary because of the 100-speed screen film combination used in the 1950s. These kilovoltage levels were obtained with single-phase equipment. When

[*]*Fuchs AW*: Principles of Radiographic Exposure and Processing. *Springfield, IL: Charles C Thomas, 1955.*

Table 9-10. Fixed vs. Variable Kilovoltage

Size	Fixed		Variable	
	mAs	*kVp*	*kVp*	*mAs*
Small	50	80	70	100
Medium	100	80	80	100
Large	200	80	92	100
Extra large	400/200	80/92	106/92	100/200

Note: Another approach to a fixed or variable kVp chart is the categorizing of patients as small, medium, large, and extra large. Centimeter measurements determine patient categories. In this table, a fixed kVp value of 80 is used with variable mAs, and a variable kVp chart is generated for a fixed mAs value. Note the adjustments in factors in both charts for the extra large patient. With the fixed kilovoltage technique, if 80 kVp were to be used for the extra large patient, 400 mAs would be required. An increase in kVp by 15% to 92 kVp would permit the use of a 200 mAs value. For example, at 100 mAs, 106 kVp would be required for adequate exposure of the extra large patient. A 15% reduction in kilovoltage to 92 kVp, to reduce scatter, would necessitate the doubling of the mAs to maintain desntiy. (See Fig. 9-1.) It is interesting to note that at this extra large level, the factors needed with either the fixed or variable kVp charts to compensate for body habitus and scatter radiation are the same—200 mAs at 92 kVp.

reviewing Fuchs' fixed kilovoltage charts, it seems that significantly less kilovoltage is being recommended now than was used by early radiographers for the same body part. The reason for this is that most modern three-phase equipment produces radiographs of comparable density and contrast at kilovoltage values approximately 10 kVp below those selected by Fuchs.

Although many radiographers report that with a fixed kVp, radiographic contrast can be maintained throughout a variety of patient sizes, this belief does not take into consideration the production of scatter radiation. In practice, there is better exposure latitude at higher kilovoltages, but contrast decreases as patient size or tissue mass increases. It is impossible to maintain the same contrast scale in the 15-cm abdomen of an emaciated patient as in the 30-cm, fluid-filled abdomen of a dense, muscular patient.

In support of fixed kVp values, however, it should be noted that when a variety of patients are examined using a fixed kilovoltage value regardless of their size, less variation occurs in the scale of contrast than when kilovoltage values are not fixed. With a variable kVp technique, a smaller patient may need 60 kVp, whereas a larger patient may require 90 kVp for adequate penetration. At 60 kVp, abrupt differences in black and white are seen; at 90 kVp, a longer scale of contrast results. This wide variation in contrast from short scale to long scale is minimized by a fixed kVp technique. Contrast can never be identically matched between similar body parts of different thickness, but a fixed kVp technique will result in images with less variation in contrast over a wider range of patient thicknesses. In practice, kVp may have to be increased for larger patients if the anatomic areas are not adequately imaged because of inadequate penetration (see Table 9-10).

There are also other technical considerations. For example, extremity techniques that require low kilovoltages (50 kVp or less) will result in images of short-scale contrast with poor soft tissue detail. Additionally, rare-earth intensifying screen speed drops off at lower kVp ranges because of the kilovoltage dependency of these phosphors. At 40 kVp some rare-earth screens lose half of their speed. When rare-earth screens are used for extremity radiography, the use of modest kilovoltage values (65–70 kVP) with an appropriate decrease in mAs increases soft tissue dilineation.

Automatic Exposure Technique

Most automatic exposure devices (AED) use fixed kVp techniques. Kilovoltage settings such as 60 kVp, 80 kVp, or 100 kVp are determined by the nature of the part being examined. When the patient is properly positioned to an AED sensor and an exposure is made, the length of the exposure is determined by a preselected density setting. Reproducible radiographs should result, regardless of variations in tissue density.

Anatomically programmed units are capable of categorizing the body into several areas and thicknesses. Individual segments of anatomy to be studied are displayed schematically on an AED program selector at the console. Kilovoltage can be selected, and, on most units, focal spot size can be determined by the radiographer. The mA value is often preselected.

Mobile radiographic techniques should be as well documented as those performed in the main department. High-quality AED systems are available for mobile radiography. An underpart exposure paddle (sensor), linked by a cable to the the mobile unit, is positioned beneath the cassette (Fig. 9-11). An interesting exercise is to review a series of radiographs of a patient in an intensive care unit over a given period of time and examine them for film quality. Many images will be under- or overexposed, although still adequate for diag-

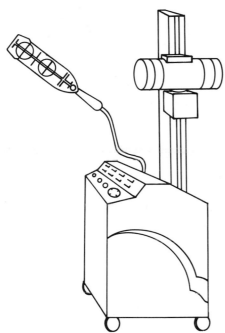

Figure 9-11
Automatic Exposure Device
for Mobile Radiography

An automatic exposure device is shown attached to a mobile radiographic unit. The sensor in the form of a paddle is placed behind the cassette and functions as an exit-type sensor. The mA and kVp settings are determined by the radiographer.

nosis. This lack of consistency sometimes prevents the radiologist from detecting small changes that occur from day to day or even hourly. An AED can help to overcome variations in density between serial radiographs.

Other Types of Technique Charts

A technique chart that uses a slide rule format was described by Kratzer.* This slide rule can be used to compensate for variations in technique, including distance, changes in grid ratio, kVp, and mAs. This method has been updated to include a computer software program.

Other computer software programs are also available. By providing a graphic display of technical factors and patient and beam positioning, these programs could replace standard technique

*Kratzer B: A technique computer. Radiol Technol 45, 1973.

charts. Elaborate computerized systems allow the radiographer to enter a description of the part to be studied along with patient information such as height, weight, age, and so on, which is used to calculate the optimal exposure for the patient and to list alternative technique options. Hard copy can be printed for wall chart or classroom use.

Many x-ray film and equipment manufacturers offer support in the fabrication of manual or computer-generated technique charts.

Standard Positioning and Projection Concepts

Technique charts should contain information regarding radiographic positioning of the patient and the projection of the central ray. One should be familiar with standard terminology for positioning and projections.* Changes in the position of the patient often affect radiographic technique. For example, in the prone position the weight of the body flattens the abdominal tissues, necessitating a decrease in the exposure factors that would be used for the supine position. Decubitus positioning of the patient for an abdominal study can result in uneven tissue thickness in the dependent portion of the abdomen. When a patient is placed in the erect position, there is an increase in tissue thickness in the lower abdomen.

Patients often are placed in oblique positions of varying degrees. A 15-degree oblique position of the body requires an increase in exposure over the anteroposterior position. A 45-degree or 60-degree oblique rotation of the same body part requires an additional increase in exposure over the 15-degree oblique position (Fig. 9-12).

As the patient position and projection of the central ray are changed, not only should the technique be adjusted, but identification labeling should be documented on the radiograph. For example, placing the patient in the supine position causes a widening of the heart and mediastinum. Proper labeling is important because, even in the erect position, poor inspiration may widen the cardiac silhouette.

*This information, available in Standard Terminology for Positioning and Projections, can be obtained from the American Registry of Radiologic Technologists, Minneapolis, Minnesota. A companion book to Producing Quality Radiographs, entitled Optimizing Radiographic Positioning (Philadelphia: JB Lippincott, 1992), describes the interdependence of radiographic positions and projections on radiographic technique.

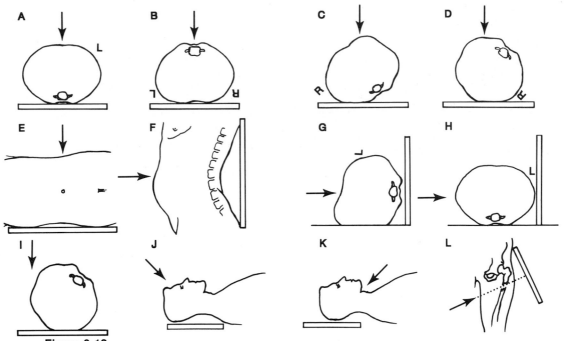

Figure 9-12
The Effect of Patient or Tube Positioning on Exposure Factors

The configuration of the body may change with changes in the position of the patient. Measurements taken in the supine position (A) for an anteroposterior projection or for a dorsal decubitus projection (H) will be greater than those taken in the prone position (B), since in the prone position there is a flattening of the soft tissues of the abdomen as they spread out bilaterally. In the oblique positions, right posterior oblique (C) and right anterior oblique (D), changes in configuration may occur as the body is rotated.

If the patient is turned to a lateral decubitus position (G), the dependent portion of the abdomen becomes thicker than the upper segment. The use of a wedge filter, with the thicker portion of the filter positioned to coincide with the upper aspect of the abdomen, may help to overcome absorption differences, particularly with obese patients.

When the patient is in the erect position (F), some of the structures within the abdomen may drop, causing differences in absorption of the x-ray beam. When the abdomen thickens or flattens, technical factors should be adjusted for conventional imaging. An AED makes these adjustments automatically.

Projections are sometimes defined by the direction of the central ray when it is not perpendicular to the film. Some variations in tube angulation are described. With the patient supine, the central ray enters anteriorly and exits posteriorly (A). In the posteroanterior position, the x-ray beam enters posteriorly and exits anteriorly (B). A lateral projection is described with reference to the side closest to the x-ray film. Illustration E represents the right lateral position with the x-ray beam entering through the left side of the patient. When the patient is in the oblique position and a central ray is used for a tangential projection, the image is seen in silhouette and the projection is described as tangential (I). This projection is often used to locate a foreign body in extrinsic tissue or to demonstrate a depressed fracture of the skull. The term axial projection is used when the x-ray beam is directed caudad (J) or cephalad (K).

Horizontal beam techniques (F, G, H, and L) require that the x-ray beam be horizontal to the floor, regardless of the position of the patient or detector. A horizontal beam projection is often used to radiograph the head of the femur in the axiolateral position (L) or for erect (F) or decubitus (G and H) imaging. (Courtesy Cullinan AM: Optimizing Radiographic Positioning. *Philadelphia: JB Lippincott, 1992)*

Chapter 10

Image Evaluation and Application of Radiographic Principles

Radiographic techniques should constantly be reviewed and updated as necessary to produce state-of-the-art images. Each radiographic image must be evaluated to determine if it is acceptable for interpretation. The previous nine chapters of this textbook have been devoted to providing the information needed to produce a quality radiograph. This chapter will address the clinical application of previously stated radiographic principles. The examination of the chest is used primarily to illustrate the application of principles of radiographic exposure and radiographic evaluation.

Information on x-ray equipment can be found in Chapter 4.

Image Evaluation

A systematic approach to image evaluation must be applied. Identifying a problem is essential to solving it; to aid in the analysis of a study a mental or printed checklist (Table 10-1) can be used to determine the following:

1. Whether a problem exists
2. The nature of the problem
3. Whether there is enough information available to make a decision
4. Whether the problem is the result of something other than a technical error
5. The alternatives and possible course of action
6. Whether a repeat examination is indicated or advisable
7. What technical considerations must enter into the changes to be made

Proper evaluation of a radiograph is impossible unless one is aware of the conditions present when the study was made. If

Angeline M. Cullinan and John E. Cullinan:
PRODUCING QUALITY RADIOGRAPHS, 2ND ED.
© 1987, 1994 J. B. Lippincott Company.

Table 10-1. Film Evaluation Checklist

Density

Overall acceptable ____ yes ____ no
If no, due to: ____ technique ____ processing
Change density by adjusting/changing:
____ mAs ____ kVp ____ screens ____ film
____ grid ratio ____ distance
____ position of patient to AED ____ collimation
____ other
Segmental increase/decrease due to:
____ extrafocal radiation
____ image undercutting ____ backscatter
____ beam attenuating cassette front/tabletop

Contrast

Acceptable ____ yes ____ no
If no, due to: ____ technique ____ processing
Long Scale ____ Short Scale ____
Change by adjusting: ____ kVp ____ grid ____ beam restriction ____ grid ratio
____ other

Recorded Detail and Visibility of Detail

Acceptable ____ yes ____ no
Poor detail caused by:
____ lack of penetration of part
____ patient motion ____ voluntary ____ involuntary
____ screen type
____ screen–film contact
____ fog: ____ chemical ____ light ____ radiation
____ safelight
____ Image geometry: ____ OFD ____ FFD
____ focal spot size
____ distortion due to: angulation of
____ part ____ tube ____ receptor

Scatter Control

Grids: ____ required ____ not required
evidence of grid cutoff or artifacts
____ yes ____ no
Collimation: ____ evident ____ not evident
evidence of collimator cutoff or misalignment
____ yes ____ no

Radiation Protection

Collimation: ____ evident ____ not evident
Shielding: ____ evident ____ not evident
____ not possible, area of interest in field
Distance: ____ FFD ____ FOD
Technique: ____ kVp range ____ mAs
Intensifying screens: ____ type ____ speed

Positioning

Departmental routine: ____ yes ____ no
Supplemental views: ____ yes ____ no
Patient centering: ____ excellent ____ acceptable
____ poor, correct by:
____ adjusting film position into alignment with central ray and/or patient area of interest

Anatomy

Area of interest demonstrated ____ yes ____ no
Correct by adjusting: ____ central ray
____ collimation ____ tube angle
____ patient position

Identification

Patient name, birthdate, sex ____ yes ____ no
ID number ____ yes ____ no
Radiographer/student ID number ____ yes ____ no
Markers used ____ yes ____ no; correct ____ yes ____ no

Artifacts or Foreign Bodies

____ increased density
____ decreased density
Caused by: ____ film ____ screen ____ cassette ____ tabletop
____ processor ____ grid
____ patient (____ internal ____ external)
____ other

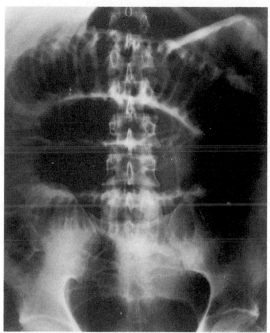

Figure 10-1
The Effect of Air-Distended Hollow Viscera on Radiographic Technique

A survey film of the abdomen shows distended loops of small bowel. The dilated radiolucent loops of bowel are easily penetrated. Since the abdomen of the patient is visibly distended, centimeter thickness measurements can be misleading. It is very easy to overexpose the film when the abdomen is distended by air-filled hollow viscera.

the technical factors selected for the study are not consistent with the recommended factors on the technique chart, the changes should be documented.

Some density or contrast limitations are the result of pathologic conditions and are not technical errors. Pathologic changes can be absorptive or nonabsorptive (Fig. 10-1). Pathology or tissue detectability is often limited by superimposed skeletal and soft tissue structures.

Evaluation Checklist

The following factors should be assessed when evaluating a radiographic image.

Protection from Radiation

The radiographic image should be evaluated for evidence of radiation protection of patient and operator, evidence of collimation, and appropriate shielding of the gonads, if applicable (Fig. 10-2). It may, however, be impossible to evaluate patient protection from looking at the radiographic image. For example, when the patient is seated at the edge of the x-ray table for a study of the hand or wrist, the x-ray beam passes through the cassette and tabletop and may strike the gonads of the patient. Although gonadal protection in the form of lead shielding or a lead apron would not be evident on the radiographic image, it should be used for all patients with child-bearing potential.

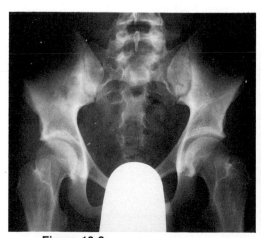
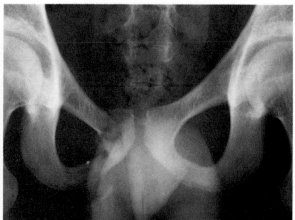

Figure 10-2
Gonadal Shielding

(Left) *Since a fracture of the pubic bones was not suspected, the gonadal area of an 18-year-old male was appropriately shielded from radiation during an x-ray exposure of the pelvis.* (Right) *A repeat examination demonstrates fractures of the right pubic bone, which had been masked by the shield.*

IMPORTANT

If filtration is removable, or if additional filtration has been added to the collimator for a specific study, the radiographer must be certain that the proper filtration has been reinserted into the collimator prior to an exposure.

Collimation should be evident in the form of unexposed borders on the radiographic image. Changes in shutter patterns, which vary the degrees of collimation, have a major effect on radiographic density.

IMPORTANT

When conventional techniques are used, an adjustment must be made in exposure factors to compensate for tight beam collimation (Table 10-2). An automatic exposure device (AED) should be capable of automatically making the necessary technical adjustments.

Extraneous, unsharp radiographic images that often appear outside the shutter pattern are generally due to extrafocal radiation and should not be attributed to scatter radiation. However, extrafocal radiation can affect overall radiographic density (see Control of Extrafocal Radiation in Chapter 5).

Size of Cassette

Part of the radiographic evaluation should concern whether the correct size cassette was used. For example, a film that is too small for an extremity examination may not permit at least one joint to be included on the radiograph or may exclude areas of adjacent anatomy needed to make the diagnosis. Extremity examinations are usually made using a single cassette divided into multiple segments by lead rubber sheeting or tight beam collimation. Multiple images exposed on the same film should be oriented in the same direction to make comparison of the views easier (Fig. 10-3).

The size of the cassette, when used with positive beam limiting devices, will determine the size of the patient area that is to be exposed. Cassettes that are too large for a study increase the potential for scatter radiation as well as for increased patient dosage.

Film Exposure

The image should be evaluated to determine if it is adequately exposed and if the part under study has been adequately penetrated. An under- or overexposed image may be the result of faulty processing or replenishment, or both. The processor should be the first consideration if images produced from multiple x-ray units appear marginal or inadequate when processed through the same

Table 10-2. The Effect of Collimation on Technical Factors

Size	Sq In	Field Size	Timer Adjustments	Heat Units
14 × 17	238	Full	1/10 sec	2400
8 × 10	80	One third	2/10 sec	4800
4 × 5	20	One twelfth	3/10 sec	7200

Starting factors: *300 mA; 1/10 sec; 80 kVp (single-phase, full-wave rectified). The time adjustment factors are approximations and are presented for the purpose of illustration only. No consideration was made for screen–film speed, kilovoltage, and so on.*

When shutter patterns are reduced to a smaller field size, an adjustment in one or more technical factors is required to maintain the original radiographic density. Because 50% or more of a full-field (238 sq in) radiograph is composed of scatter, an adjustment in technical factors must be made to compensate for the decrease in radiographic density owing to the reduction in scatter radiation. Conversely, if field size is increased, a reduction in technical factors is necessary to maintain the original radiographic density.

When evaluating a radiograph made with a conventional technique, if a repeat examination is necessary, any one of several technical adjustments can be selected by the radiographer. A change in exposure time not only increases the possibility of patient motion, but may necessitate the need for a large focal spot, and may tax the anode thermal capacity of the x-ray tube.

When an automatic exposure device (AED) is used with a reduction in field size and the mA or kVp settings are not adjusted, the exposure time will be prolonged until a preselected density is reached. Note the increase in heat units associated with an increased in exposure times.

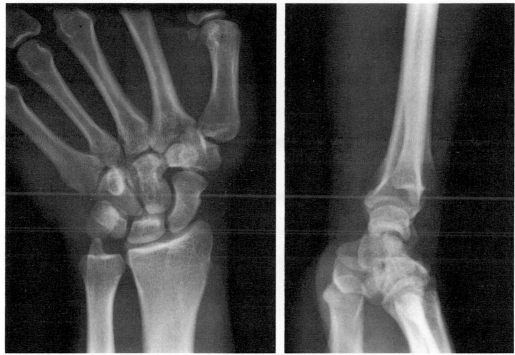

Figure 10-3
Radiographic Orientation of Part to Cassette

Posteroanterior and lateral views of the wrist have not been properly oriented from top to bottom. This arrangement not only is esthetically unacceptable but also may interfere with diagnosis.

automatic processor. The processor temperature should not be lowered to minimize the effect of an inherent high-contrast radiographic film or to compensate for a film with a high gross fog. When the processor temperature is lowered, an increase in exposure factors is needed to make up for inadequate film processing; the undesirable result is increased potential for additional radiation to both patient and operator. Faulty replenishment rates or chemical concentration, or both, also affect the quality of the radiographic image.

Presence of Image Blur

The presence of image blur should be noted. Image blur is usually easy to identify (Fig. 10-4); the source of the blur may be difficult to isolate. Tube crane vibration, faulty Bucky locks, and cassettes not securely fastened in the Bucky tray, particularly when used for upright radiography, should be considered. Cardiac and peristaltic motion can also influence image sharpness. The ability of the patient to cooperate often determines the length

of the exposure. Immobilization techniques can help to overcome motion, although compression may be contraindicated in selected examinations. (Some contraindications are listed in Chapter 4.)

IMPORTANT

The use of short exposure times with high-speed screen film systems requires strict adherence to a technique chart. Minor adjustments in exposure times can result in significant changes in radiographic density.

Motion can be used to advantage with certain body parts (Fig. 10-5).

Whenever possible, minimal tube angulation should be used to avoid the parallax effect associated with dual-emulsion film.

The distortion of anatomic structures is sometimes desirable. The barium-filled colon is used as a clinical example. On the conventional anteroposterior projection, there is a foreshortening of the

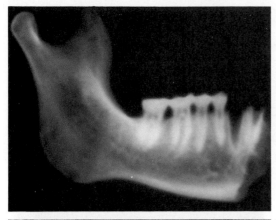

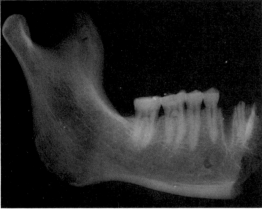

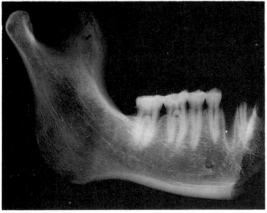

Figure 10-4
Image Blur

Of three radiographs of a dry mandible the least sharp image is easy to identify, since the radiograph appears blurred at a normal viewing distance (top). (Middle) A low-contrast image minimizes the differences between densities and so reduces visibility of detail. (Bottom) Appropriate geometric considerations combined with adequate contrast result in a visibly sharper image. (Reprinted courtesy Eastman Kodak Company.)

sigmoid portion of the colon. When the tube is angled 35 degrees cephalad in the anteroposterior projection, the rectosigmoidal area is elongated to better visualize this area (Fig. 10-6).

The examination of the abdomen for an opaque foreign body demonstrates the divergent effect of the x-ray beam on a foreign body even though the x-ray tube is not angled (Fig. 10-7).

Sharpness will also vary from cathode to anode as a result of the change in the shape of the projected focal spot.

If a magnifying glass is used to view a radiograph, an image may appear to be unsharp. This is due in part to the parallax effect of dual-emulsion film and is particularly obvious with tube-angled techniques.

Presence of Scatter Radiation

The radiographic image must be evaluated for scatter radiation or other types of fog, including the identification of all sources of supplemental density, such as that seen with image undercutting.

Grid and Focal Range Selection

The selection of the grid ratio and focal range is generally predetermined by departmental preference. The image is evaluated for grid cutoff and for the use of the proper grid relative to the kVp level selected. The focal range at which the x-ray beam is centered to the grid is very important. The use of the wrong FFD, for example, a 40-inch FFD for a chest radiograph with a grid focused at 72 inches, will produce bilateral grid cutoff on the image. Both costophrenic angles may appear underexposed with a loss in recorded detail (Fig. 10-8). When evaluating the image this loss of density and detail should not be attributed to poor screen contact or pathology.

Presence of Grid Artifacts

The presence of grid artifacts should be noted. Grid damage or the capturing of a grid in motion by the use of short exposure times can produce changes in the radiographic image that blend into the superimposed radiographic anatomy. These subtle changes can mask both normal radiographic anatomy and pathology. When grid artifacts are suspected, the radiograph should be positioned so that the image of the grid pattern is viewed horizontally. Stepping back from the viewbox when evaluating the image may make it

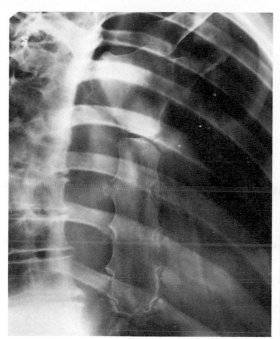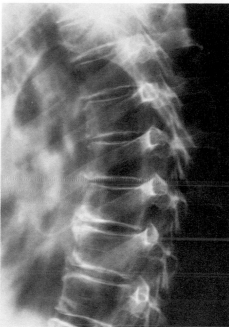

Figure 10-5
The Use of Motion During Radiography of the Sternum and Thoracic Spine

(Left) *The sternum is difficult to image radiographically because of superimposed pulmonary structures. The patient, in a prone oblique position, is instructed to breath rhythmically during the exposure. An extended exposure time is used with a low mA setting to erase pulmonary vasculature.* (Right) *The thoracic spine is also difficult to image radiographically in the lateral position because of superimposed pulmonary structures. The patient is instructed to breath rhythmically during the exposure. An extended exposure time is used with a low mA setting to erase pulmonary vasculature. Note that the ribs also moved during the exposure and are almost completely blurred out.*

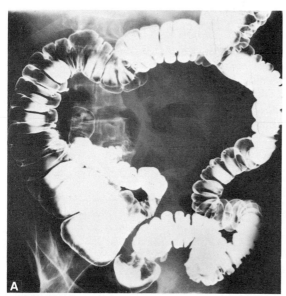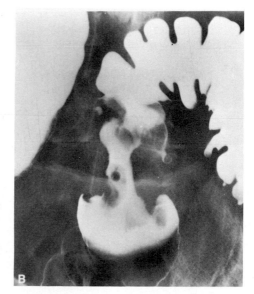

Figure 10-6
Deliberate Distortion of Anatomic Structures

(A) *A barium-filled colon is shown with narrowing near the rectum. Because the rectosigmoidal area was foreshortened in this projection another image will be needed, made at an angle.* (B) *The tube is angled 35 degrees cephalad to elongate the rectosigmoidal colon adequately to demonstrate the disease process.*

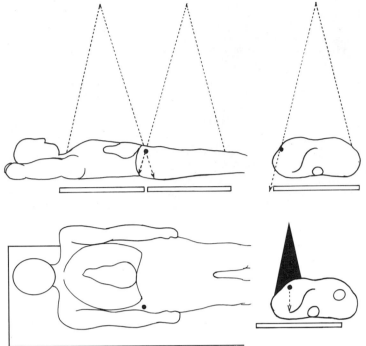

Figure 10-7
The Effect of the Divergent Beam on the Radiographic Image

The illustrations show a patient with a foreign body (black dot) in the anterior right upper quadrant of the abdomen. This dot represents a bullet lodged near the upper anterior portion of the liver. An entrance wound was noted in the anterior portion of the thorax; no exit port was evident. Since it was impossible to determine the path or location of the bullet, survey radiographs of the thorax and abdomen were required. The divergent effect of the x-ray beam used for the thorax examination projected the bullet caudally. When the abdominal image was obtained (top, left), the divergent beam projected the bullet cephalad. A transverse section of the abdomen (top, right) shows the divergent x-ray beam projecting the bullet laterally, away from the detector.

The patient is shown in the supine position to demonstrate the relation of the foreign body to the abdomen and thorax. For this metallic structure to be visualized, the central ray must pass through the object, with the cassette appropriately placed to avoid the divergent effect of the x-ray beam (bottom, right). The central ray must bisect the area containing the foreign body in order to accurately record the relation of the bullet to adjacent anatomic structures. After survey images of the thorax and abdomen are made, radiographs of the thoracolumbar junction must be considered. The cassette must be placed at the level of the right diaphragm, with the patient positioned so that the central ray enters the right upper quadrant just below the right costophrenic angle.

Figure 10-8
Grid Cutoff

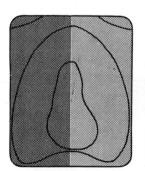
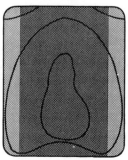

(Left) When an x-ray tube is positioned off-center (to the left) to a focused grid, a difference in radiographic density can be noted on one side of the radiograph. The darker areas represent the portions of the radiograph that received an adequate amount of x-ray exposure. The lighter areas represent the effect of grid cutoff.

(Right) If the wrong FFD were used, for example, a 40-inch FFD with a grid focused for a 72-inch FFD, radiographic density would diminish bilaterally. One- to 2-inch segments of both lateral aspects of the chest radiograph would appear underexposed.

easier to identify grid banding artifacts. A simple test to determine the presence of grid damage is suggested in Chapter 5.

Patient Condition

When evaluating an image, the condition of the patient and the purpose for the examination must be taken into consideration. A deviation from departmental routine may sometimes be required. For example, when evaluating the abdomen in the decubitus position for free air, the patient's right side should be superior and the left side should be inferior, so that air in the fundus of the stomach or the splenic flexure of the colon is not superimposed on the free air. In theory, the right upper quadrant should be devoid of gaseous shadows.

Viewing Conditions

Viewing conditions influence the evaluation of an image. Viewboxes at the quality control station or automatic processor should be similar in light intensity to the viewboxes used for interpretation. Ambient light that reflects off the surfaces of the images on the viewbox can influence the perception of technical quality and may result in a request for a repeat examination.

Image Identification

Patient data, operator identification, and other related information should be evident on the image. Information should be documented using precise technical and medical terminology. Jargon is not appropriate on a medicolegal document. For example, when examining the supine abdomen in the anteroposterior position, the term "flat plate of the abdomen" or "KUB" is often used. Flat plate of the abdomen is a term derived from the use of emulsion-coated glass plates prior to the development of cellulose acetate film base in the mid-1920s. The term KUB refers to an evaluation of the kidneys, ureters, and bladder. A more descriptive term is scout or survey radiograph of the abdomen.

The labeling of the radiographs and documentation of technical factors can become a medicolegal issue. Radiographers may be called on to substantiate their role in the making of a radiograph.

Positioning

When a unique or seldom-requested radiographic position is evaluated (Fig. 10-9), a positioning guide or textbook should be reviewed for tube angulations or part positioning, since a minor error in tube–part alignment may fail to produce the intended image.

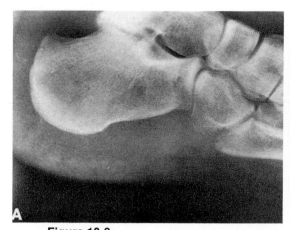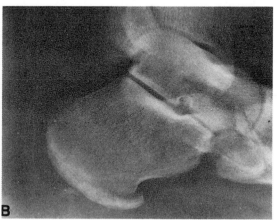

Figure 10-9
Perpendicular vs. Angled X-ray Beam Study
(A) A conventional radiograph of the calcaneus demonstrates normal anatomic relations. (B) A dual tube angulation technique (25 degrees caudad, 25 degrees to the toes) with the foot in the lateral position distorts the osseous structure of the foot and ankle while demonstrating the talocalcaneal joint. Of interest, there is a fracture of the inferior portion of the calcaneus, demonstrated only on the dual tube angle projection.

Repeat Examinations

A marginal-quality radiograph should not be accepted for interpretation unless the patient's condition or age contraindicates reexamination. The arbitrary disposal of a radiograph prior to the evaluation of the entire study should be avoided. A radiologist may find some information on a less-than-optimal image that might be helpful in diagnosis, and the quality control technologist can often include these images in a technical teaching file.

Just as a clinical history is necessary when a radiographic examination is ordered, a technical history is needed before a repeat examination is attempted. If previous radiographs are available, they can be used to establish an alternative technique if needed.

Before repeating a radiograph, one should determine whether proper technical factors were used. Good technical practice dictates that the number of variables in the repeat study be limited. If possible, repeat examinations should be made by the same radiographer, using the same equipment, under the same conditions. For example, if the lumbar spine was evaluated and was determined radiographically to be osteoporotic (Fig. 10-10), a lower kVp value could be used with increased mAs to augment subject contrast. If the radiograph were to be repeated for a positioning error, a second radiographer assigned to the repeat examination may correct the positioning error but, if unaware of the previous technique adjustment, may make an improper technical factor selection. If it can be established that the technical factors were correct and the cause of the poor quality radiograph cannot be identified, a consultation with a quality control supervisor or radiologist is in order before the study is repeated.

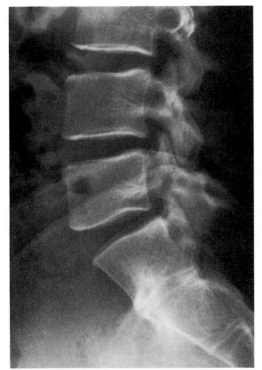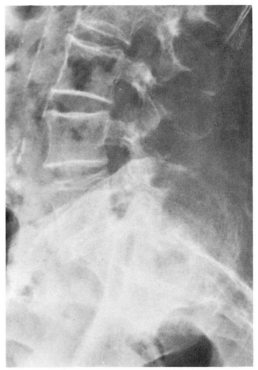

Figure 10-10
The Effect of Pathology on Subject Contrast
(Left) A lateral lumbar spine view demonstrates the normal osseous anatomy of a young adult. Both radiographic contrast and detail are excellent. (Right) An osteoporotic lumbar spine of an 85-year-old patient is shown in the lateral position. Note the lack of subject contrast. Osseous detail is difficult to demonstrate in an osteoporotic spine unless a low kVp, high mAs technique is used to augment subject contrast. Note the presence of calcification in the abdominal aorta.

A repeat analysis program is discussed in Chapter 14.

Application of Principles of Exposure

Radiographic contrast is subjective. Although overall density and contrast should be adequate, it is important to evaluate the specific part or segment of the area under study. For example, a 35-degree cephalad-angled exposure of the sigmoid colon may adequately demonstrate disease of the colon near the rectum but may not penetrate adjacent portions of the colon, such as the cecum (see Fig. 10-6). Although this radiograph may be of excellent quality for its intent, an additional radiograph would be needed to adequately visualize the remainder of the barium-filled colon.

In Figure 10-11 two lateral views of the skull are shown for image evaluation. Both short-scale and moderate-scale contrast are evident in these images.

Since the posteroanterior projection of the chest is the most frequently performed radiologic examination, the remainder of this chapter will be devoted to the application of radiographic principles of exposure to chest radiography.

The Chest X-ray

Comparison films of the chest are often difficult to evaluate unless images of comparable quality are available. In facilities where many patients are examined for specific pulmonary diseases such as pneumoconiosis, the quality of chest images is almost always consistent. Every effort must be made

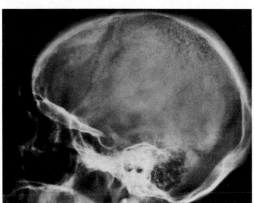
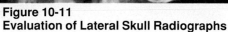
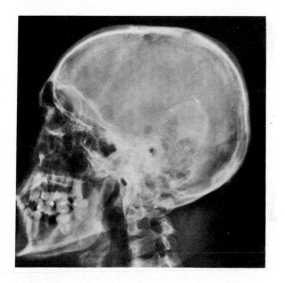

Figure 10-11
Evaluation of Lateral Skull Radiographs

Radiographs should be systematically analyzed to determine if they are technically acceptable. Using the checklist provided in Table 10-1 and the information that follows, the reader is asked to critique the images shown. A lateral skull view (left) is presented for evaluation with a second image (right) for evaluation and comparison.

The radiograph on the left was made with a 400-speed screen film combination, a 0.6-mm focal spot, a 40-inch FFD, and a 12:1 ratio moving grid, with 80 kVp at 20 mAs. The factors required to expose the vault of the skull will overexpose the aerated sinuses and soft tissue of the scalp.

The lateral skull view on the right was made on a dedicated head unit with a 200-speed screen film combination, a 2.0-mm focal spot, a 36-inch FFD, and an 8:1 ratio moving grid. The kVp value was 75 at 20 mAs (400 mA at 1/20th of a second). Note that the sinuses and facial bones are not overexposed, but the bony vault of the skull is underexposed. A faint "corduroy" pattern caused by the capturing of the grid in motion can be seen superimposed on the bony vault of the skull. To better visualize the grid pattern, rotate this illustration 90 degrees, so that the grid lines are horizontal to the floor.

to follow established chest techniques, since technical changes made by the radiographer may affect the diagnosis and perhaps the treatment of the patient.

The making of a chest radiograph requires careful attention to the basics, from technical factor selection to processor control. The simple posteroanterior chest examination uses a high level of technology. Evaluation should include the following questions:

1. Was the study performed with the patient erect, recumbent, posteroanterior or anteroposterior?
2. Is the patient rotated? Are the clavicles horizontal? Are the medial ends of the clavicles symmetric in appearance? Is the relation of the sternoclavicular joints to the thoracic spine symmetric?
3. Are the apices imaged?
4. Are the costophrenic angles imaged?
5. Is there tracheal displacement?
6. Are the scapulae clear of the lung fields?
7. Was the exposure made on full inspiration?
8. Are the densities of both lung fields equal? If not, is this due to pathology, unilateral grid cutoff, or some type of artifact?
9. Is there evidence of motion?
10. Is there evidence of beam collimation?
11. Is the radiograph properly identified?

Two posteroanterior views of the chest are shown for evaluation by the reader (Figs. 10-12 and 10-13).

The Effect of Positioning

More of the contents of the thoracic cage can be imaged with the patient in the erect position. The patient is better able to cooperate, particularly

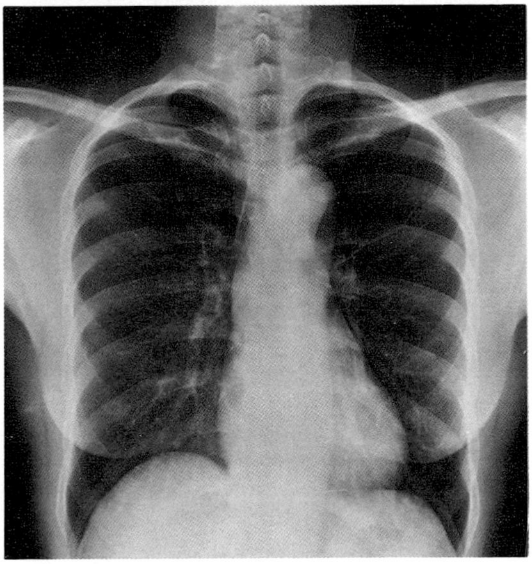

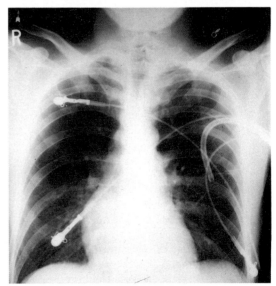

Figure 10-12
Evaluation of a Conventional
Posteroanterior Chest Radiograph

Using the checklist provided in Table 10-1 and the suggestions in the text, the reader is asked to critique the image shown.

This posteroanterior view of the chest was made in the erect position with a 72-inch FFD. A 250-speed screen film system using a latitude film and a 1.5-mm focal spot was used with a 10:1 stationary grid, 125 kVp (three-phase, 12-pulse), and automatic exposure timing. As part of the chest evaluation process, compare this image with Figure 10-13, a bedside chest examination.

Figure 10-13
Evaluation of a Bedside Chest Radiograph

Using the checklist provided in Table 10-1 and the suggestions in the text, the reader is asked to critique the image shown.

A posteroanterior chest was imaged in the upright position at the bedside using a 72-inch FFD. The increased FFD was made possible because of a 400-speed, rare-earth screen film system using a high-contrast film and a 1.2-mm focal spot. A non-grid exposure at 85 kVp (single-phase, full-wave rectified) was used. Note the lack of radiographic information in the mediastinum. Compare this image with a conventional high kVp, grid chest radiograph in Figure 10-12.

with regard to breathing. The abdominal organs do not press against the diaphragm and cause compression of the lung fields, and the heart is shown in its true configuration. The posteroanterior projection permits rotation of the scapulae, taking advantage of the divergent effect of the x-ray beam to project the scapulae off the lung fields. Females with large breasts should be asked to displace their breasts laterally to lessen the filtering effect of breast tissue.

For the posteroanterior erect chest examination, the patient should be positioned with the body weight distributed equally on both feet. The back of the hands should be placed on the hips, with the elbows flexed slightly and the shoulders rotated forward, against the image receptor. If the shoulders have not been rotated sufficiently, the scapulae will be superimposed on the lateral aspects of the lungs. The chin should be raised and placed at the top of the image receptor. If the chin is markedly elevated, however, the occipital portion of the skull may be projected into the apical area of the chest. The chest of a kyphotic patient should be centered with the chin elevated as high as possible, even though the inferior portion of the mandible may appear on the radiograph.

Air as a Contrast Medium

Radiography of the chest should be made on full inspiration, using the air as a contrast medium. When the lungs are completely expanded, vascular markings are easier to see and small lesions within the chest may be demonstrated. There is an increase in subject contrast and the mediastinum is well outlined. Since the expanded lungs are more radiolucent, less exposure is required than for an image obtained during an expiration phase.

The cardiothoracic ratio changes on expiration. The heart will appear wider, and the lung markings will be compressed closer together; the lung fields will appear to be more radiodense (Fig. 10-14).

Valsalva's maneuver, which consists of forced expiration against a closed glottis, should be avoided. This maneuver lowers the flow of venous blood to the heart, reducing cardiac output and producing changes in the appearance of the heart size and vascular markings of the lungs. Occasionally, a radiograph may be requested that uses Valsalva's maneuver. If an enlarged lymph node is suspected in the hilar area, it should be more obvious on an image made with Valsalva's maneuver, since the hilar blood vessels decrease in size.

In the anteroposterior projection, the heart, which is primarily anterior, appears enlarged and is superimposed on adjacent pulmonary structures.

Because stability of the patient during the procedure is essential, the use of an overhead arm support for the lateral position is helpful. A laser positioning device can also be helpful.

Technical Factors

When technical factors are selected for a radiographic examination, kVp and mAs are the first priority. With chest radiography, the choice of a grid or non-grid technique will influence the choice of kVp and mAs. A grid is ordinarily used for body parts measuring more than 10 cm in thickness. The chest, because of its radiolucent nature, is an exception to this rule, and an acceptable image can be obtained with or without a grid.

Non-grid Technique

The use of lower kVp values of approximately 85 kVp for non-grid chest studies produces relatively high-contrast images. Although the lung fields are often satisfactorily exposed, mediastinal details are difficult to demonstrate with this type of technique. Non-grid techniques are popular for mobile or bedside radiography because of grid-focusing difficulties and the limited output of mobile units.

Grid Technique

For chest radiography in the upright position, a full-field (14 × 17 inches) grid should be positioned with its lines running perpendicular rather than parallel to the floor. When a smaller patient is centered to the grid or Bucky, the x-ray beam can be positioned to the patient without grid cutoff. If the grid were positioned with its lead lines running parallel to the floor, the x-ray tube would have to be centered equidistant from the top and the bottom of the grid. The center of every chest examined would have to be exactly 7 inches from the top and bottom of the cassette.

Selection of Grid Ratio and kVp

High kVp–high-ratio grid techniques used with chest radiography accentuate the differences between the heart and the lungs. Soft tissues of the thorax are easily seen, particularly those struc-

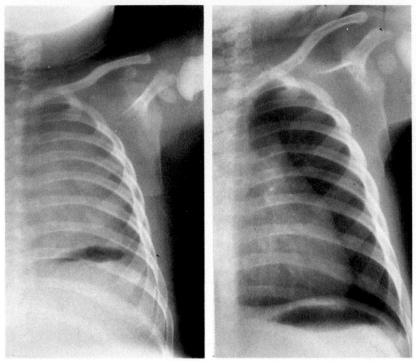

Figure 10-14
Inspiration vs. Expiration, Infant Chest Study
(Left) *The left side of a chest radiograph of an infant is shown at full expiration. Note the lack of normal lung markings and the illusion of massive pulmonary disease. The diaphragm is not seen, and the heart appears enlarged.* (Right) *A repeat radiograph of the same infant was made at full inspiration, with the left diaphragm seen at the level of the tenth posterior rib. The same technical values were used for both exposures. (Courtesy of the Department of Radiology, Rochester General Hospital, Rochester, NY)*

tures in the retrocardiac area or those that are superimposed on vertebral or rib shadows.

Grid ratio and grid focal range must be matched to the kVp level selected for chest radiography. If a high-ratio grid is used with a low to modest kVp value, the mediastinum may not be adequately penetrated. The radiolucent lungs and dense mediastinum and osseous structures may mask a small pulmonary nodule; it could be superimposed on a rib or "lost" in the blackened lung fields associated with low-kVp, high-mAs techniques. As kVp is lowered, a lower-ratio grid must be used (Table 10-3).

Air-Gap Technique

In most situations, unless the chest is similar to the abdomen in thickness and density, the use of an air gap for scatter cleanup in chest radiography is an acceptable substitute for a high-ratio grid

(Fig. 10-15). McInnes states that a 6-inch air gap is roughly equivalent to a 6:1 ratio grid.*

When using the air-gap chest technique, with the patient positioned 10 or 12 inches from the image receptor, an increased FFD of 10 or 12 feet becomes necessary to avoid image enlargement.

The scatter radiation produced by a patient with an enlarged heart or a fluid-filled thorax would be difficult to overcome using an air-gap technique.

Single- vs. Three-Phase Values

There is a considerable difference in radiographic density and contrast when comparing images made using single- versus three-phase equipment. Since three-phase x-radiation is almost ripple free

*McInnes J: The elimination of scatter radiation. Radiography 36:141–142, 1970.

Table 10-3. Generator/kVp/Grid Considerations for Chest Imaging

Generator Type	kVp Range	Recommended Grid Ratio	Optional Grid Ratio
Single-phase	100–114	6:1 or 5:1	8:1
	115–134	8:1	10:1
	135–150	10:1	12:1
Three-phase, CP or HF*	100–114	8:1	10:1
	115–134	10:1	12:1
	135–150	12:1	

The kVp range and grid ratio must be matched to the output of the x-ray generator. As kVp is lowered, grid ratio must be lowered.

*For practical purposes, three-phase, constant potential (CP) and high frequency (HF) output are considered similar.

as opposed to single-phase x-radiation, which has a 100% ripple factor, technical adjustments are often required to maintain image quality, particularly if a specific radiographic density and scale of contrast is desired. Identical kVp values (single-phase vs. three-phase) will produce a visible difference in density and the scale of contrast. If the same kVp and mA setting is used, the three-phase image will exhibit a longer scale of contrast than the single-phase image. Constant potential and high-frequency generators perform similarly to three-phase, 12-pulse equipment; a shorter exposure time can be used. This shortening of exposure time, however, can adversely affect the minimal response time of an AED and can require an adjustment in the mA value. Minimal response time is discussed in Chapter 2.

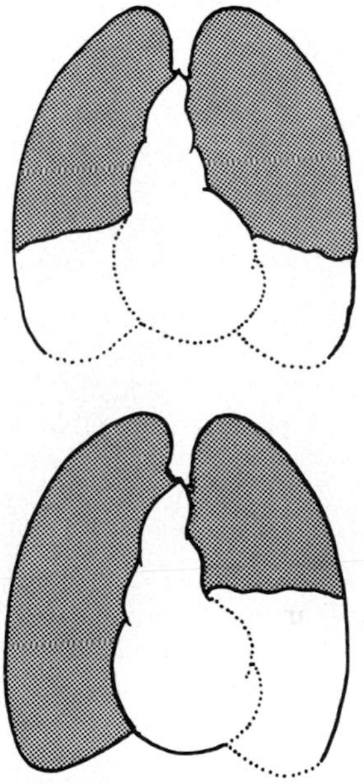

Conventional and Automatic Exposure Controls

The use of an exposure time of 10 msec (⅟₁₀₀th of a second) or less is recommended for the examination of the chest to overcome the motion of the heart. However, the limitations of an AED must also be considered. If a radiographic image of the chest is not acceptable owing to under- or overexposure, the position of the patient relative to the AED sensor should be evaluated. The patient may have been positioned off-center to the sensor, or an incorrect sensor may have been selected.

Another problem is image undercutting, which occurs in the lateral position when the unattenuated primary beam strikes a major portion of the receptor surface, causing the AED to terminate the exposure prematurely.

Figure 10-15
Limitation of the Air-Gap Technique
Schematic representations of the chest include (top) an enlarged heart with diffuse pulmonary disease bilaterally and (bottom) fluid in the left thorax. The use of an air-gap technique for chest radiography is usually an adequate replacement for a grid technique. When an enlarged heart or fluid constitutes a major part of the thorax, a high-ratio grid or Bucky is recommended with a high kVp technique.

IMPORTANT

If an image is of poor quality because of an improperly functioning AED, a repeat examination will yield an image of equally poor quality.

Careful attention must be paid to the degree of inspiration, particularly when using an AED. An AED can produce images of comparable density regardless of the degree of inspiration or expiration. The radiograph made with poor inspiration may give the illusion of an enlarged heart (see Fig. 10-14). For example, an enlarged heart or bilateral pleural effusion may cause the AED to remain activated until a preselected degree of film blackening is produced (Fig. 10-16).

The increase in radiographic density that is associated with pulmonary emphysema resulting from hyperventilated lungs can cause the diaphragms to be pushed downward, and it may necessitate an exposure shorter than the minimal response time of the AED. Lowering of the kVp should be avoided, since this will cause the lungs to appear darker and osseous structures to be more prominent. Additionally, vascular details may be obscured and mediastinal structures not adequately penetrated.

A 400-speed screen film combination may require exposure times shorter than the minimal response time of the AED. The use of high kVp values, up to 150 kVp, further complicates this problem. An adjustment in mA can sometimes overcome the limitations of the minimal response time, as previously discussed in Chapter 2.

X-ray Film Latitude

It is difficult to adequately expose the lungs while simultaneously visualizing mediastinal anatomy. If structures are adjacent to tissues of differing densities they will be visible on the radiograph. For example, the cardiac shadow is easily visualized because it is silhouetted against the lung fields. The dense blood-filled heart, however, is similar in radiopacity to the descending aorta and thoracic spine. These structures are imaged on conventional radiographic film at or near the toe of the sensitometric curve (Figs. 10-17 through 10-

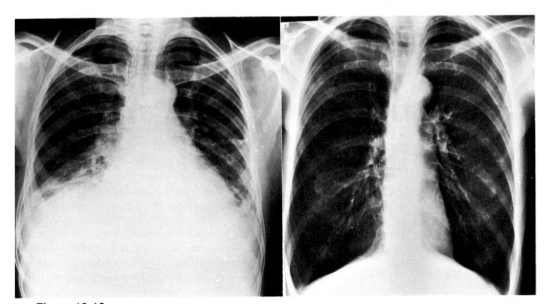

Figure 10-16
The Effect of Pathology on the Radiographic Image
Pathologic changes can influence radiographic density. (Left) A chest radiograph of a patient in congestive heart failure reveals bilateral pleural effusion. Note the prominent pulmonary vessels in the hila and upper lung fields. (Courtesy of Thompson TT: Primer of Clinical Radiology. Boston: Little, Brown and Company, 1973)

(Right) A second chest image is shown of a patient with pulmonary emphysema. Note the elongation of the heart causing a disproportionate cardiothoracic ratio. Nipple shadows can be seen in both lung fields. A nipple localization technique is described in this chapter. (Courtesy of the Department of Radiology, Rochester General Hospital, Rochester, NY)

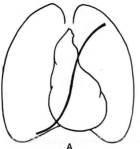 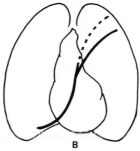 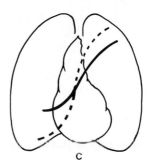

A　　　　　　　　　B　　　　　　　　　C

Figure 10-17
Sensitometric Representation of Chest Films
Sensitometric representations of three types of radiographic films for the chest are illustrated. (A) A high-contrast film will image vascular details within the darkened lung fields but will often fail to demonstrate mediastinal structures (imaged near the toe of the sensitometric curve). (B) A latitude x-ray film can be used to reduce film blackening of the radiograph in the areas of the lungs. The dashed extension of the curve represents the high-contrast film (A). (C) An extended latitude film will also minimize blackening of the lung fields. Note the filled-in toe of the sensitometric curve, which permits imaging of the mediastinal structures without an increase in x-ray exposure to the patient. The dashed line represents the high-contrast film (A). Extended latitude film was designed specifically for chest radiography because it provides an extended scale of contrast. This type of film or latitude film (B) is recommended with a high kVp technique for chest radiography. It is not recommended for iodinated contrast studies or osseous evaluation. (See Chapter 6 for dual-receptor, zero-crossover chest imaging technology.)

19), where very little separation of the superimposed tissues can be demonstrated.

A compensatory filter is often used in an attempt to overcome these differences in tissue density (see Fig. 10-18). Filters are used as close to the x-ray source as possible and are usually mounted on the external tracks of the collimator. Most filters used for chest radiography differ from wedge or trough filters by having an opening in the center to permit the full x-ray exposure to penetrate the dense mediastinum while attenuating the radiation used to image the lung fields. Since the opening in the filter is a predetermined size, it cannot match the mediastinal configuration of every patient examined. A filter has not been designed that can accommodate the narrow cardiac silhouette often associated with the emphysematous chest as well as the enlarged heart (see Fig. 10-16), fluid in the lung, or a pulmonary mass (see Fig. 10-18).

To solve this dilemma, sensitometric characteristics of x-ray film have been modified specifically for chest radiography, eliminating the need for compensatory chest filters. The use of an extended latitude film with a sensitometrically "filled-in toe" can help to demonstrate the air–soft tissue interface of the mediastinum (Fig. 10-20). A conventional, high-contrast sensitometric curve is compared to latitude and extended latitude sensitometric curves in Figure 10-17. For conventional chest radiography, new dual-receptor, zero-crossover intensifying screens and film are recommended. (See Chapter 6, Fig. 6-10.)

Horizontal Beam Technique

Most x-ray tube stands and ceiling-mounted cranes permit rotation and angulation of the x-ray tube for horizontal beam projections.

A horizontal beam technique is often used to advantage to evaluate the chest (Fig. 10-21), sinuses, or abdomen. Fluid in the thorax as well as in the sinuses and hollow viscera will "level" with the floor when the patient is placed in the erect or decubitus position. Horizontal beam studies of the chest or abdomen can also demonstrate free air under the diaphragm, which may be due to either a ruptured hollow viscera or a penetrating wound of the abdomen.

If the patient cannot be placed in the full upright position, the x-ray beam should still be positioned horizontal to the floor to demonstrate an air–fluid level. The x-ray tube should not be angled perpendicular to the semi-elevated patient if a fluid level must be demonstrated (see Chapter 4, Fig. 4-10). With a transverse measurement of 14 inches, a dedicated chest unit can accommodate

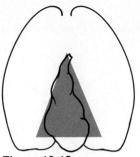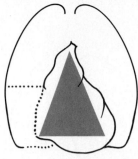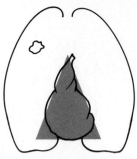

Figure 10-18
A Compensatory Filter for Demonstrating Mediastinal Densities

It is difficult to produce adequate film blackening in the mediastinal area with conventional postero-anterior chest techniques without overexposing the lung fields. A compensatory filter is occasionally used to image the mediastinum. Metallic or lead-acrylic filters, shaped to conform to a typical postero-anterior chest configuration, are used in the external tracks of a collimator. The filter shown permits 100% of the x-ray generated to pass through its central opening. The filter material holds back one half, or more, of the x-radiation to avoid overexposure of the lungs.

A single-size opening in a filter is not adequate for all types of body habitus or disease processes. (A) With an emphysematous chest, the opening in the filter does not permit proper exposure of the inferior portion of the heart. (B) When an enlarged heart is evaluated with this filter, much of the cardiac silhouette extends beyond the filter opening. In this example, there is a significant amount of fluid in the right lung, which requires additional penetration rather than filtration of the x-ray beam. (C) Even if the opening in the filter were to match the mediastinal configuration, a lesion in the right upper lung may not be adequately penetrated by the x-ray beam.

Most filters of this type require a twofold or greater increase in the amount of exposure ordinarily needed for a conventional posteroanterior chest image to adequately penetrate the mediastinum.

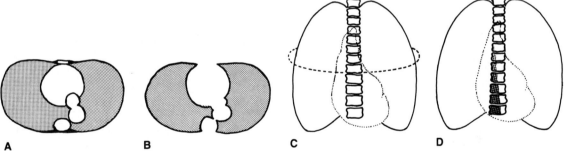

A   B   C   D

Figure 10-19
Mediastinal Air–Soft Tissue Interface

With conventional radiographic film, mediastinal air–soft tissue interfaces are difficult to demonstrate because of sensitometric limitations (see Fig. 10-17). The mediastinal structures approximate the absorption characteristics of the abdomen.

(A, B) A transverse anatomic section of the chest is illustrated; the lung fields are shaded. In a posteroanterior examination, the x-ray beam enters the posterior portion of the thorax and passes through the ascending aorta and the blood-filled muscular heart, exiting through the sternum. Note the amount of air in the right lung field, behind the heart, anterior to the thoracic vertebrae. The lung fields only are outlined in B. The transverse section is represented by the dashed line in C.

(C, D) When evaluating a conventional posteroanterior chest image, some radiographers suggest that the vertebral bodies should be visible through the dense cardiac silhouette. As the heart widens at its inferior portion, the vertebral bodies and interspaces are more difficult to visualize. Aerated lung tissue behind the heart, adjacent to the soft tissue structures (air–soft tissue interface), should be visible within the mediastinum. Since there is lung tissue on the right side of the chest between the heart and thoracic spine, more x-radiation should pass through the aerated lung, imaging the right side of the vertebral bodies to a greater degree than the left (D). This air–soft tissue interface is difficult to demonstrate because it is imaged near the toe of the sensitometric curve with conventional x-ray film. The use of an extended latitude x-ray film helps to overcome the differences between the aerated lungs and the dense mediastinum. (See Fig. 10-20 and Chapter 6, Fig. 6-10, for dual-receptor, zero-crossover chest imaging technology.)

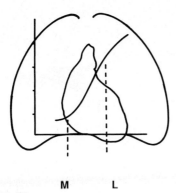

M   L

Figure 10-20
Sensitometric Characteristics of
an X-ray Film Designed for Chest Radiography

A schematic of a chest x-ray is superimposed on a sensitometric curve. The vertical axis illustrates increased density; the horizontal axis illustrates increased exposure. Exposure is expressed logarithmically. M labels the portion of the sensitometric curve that images the mediastinum; L labels the portion that typically images the blackened lung fields. Note that the mediastinum is imaged near the toe (inferior portion) of the sensitometric curve. The lungs are imaged in the ascending (straight line) portion of the curve. Density differences in the mediastinum should be better seen with this type of film because of the "filled-in" sensitometric toe.

the chest of most patients in the lateral position on a litter (Fig. 10-22).

Modifications of the horizontal beam technique have been developed to demonstrate free fluid within the thoracic cavity.*

The Effect of Patient Pathology

Special positions or projections are often required for certain disease processes. When free air is present in the pleural cavity as a result of a pneumothorax, there may be an absence of lung markings in the space between the visceral pleura and the parietal pleural. Air can enter the pleural space in several ways, for example, by a penetrating injury from a sharp edge of a fractured rib, a spontaneous pneumothorax, and so on. The presence of free air in the pleural space can cause a collapse of the lung.

Expiration radiography of the chest is indicated when a pneumothorax is suspected. A radiograph made during expiration in the lateral decubitus

Moller A: Pleural effusion, use of the semi-supine position for radiographic detection. Radiology 150:245–249, 1984; and Tocino IM: Pneumothorax in the supine patient: Radiographic anatomy. RadioGraphics 5:557–586, 1985.

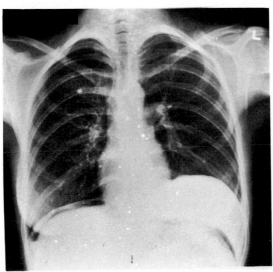
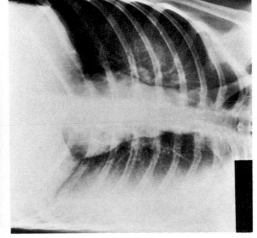

Figure 10-21
Horizontal Beam Radiography of the Chest

(Left) *A conventional posteroanterior chest film is made with the left diaphragm elevated. This increase in radiopacity in the left base represents fluid. (Right) The patient was placed in the lateral decubitus position, left side down, and the fluid gravitated to the dependent portion of the chest. The use of a horizontal beam projection enables a radiologist to differentiate between pleural thickening and free fluid. Note the presence of free air beneath the right diaphragm in both projections, due to the fact that these images were both made following recent abdominal surgery. (Courtesy of the Department of Radiology, Rochester General Hospital, Rochester, NY)*

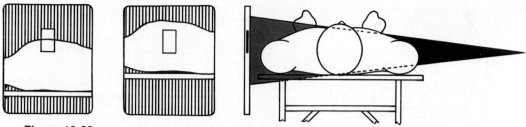

Figure 10-22
Horizontal Beam Radiography of the Chest of
a Recumbent Patient in the Lateral Position

When a patient cannot be moved from a litter for a lateral chest radiograph, a horizontal beam radiograph can be made with the patient appropriately positioned to the lateral sensor of an automatic exposure device. The chest should be positioned so that it covers the lateral sensor (center and right). If the chest is positioned so that a portion of the lateral sensor is struck by the primary beam (left), an underexposed radiograph will result, because the AED will prematurely terminate the exposure.

An x-ray tube mounted in the ceiling of a chest room can be used with a grid cassette for a supine study of the chest of a patient on a litter (see Chapter 4, Fig. 4-6).

position, with the suspected side elevated, can be helpful when evaluating the chest for a minimal pneumothorax. Owing to the effect of gravity, the elevated lung will pull away from the lateral chest wall.

IMPORTANT

Expiration images made for a minimal pneumothorax should be obtained using manual technical settings. If an AED were used, the predeter-

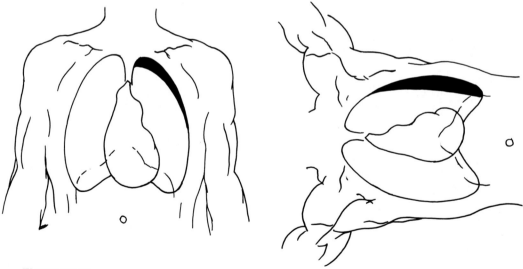

Figure 10-23
Demonstration of a Minimal Pneumothorax

(Left) On a schematic representation of the chest in the posteroanterior erect position, the blackened segment of the left lung represents a minimal pneumothorax; the space between the distal and parietal pleura is occupied by free air. (Right) A small pneumothorax is easier to visualize when the patient is placed in the lateral decubitus position with the suspected side elevated.

Radiographs should be taken on expiration, since free air trapped within the thorax will maintain its radiolucency while the lungs will become relatively radiodense. The use of an automatic exposure device with the expiration technique is not recommended, because an AED is calibrated to produce a preselected film blackening, which may mask a minimal pneumothorax.

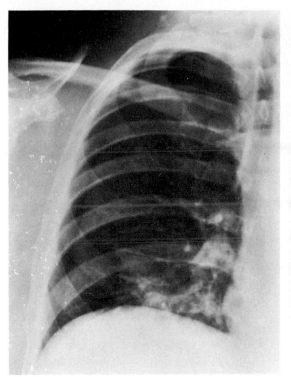 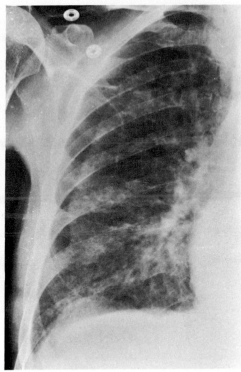

Figure 10-24
Pneumothorax vs. Skin Fold

(Left) *The right side of a chest is imaged at full expiration, demonstrating a pneumothorax. Note the lung has decreased in size and the diaphragm is elevated. There are no peripheral lung markings in the area of the collapsed lung. When a minimal pneumothorax is suspected a radiograph should be made at expiration in the lateral decubitus position with the suspected side elevated (see Fig. 10-23).*

(Right) *The right side of a chest is viewed with the patient in the anteroposterior supine position. Note the thickened edge of a posterior skin fold, caused as the patient was pulled across the table. (Courtesy of the Department of Radiology, Rochester General Hospital, Rochester, NY)*

mined density settings could mask a minimal pneumothorax (Figs. 10-23 and 10-24).

A skin fold may give the impression of a pneumothorax or pleural thickening (Fig. 10-24). Loose skin folds can produce this edge effect when a patient is moved across the tabletop. Breast shadows in younger patients can also simulate a pneumothorax.

An overexposed radiograph may be necessary to demonstrate the position of a pacemaker lead, to evaluate the battery of a pacemaker, or to determine the location of gastric tubes within the esophagus and superimposed on the mediastinum.

The nipples of a patient can simulate a pulmonary lesion (see Fig. 10-16). External markers should be applied to the chest before a repeat image is made to identify the nipple shadows. A paper clip straightened full length and then formed into a circle (approximately 1 in in diameter) can serve as a marker, with the nipple positioned in the center of the circle. If the suspected lesion is a nipple, it should appear in the center of the metallic ring on the repeat radiograph. Slightly oblique projections, 5 to 10 degrees, are also helpful, since a slight rotation of the thorax will cause a pulmonary mass to shift right or left in relation to the metallic ring. This localization technique can also be used to radiographically identify moles or warts on the surface of the body that may be projected into the lung fields and give the illusion of pulmonary lesions.

Occasionally lead shot is taped to a patient's skin to radiographically identify an area of in-

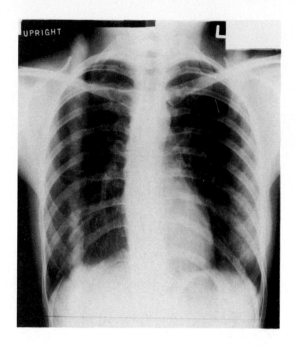

Figure 10-25
External Artifact on a Radiographic Image

Hair, ribbons, rubber bands, externally applied medications, oils, powder, or an excessive amount of deodorant may be imaged on a radiograph. In this posteroanterior chest film, hair braids are superimposed on the lung fields. The braids were concealed by the patient's gown and were not apparent to the radiographer. The right braid was anterior to the chest, in contact with the image receptor; the left braid was draped over the posterior chest (increased OFD). Although the braid on the right side of the chest is obvious, the braid artifact on the left side of the radiograph simulates a unilateral grid cutoff, owing to the increase in image blur associated with an increased OFD.

terest, for example, a suspected rib fracture or a mass.

IMPORTANT

Some patients are reluctant to remove any type of identification marker applied in a radiology department. The metallic markers, if left in position for an extended period of time, may break through the skin and cause an inflammatory process. It is important to remove localization markers from the patient's skin after it has been determined that the radiographs are technically acceptable.

Clothing artifacts can produce confusing radiographic densities. Some synthetic fibers can simulate the small, rounded opacities associated with pneumoconiosis. Flame-retardant children's sleepwear may produce radiographic artifacts because of changes in the surface properties of the fabric. Laundering processes, including starch, may also produce artifacts in clothing. These external artifacts should be considered when evaluating a radiograph. An artifact-free gown should be substituted for patient clothing.

Hair should be raised away from the shoulders to avoid extraneous shadows in the upper portions of the lungs (Fig. 10-25). Ribbons, rubber bands, externally applied medications, oils, powder, or an excessive amount of deodorant may also appear as external artifacts on the image.

Chapter 11

Dedicated Radiographic Equipment and Techniques

Although they may be routine procedures in many x-ray facilities, the procedures described in this chapter—stereoradiography, tomography, angiography, direct roentgen enlargement, and mammography—are specialized techniques.

Stereoradiography

Three-dimensional structures viewed on a two-dimensional radiograph lack depth, the third dimension. In order to produce radiographs that give the illusion of depth, two slightly different projections must be made. The patient must remain in exactly the same position for both exposures. These dual images, when viewed through a pair of lenses, form a three-dimensional image.

To produce a stereoscopic image, the tube is moved off-center a predetermined distance for the first exposure. After the first exposure but before the second, the tube is moved an equal distance past center in the opposite direction. The tube shift can be either manual or automatic. It is important that the tube shift be made in the direction of the grid lines to avoid grid cutoff (Fig. 11-1).

The interpupillary distance and the distance at

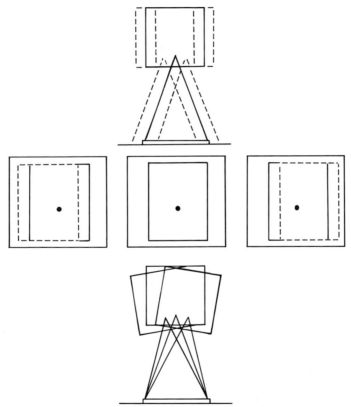

Figure 11-1
Tube Alignment for Stereoradiography

(Top) A three-dimensional effect can be produced with conventional radiography by shifting the x-ray tube off-center an equal distance between each exposure. The patient must remain in the same position for both exposures. To avoid grid cutoff when using a grid or Bucky, the tube must be moved from top to bottom, not from side to side. (Center) The shutter pattern must be elongated, or else tight beam collimation will result in image cutoff on both images. (Bottom) A slight tube tilt toward center for both exposures is recommended. (Courtesy Cullinan AM: Optimizing Radiographic Positioning. Philadelphia: JB Lippincott, 1992)

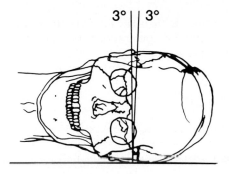

3° | 3°

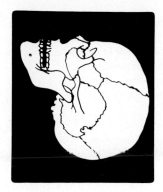

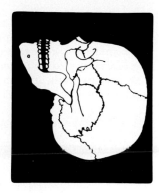

Figure 11-2
Stereoradiography

(Left) For stereoradiography of the skull in the lateral position, the x-ray tube is angled 3 degrees caudad and 3 degrees cephalad. (Center and right) When viewed, these images must be placed together sideways in the viewer to produce a three-dimensional effect. (Modified from Cullinan AM: Optimizing Radiographic Positioning. Philadelphia: JB Lippincott, 1992)

which stereo images are viewed are directly related to the degree of stereo shift and the FFD.

$$\frac{\text{interpupillary distance}}{\text{viewing distance}} = \frac{\text{tube shift}}{\text{FFD}}$$

The distance between the pupils of the eyes is approximately 2.5 inches; the viewing distance for stereoradiography is usually about 25 inches. This is a 1:10 ratio. If a 40-inch FFD were used, the total tube shift required would be 4 inches—2 inches to either side of the midline. For chest images taken at a 72-inch FFD, a total tube shift of 6 inches (or 3 inches to either side, up and down) is required.

Stereo images must be simultaneously viewed on a special stereoscopic viewer in which the images are reflected by a mirror system. The mirrors are arranged so that each eye sees only one image (Figs. 11-2 and 11-3). The brain converts both images into a single image, giving the illusion of depth.

Stereoradiographs are used to separate superimposed anatomic structures. Tomography is another radiographic method used to radiographically separate anatomic structures.

Tomography

Tomography is the generic term selected by the International Commission of Units and Standards to designate all systems of body section radiog-

raphy. Tomography is derived from the Greek word *tomos*, meaning a cut or section. This type of sectional radiography should not be confused with computed tomography (CT), discussed in Chapter 12.

Planigraphy, stratigraphy, and laminography are other terms used to describe radiographic studies in which radiographic equipment is used to blur out superimposed body structures on a radiograph. Conventional tomography can be linear as well as pluridirectional.

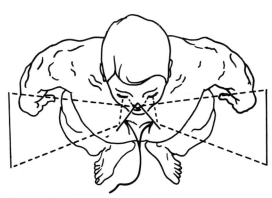

Figure 11-3
Viewing Stereoradiographs

A stereoscope contains lenses, prisms, and mirrors. The radiographs should be placed on the stereo viewboxes in the same position as they were made. The right eye views the radiograph taken with tube shift to right of center; the left eye views the radiograph taken with tube shift to left of center, and the brain forms a single three-dimensional image.

A typical tomographic unit is connected mechanically to an adjustable fulcrum. The fulcrum can be moved to a predetermined level known as the *focal plane* prior to the making of an exposure. This permits levels of the body to be selected for tomographic evaluation. The tube moves in op-

TUBE

10°

40°

CASSETTE

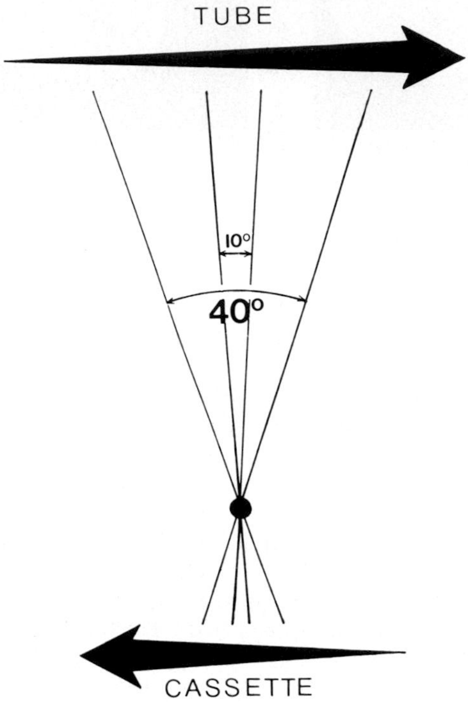

Figure 11-4
Basic Concept of Linear Tomography

The x-ray tube and radiographic cassette move in opposite directions during linear tomography. The black dot *in this illustration represents the pivot point or fulcrum of the x-ray beam. The position of this fulcrum determines the focal plane. The exposure angle determines the thickness or thinness of cut. An increased exposure angle of 40 degrees represents a thin cut, approximately 1 mm in thickness. The narrow exposure angle of 10 degrees represents a thicker cut, approximately 1 cm in thickness.*

Tomographic exposure angles of 10 degrees or less result in zonograms. The tube and cassette move in straight parallel lines and, as a result, shadows of rodlike objects parallel to the direction of the tube motion may not be completely erased. Rodlike structures above or below the focal plane will produce parasitic linear streaks (see Figs. 11-7, 11-8, and 11-14). Streaking can be minimized if the tube–cassette motions cross the long axis of the structure at right angles, or in some tangential fashion (see Fig. 11-8).

posing directions to the x-ray film. Electronic systems using microcomputer principles eliminate the need for mechanical linkage.

Terminology

In order to discuss tomography, the terms commonly used as imaging parameters should first be described.

TUBE-FILM OR TUBE-CASSETTE TRAJECTORY. The moving of the x-ray tube and cassette in opposite directions blurs superimposed anatomic details above and below the focal plane (Fig. 11-4). Any structure that is positioned parallel to the motion of the tube and film is difficult to blur out.

Several tube-film trajectories are possible (Fig. 11-5): linear, circular, and pluridirectional.

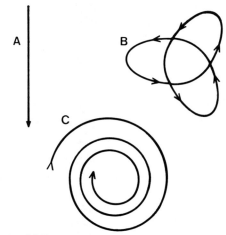

A   B

C

Figure 11-5
Typical Tube–Cassette Movements

Several types of tube–cassette travel patterns are used for tomography, the most popular being linear (A). The radiographic tube is made to move in a linear direction and the cassette in the opposite direction, about a pivot point or fulcrum. The more complex the tube–cassette trajectory, the better the separating capacity (cleanliness of cut).

One of the first complex pluridirectional devices used the hypocycloidal movement (B). This motion has an asymmetric cloverleaf trajectory, about five times longer than a linear path. The descending spiral pattern (C) is an elongated motion that provides an increased exposure angle with improved separating capacity. Some other types of tube–cassette patterns include eliptical, circular, and sinusoidal.

1. The trajectory is linear when the tube and film move in parallel lines (see Fig. 11-4). With linear motion, the long axis of an anatomic structure will not blur out, and striations or linear artifacts may appear in the tomographic image (Figs. 11-6 to 11-8). Even structures out of the focal plane may not be completely erased. When using a linear tomographic unit, the body part should be positioned so that its long axis is not parallel to tube-film motion. The tube-film motion should cross the long axis of the area under study at a right angle or at least in some tangential fashion (see Fig. 11-8).

2. A circular motion is used to minimize phantom imaging (see definition of separating capacity). Occasionally a small circular anatomic structure within the patient will appear as a larger circular phantom image on the radiograph.

3. Complex pluridirectional motions produce a better blur effect with less phantom imaging when compared with linear tomographic motion. Some pluridirectional motions include circular, elliptical, spiral, and hypocycloidal. Long exposure times, from 6 to 9 seconds, are required for complex tube-film patterns (see Fig. 11-5). Pluridirectional tomographic units may also be used to produce linear tomographic images.

All tube film patterns produce some type of phantom imaging artifact. As complex tube patterns such as hypocycloidal motion are used, the probability of phantom imaging is reduced but never completely eliminated. The anatomic structure to be imaged influences the type of tube-film trajectory selected.

OBJECTIVE PLANE. This is the plane in which all points of a radiographic image or section will be sharply imaged by the image receptor. It is the plane of maximal focus in a tomogram (Fig. 11-9).

FOCUS PLANE DISTANCE. This is the distance between the x-ray source and objective plane, also known as the source plane distance.

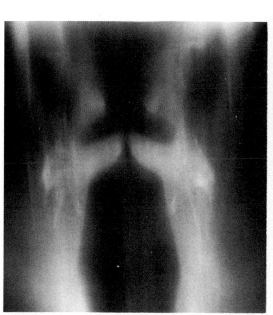
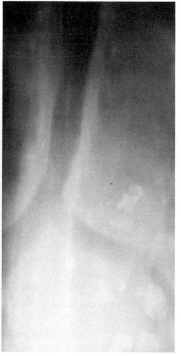

Figure 11-6
Linear Sections of the Larynx and Trachea

(Left*) A linear tomographic section of the larynx was made at a 20-degree exposure angle. Parisitic streaks are minimized by the shortened tube–cassette trajectory. (*Right*) An extended exposure angle of 40 degrees was used to image the trachea and mainstem bronchi.*

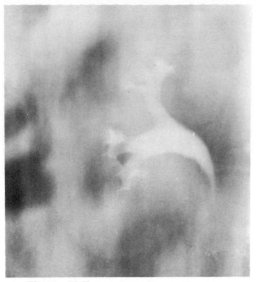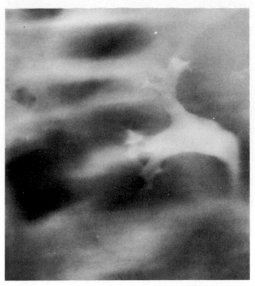

Figure 11-7
Streaking Artifacts Associated with Linear Tomography

Poor separating capacity often occurs with linear tomography. The structures above and below the focal plane, particularly those parallel to the tube–cassette motion, can never be completely obliterated. (Left) With the patient in the supine position, a linear tomographic section was made with the x-ray tube and cassette moving lengthwise (top to bottom) to the kidney. (Right) The patient was repositioned so that the linear tube–cassette motion would cross the kidney. Linear streaking is again demonstrated parallel to the tube–cassette trajectory. Complex pluridirectional motions minimize phantom imaging and thus improve separating capacity. (See Fig. 11-8E.)

IMPORTANT

This plane should not be confused with the term focus object distance (objective plane), since the plane of interest could be at any depth within the object.

PLANE FILM DISTANCE. The plane film distance is defined as the difference between the objective plane and the detector as determined by the position of the fulcrum and the image receptor.

FOCAL FILM DISTANCE (FFD). The focal film distance, the distance between the x-ray source and the detector, can also influence the thickness of a tomographic section. In practice, the FFD is rarely changed. If the FFD were decreased, the exposure angle would increase (Fig. 11-10).

SEPARATING CAPACITY. Separating capacity is defined as "cleanliness of cut." Complex tube-film trajectories have a greater effect on the separating capacity of the sections. The more complex the tube-film pattern, the greater the probability of reduced phantom imaging (see Fig. 11-5).

THICKNESS OF SECTION. The position of the fulcrum determines the layer to be sectioned. The

thickness of the section is controlled primarily by amplitude—the distance that the x-ray tube travels during the actual radiographic exposure.

IMPORTANT

The x-ray tube must be in motion before and after the exposure. Only the time in which an exposure is being made is considered amplitude. The longer the x-ray tube travels (during exposure), the thinner the tomographic section (Fig. 11-11).

EXTENDED-ANGLE TOMOGRAPHY. Extended-angle tomography uses an exposure angle of 40 to 50 degrees, whereas narrow-angle tomography (zonography) is achieved with an exposure angle of 10 degrees or less (Figs. 11-11 and 11-12). The thicker cut can be used to radiographically lift out thick layers of anatomy from their surroundings (Fig. 11-13). The thinner cut made with an extended exposure angle is used for definitive tomography (Figs. 11-14 and 11-15). For example, to tomographically evaluate the kidneys, a zono-

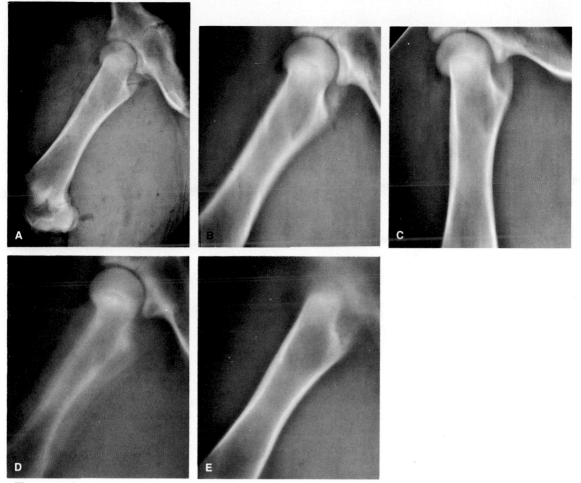

Figure 11-8
Comparison of Linear and Complex Pluridirectional Tomography

When evaluating tomographic motions for thinness or separating capacity, or both, a suitable phantom is required. A phantom composed of dried bones encased in plastic will produce adequate images with regard to resolution and sectional thickness, but unfortunately very little scatter radiation.

The phantom used in this illustration (bone, flesh, muscle, and other scatter-producing tissue) is the thigh of an animal. The femur measured approximately 12 inches in length, and the overall specimen, a processed ham weighing about 20 lb, was easy to handle. (A) A conventional radiograph of the ham exhibits good bony detail.

Four tomographic images using different tube–cassette motions were made. (B) A linear study of the thigh in abduction shows the relation of the head of the femur to the acetabulum. Note the parasitic streaking through the shaft of the out-of-focus femur. (C) The femur was then adducted so that it paralleled the tube–cassette motion pattern. It appears that the shaft of the femur is now in plane; however, this is not true. Since the femur is positioned in the direction of the tube–cassette motion, full erasure above and below the focal plane is not possible. Whenever a linear anatomic structure is visualized parallel to the tube–cassette motion, an accurate focal plane cannot be guaranteed. The radiographer may believe that the proper focal plane has been selected, and yet the information in the original conventional image that suggested the need for tomography may not be visible in the tomographic section. The tomographic study should be repeated with the tube–cassette motion crossing the long axis of the structure at a right angle or at least in some tangential fashion.

A hypocycloidal tube–cassette pattern was used for the remaining images. (D) With the focal plane still at the original level, a section was made. A phantom image (doubling effect) of the shaft of the femur is caused by the femur being out of plane. This type of artifact is associated with a hypocycloidal trajectory. (E) The focal plane was readjusted to a higher level in an attempt to place the shaft of the femur in sharp focus. Note the sharp cortex, the artifact-free medulla, and the absence of the head of the femur due to the excellent separating capacity of the hypocycloidal movement. The head of the femur appears to have been surgically excised.

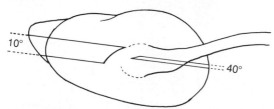

**Figure 11-9
Objective Plane: Extended-Angle Tomography vs. Zonography**

An extended-angle (40 degrees) tomographic study produces a relatively thin objective plane or section. Thin-cut sectioning is used for definitive tomography. The increased amplitude used with extended-angle tomography produces a thin objective plane with maximal blur above and below the area being examined. With linear tomography, the extended tube angle produces parasitic streaking.

The zonographic cut (10 degrees or less) yields a relatively thick section, approximately 1 cm across. A thick cut is used to lift out thick layers of anatomy from their surroundings (see Figs. 11-14 and 11-16). With linear zonography, the narrow-angle study results in less parasitic streaking than the thinner section and a higher degree of radiographic contrast, since less tissue is being exposed to x-radiation (see Fig. 11-11).

graphic cut would produce a layer thickness of approximately 1 cm, a gross radiographic specimen. An extended-angle cut would produce a layer of approximately 1 mm, a radiographic biopsy (see Figs. 11-9, 11-14, and 11-15).

Multiple sections may be needed to completely image an area of pathology (Figs. 11-15 to 11-17).

Basic Technical Considerations

Dosage

Tomographic studies require an increase in exposure factors. One practical method of reducing radiation exposure to the patient is the use of rare-earth imaging systems, 400 speed or greater. When examining the skull, particularly in the anteroposterior position, there is the risk of a cataractogenic radiation dose to the cornea. A radiation cataract can develop after an exposure of 200 rad. A protective eye lens shield made of lead glass with a roentgen ray absorption equivalent to 1 mm of lead is suggested for skull x-ray examinations. The glasses are transparent so that the pupils of the patient's eyes can be observed. The shield covers the eye lens for both the lateral and

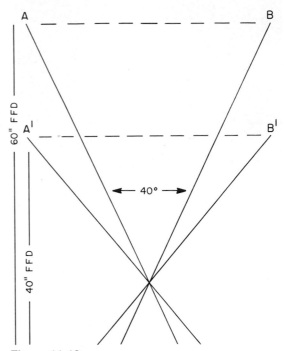

**Figure 11-10
Thickness of Section**

The thickness of a tomographic section is controlled primarily by amplitude. Amplitude describes the distance the x-ray tube travels during the actual radiographic exposure (from A to B, at a 60-inch FFD, and from A[1] to B[1] at a 40-inch FFD). The greater the amplitude, the thinner the cut; the lesser the amplitude, the thicker the cut. Note that tube travel is exactly the same in both examples at both focal film distances, A to B or A[1] to B[1]. When the FFD is lowered, the exposure angle is extended, even though the same amplitude is used. Increased amplitude and decreased FFD result in the thinnest possible cut.

anteroposterior projections, reducing lens dose to about 1/10th of that of a nonshielded study.* The disadvantage of an eye lens shield is that its use may result in pronounced parasitic streaks on a linear tomographic study.

Dosage to the lens of the eye can also be reduced by placing the patient in the prone position to allow primary radiation to enter the posterior portion of the skull and remnant radiation to exit through the eyes. The use of the posteroanterior projection approximates the dosage to the lens of

---

*For additional information on this technique see Bergstrom K, Hakan J: Eye lens-shield for the patient in diagnostic radiology. Australas Radiol 21:385–386, 1977.

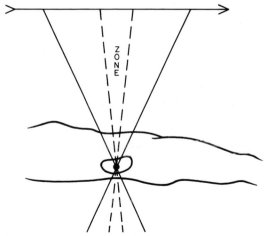

Figure 11-11
Extended-Angle Tomography vs. Zonography

An extended-angle tomographic section is represented as a solid line. With this increased amplitude, the exposure angle is increased and thinness of cut is maximized. With a narrow-angle tomographic section (zonogram), represented as a dashed line, a thicker cut results. A clinical example of extended-angle versus narrow-angle tomography is shown in Figure 11-14.

the eye attained when the anteroposterior projection is used with lens shielding (Fig. 11-18).

Tight beam collimation can lessen the dosage to surrounding tissues.

Contrast and Resolution

Tight beam collimation can minimize the effect of scatter radiation on radiographic contrast. Motion in the mechanical linkage of the equipment or voluntary or involuntary patient motion can affect recorded image detail.

Cassette Selection

The same screen film combination should be used, in the same type of cassette, when multiple consecutive exposures are made. If screens are mounted within cassettes at slightly different levels, they can create a focal plane problem, particularly during thin-section tomography. Cassette fronts can also vary in their x-ray absorption properties, thereby producing changes in radiographic density.

Multiscreen or book cassettes are sometimes used for simultaneous multilevel tomographic studies. These book cassettes hold from three to

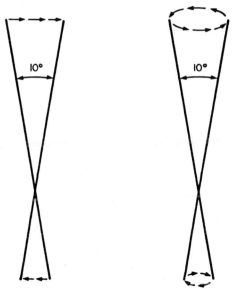

Figure 11-12
Zonographic Tube–Cassette Motion

Zonography is a form of narrow-angle tomograpy. Regardless of the type of tube–cassette motion, whether linear (left) or circular (right), zonography is accomplished with an exposure angle of 10 degrees or less. With the narrow exposure angle, a thicker layer is lifted from the body. Areas such as the facial bones can benefit from zonography. With linear zonography there is a reduction in parasitic streaking. The striations are shorter in length than those generated with extended-angle linear tomography. Zonography exhibits better radiographic contrast when compared with extended-angle tomography, since less tissue is exposed to primary radiation; with the narrow exposure angle, less scatter radiation is generated.

seven pairs of intensifying screens and are used to simultaneously expose three to seven sheets of x-ray film with a single exposure. These images are often of marginal quality, and this technique has not been well accepted. With kVp remaining constant, a seven-cut book cassette requires about two and one half times the mAs value of a single cut.

A special book cassette with four sets of intensifying screens, spaced approximately 1 mm apart, is known as a *plesiocassette*. The exact 1-mm spacing of the intensifying screen pairs in the plesiocassette produces four equidistant radiographic images with one exposure.

Intensifying screens used in book cassettes must be carefully balanced to produce comparable densities. For example, the first screen pair is very

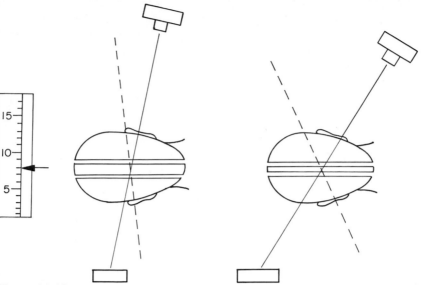

DECREASED AMPLITUDE   INCREASED AMPLITUDE

Figure 11-13
Amplitude and Thinness of Section

The shorter the travel of the x-ray tube during the x-ray exposure (decreased amplitude), the thicker the tomographic section. The longer the travel of the x-ray tube (increased amplitude) during the radiographic exposure, the thinner the tomographic section. (Left) With the fulcrum set at 8 cm from the tabletop to image the skull in the lateral position, a decreased amplitude of 20 degrees or less will result in a thick section. (Right) Increased amplitude of 40 degrees or greater will result in an extremely thin section.

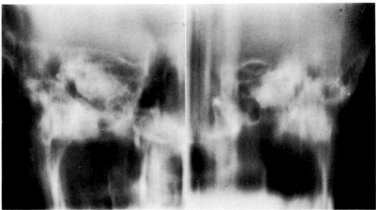

Figure 11-14
Tomography of the Petrous Ridge

Separate exposures were made of the petrous ridges to demonstrate extended-angle tomography (50 degrees) versus narrow-angle zonography (10 degrees). (Left) The entire petrous ridge is almost completely disengaged from the skull in the zonographic study. It has been radiographically removed from its surroundings. (Right) When a 50-degree exposure angle is used a thin, approximately 1.0-mm section is available for diagnosis. With this technique the hearing structures housed within the petrous ridge can be evaluated.

Zonography looks within the skull and lifts out the petrous ridge; increased-angle tomography looks within the petrous ridge, within the skull. Zonography represents a gross radiographic specimen; extended-angle tomography results in a radiographic biopsy.

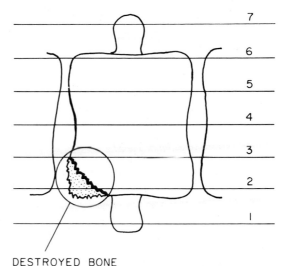

Figure 11-15
The Need for Multiple Sections

A 7-cm segment of the lumbar vertebra in the lateral position is used to demonstrate the need for multiple-section tomography. Unless an adequate number of sectional images are made, a questionable finding on a conventional image may be ignored because of an apparently normal tomographic study. The pathology in the lumbar spine would be demonstrated on section 2. If images were only made at levels 3 to 6, they would show normal bone and could be misleading.

DESTROYED BONE

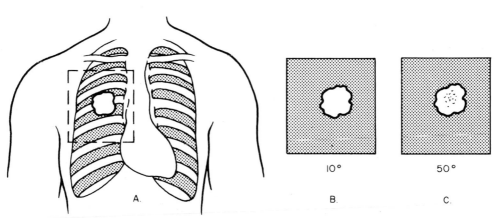

Figure 11-16
Narrow-Angle vs. Extended Tomography

The decision of thick or thin sections needs to be made before beginning a tomographic examination. (A) A chest image shows a lesion in the right lung, which requires tomography for additional diagnostic information. If one intends to simply erase the image details of other structures in the path of the beam, zonography is suggested. (B) With zonography, the lesion is lifted out of the chest as a relatively thick cut (approximately 1 cm). (C) If the internal composition of the lesion is to be evaluated, extended-angle tomography may be required. Note that the calcific flecks in the extended-angle cut are not visualized in the narrow-angle section (B).

The zonogram yields a full centimeter of tissue, whereas the extended-angle image demonstrates only a millimeter of tissue. If the chest measures 25 cm in the anteroposterior position, 25 zonographic cuts would be required to visualize the entire chest. If extended-angle tomography is used, 250 cuts would be required. Often, the number of radiographs is confused with the amount of information. Rather, it is important to evaluate the conventional radiograph prior to a tomographic study and to localize the area to be sectioned (see Fig. 11-20) to minimize dosage to the patient, examination time, and film usage.

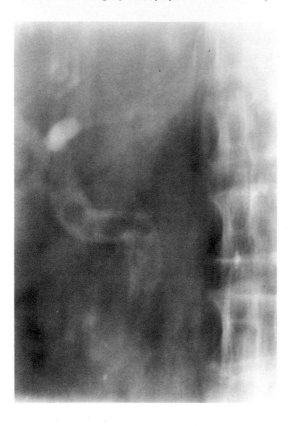

Figure 11-17
Tomographic Section of an Intravenous Cholangiogram

An extended-angle linear tomographic section was made of the biliary system after intravenous injection of an opaque contrast agent. Some linear parasitic streaks can be seen.

The common hepatic duct and the common duct are in good focus. Note the radiolucent defects within the opacified biliary system. Unfortunately, the distal end of the common duct, as it enters the ampula of Vater, is not in focus. Additional cuts must be made to visualize this portion of the anatomy. Often a radiolucent calculus will be lodged at the distal end of the common duct, producing a "check valve" effect. Because of the lower contrast level associated with an intravenous opaque medium, moderate to low kilovoltage must be used with high mAs values to produce radiographic contrast. Since this is a relatively thin section, radiographic contrast is further reduced. The x-ray beam has to traverse considerably more tissue for an extended-angle tomogram than for a conventional radiograph. Ultrasonography and computed tomograpy are more commonly used to evaluate the biliary system.

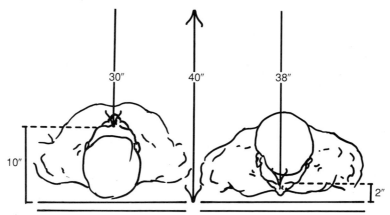

Figure 11-18
Patient Positioning for Dosage Reduction

Dosage to the lens of the eye can be reduced by placing the patient in the prone position (right), which allows primary radiation to enter the posterior skull, with remnant radiation exiting through the eyes. Not only is the FOD to the orbits increased in this position (38-in FOD), the primary beam is severely attenuated by the skull. In the anteroposterior position (left), the unattenuated x-ray beam enters the eyes at an approximate 30-in FOD.

slow, and the last screen pair is very fast. This variation in screen speed is not a problem with calcium tungstate screens; however, newer rare-earth screens, with their high absorption potential, are not practical for book cassette tomography. The first pair of rare-earth intensifying screens may absorb a high percentage of the primary beam, leaving little or no radiation available for the remaining screen pairs.

Patient Positioning and Level Determination

Body section radiography is often limited to the anteroposterior and posteroanterior positions. If a specific lesion is better demonstrated in a standard oblique or lateral position, the tomographic study should be made in that position.

For level determination a scout tomographic section should be made at what seems to be the appropriate level (Fig. 11-19). At the same time, a second section should be made either 2 cm in front of or behind the initial cut. Both scout radiographs should be viewed immediately. Two sections should be taken because even if the first section demonstrates that the lesion is in plane, one cannot be certain whether the tomographic cut was made through the center, anterior, or posterior segment of the lesion. Evaluation of the second scout image will help to determine if the lesion is in sharp or poor focus, or not in focus at all.

If the lesion is seen in both the frontal and lateral projections, level determination is relatively easy (Fig. 11-20).

The second section also serves another purpose, that of factor determination.

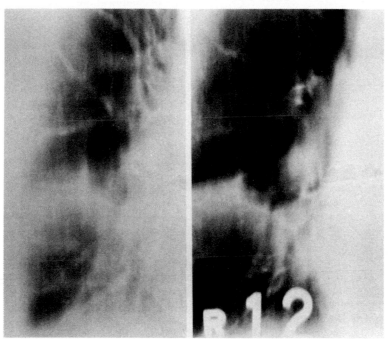

Figure 11-19
Level Determination and Technique for Tomography
Two scout images can often expedite a tomographic study. (Left) The first image is made at a predetermined level, such as 10 cm from the tabletop, with specific technical factors, for example, 55 kVp. (Right) The second scout is made either 2 cm above or below the level of the first image. A 12-cm section with a 10-kVp increase over the first image demonstrates a wedge-shaped area, sharply defined, in the parahilar region. Level determination can be more accurately established with successive sections being made on either side of the 12-cm level. Technical factors can be adjusted after comparing the densities of both scout images.

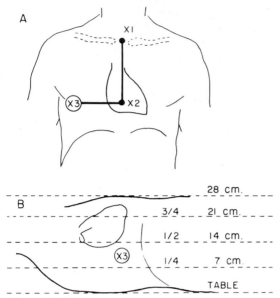

Figure 11-20
Tomographic Localization Technique

(A) *The lesion in question (×3) is seen at the lateral aspect of the right lung field on a posteroanterior chest radiograph. A wax crayon mark is made on the radiograph at the sternoclavicular joints (×1). A second mark (×2) is made in the midline at the level of the suspected lesion. These measurements are transferred to the chest of the patient. The chest is then measured at ×3, and in this example is found to be 28 cm in the frontal measurement. (B) On the lateral radiograph, which has been divided into four segments of 7 cm each, the lesion (×3) is localized in the second section, between 7 cm and 14 cm. Scout cuts are made at 9 cm and 11 cm for level determination. (See Fig. 11-19.)*

Factor Determination

There are some basic guidelines to be followed when formulating starting factors for body section studies. Zonographic sections use technical factors that approximate conventional exposures. For extended-angle tomography, the average section requires an approximate 50% increase in mAs over the conventional radiograph, if the original kVp is maintained. For example, if an intravenous urographic image required 70 kVp at 30 mAs, a tomographic sction at the same kVp would require 45 mAs.

Two technical decisions can be made from two scout radiographs: level determination and factor determination (see Fig. 11-19). The second scout image, 2 cm from the first scout, should be exposed at the same mAs value as the first scout, but with a 10 kVp increase. Making two exposures to

determine level and technique is preferable to making a series of over- or underexposed tomograms.

IMPORTANT

When conventional techniques are converted for tomographic studies, there should be no change made in the field size of the x-ray beam, the type of collimator used, the FFD, the grid ratio, or the speed of the screen film combination selected. Any variation in the aforementioned requirements would necessitate additional technical adjustments.

Angiography

Increased benefits to the patient by way of diagnostic information must be balanced against the risk of complications. Many radiographers work a lifetime in angiography and witness only a few complications; nevertheless, problems with contrast material, anesthesia, electrical and mechanical hazards must be considered. Hospital and departmental protocol for emergency care should be documented, posted, and made part of a continuing education program.*

Angiographic studies require the use of serial film or cassette changers to transport the film or cassettes when a series of radiographs are to be made in a short period of time (Fig. 11-21).

Serial angiograms are often exposed, alternately or simultaneously, in the anteroposterior and lateral planes to eliminate the problems created by vessel overlap. A distinct advantage of film changers or cassette changers is that both use large-size x-ray film. A major benefit with the biplane procedure is that only a single dose of a contrast medium is needed to image the vascular anatomy in both planes. However, simultaneous biplane exposures do compound the effect of scatter on the radiographic images.

Serial Film or Cassette Changers

A serial film study is made by exposing radiographs at predetermined intervals. If more than one radiograph per second is made, the procedure is known as a *rapid serial study.*

The scope of special vascular imaging technology is documented in Curriculum Guide for Special Vascular Imaging Technology. *Albuquerque, NM: American Society of Radiologic Technologists, 1978.*

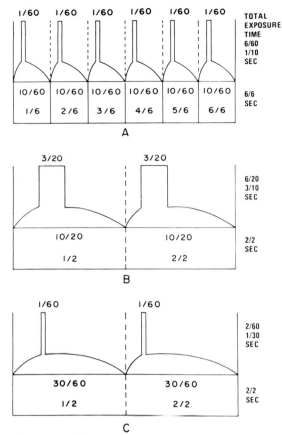

Figure 11-21
Exposure Rate per Second

Some angiographic studies are made at a rate of six to 12 frames per second. (A) When making six images per second with an exposure of 1/60th of a second, the total time of exposure is 6/60th of a second or 1/10th of a second. The delay between individual frames is 9/60th of a second. (B) When exposing two frames per second, with a time of 3/20th of a second, the total time of exposure is 3/10th of a second. The delay between exposures is 7/20th of a second. Compared with A, this delay between frames is 2 1/3 times longer. (C) If an exposure of 1/60th of a second is used to overcome motion in a two-frame-per-second study, the increased time delay between frames is 29/60th of a second. When compared with A, less information may be imaged. The radiographic detail in the individual frames will exhibit less image blur than those imaged in B.

Serial film and cassette changers include the following (Fig. 11-22):

Multiple cassette changer
Cut film changer
Roll film changer
Full-length cassette changer

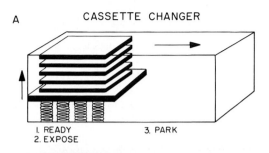

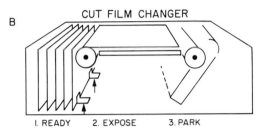

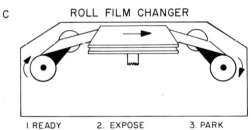

Figure 11-22
Serial Film and Cassette Changers

The basic mechanical concepts of serial cassette and film changers are illustrated. (A) A cassette changer holds 12 (11 × 14 inch) cassettes and can be operated as fast as two frames per second or as slow as one frame per two seconds. The cassettes have a thick layer of lead beneath the back intensifying screen to prevent the leakage of radiation to underlying cassettes. The cassettes are positioned on top of each other in a ready position and are elevated to an expose position by a spring-operated tray. When an exposure is made, a chain mechanism pulls the exposed cassette into a park chamber and the cycle is repeated. (B) Cut film changers use film magazines to hold 30 sheets of film (14 × 14 inch). Ejection fingers flip the film upward from the sending cassette into a pair of intensifying screens; the screens close and an exposure is made. After the exposure, the screens open and the film is transported into a receiving magazine. (C) Most roll film changers have a maximal exposure capability of six (11 × 14 inch) frames per second. A roll of film 60 feet in length can be advanced into a pair of intensifying screens and an exposure can be made. When the screens open, the film is advanced to a take-up roll. A 12-frames-per-second roll film changer is also available.

Multiple Cassette Changer

A multiple cassette changer uses large-sheet x-ray film (11 × 14 inches) with cassettes that are stacked in a "ready" position. There is extra-thick lead foil in the back of each cassette to minimize the "punch-through" of x-radiation to succeeding cassettes. If large field radiographs are made with this unit, there may be a slight penetration of the next cassette by an unattenuated primary beam when each exposure is made. For example, when an anteroposterior skull projection is made on film 1, part of film 2 may be exposed by the unattenuated frontal x-ray beam. When film 2 is processed, an outline of the skull may be seen, but the area where the Towne view of the skull should have been recorded will be clear. The skull acts as a primary beam shield, preserving the sensitized emulsion of the underlying frame from x-ray exposure. This faint outline of the skull is not a problem as long as the same position of the patient is maintained. When frame 2 is exposed, frame 3 receives an outline of the skull, and so on throughout the entire serial run.

IMPORTANT

If 12 cassettes are loaded into the exposure magazine and 6 are used for the anteroposterior study, when the unit is turned into the lateral position, frame 7 will have an outline of the frontal view of the skull. The lateral borders of the blackened anteroposterior film will superimpose on the lateral view of the first frame in the lateral series.

When an exposure is made, the cassette is pulled by a moving chain into a "park" position, and a spring mechanism elevates the next cassette to the "expose" position (see Fig. 11-22). The movement of these heavy cassettes can create a vibration in the unit. However, the unit has an excellent "dampening" effect and can be used without motion interference if a few simple precautions are observed. When the first film is exposed, the cassette leaves the expose position and falls into the park chamber. This rapid shifting of the heavy cassette causes the unit, the strap, and the patient's head to vibrate. The unit quickly dampens and motion ceases. Unfortunately, if the patient is strapped to the cassette changer, the head may still move.

The skull should not be strapped directly to the cassette changer in the anteroposterior mode. A radiolucent extension board should be used to support the head independently of the cassette changer during cerebral angiography. Any restraining devices should be attached to the extension of the radiographic table. The changer should then be raised into contact with the headboard.

A four-per-second exposure capability can be achieved using lightweight, 14 × 14 inch, carbon fiber–reinforced, vacuum-type cassettes. (A two-per-second changer [12-cassette maximum] was introduced about 50 years ago and is no longer in common use.) These cassettes can also be loaded with smaller size films for pediatric angiography or selective arteriography. Instead of using a typical rigid metal cassette that relies on some type of hinge or lock to achieve mechanical pressure, the vacuum cassette uses atmospheric pressure to produce exceptional screen film contact. The intensifying screen, film, and lead backing for the cassette are placed in the open end of a lightproof, black, plastic envelope that is sealed on three sides. In the darkroom, a vacuum sealing unit is used to create a vacuum in less than 5 seconds. The sealed, loaded cassettes, stacked in the changer, are elevated after each exposure is made. A push bar moves forward, thrusting the exposed top cassette into a pair of rollers that draw it into the adjacent receiving chamber. This process can be repeated about 20 times, up to 4 times per second. The size and overall rigidity of the units helps to eliminate vibration.

Any brand, speed, or combination of intensifying screens can be used with a vacuum cassette changer, which can be computer programmed to automatically control every phase of the operation. Exposures can be made, the power syringe triggered, and the tabletop moved automatically. The computer can vary exposure times, frame intervals between exposures, and kilovoltage settings.

Cut Film Changer

A cut film changer (see Fig. 11-22) uses a film magazine that is preloaded with 30 sheets of film in the darkroom before the angiographic study. When activated, a mechanical device advances the film from the preloaded magazine into a pair of intensifying screens. The screens close and an exposure is made. The exposed film is then advanced to a receiving cassette, which can be removed from the changer and taken to the darkroom for processing.

Each film in the loading magazine is separated by a wire frame. The magazine, with its lid and

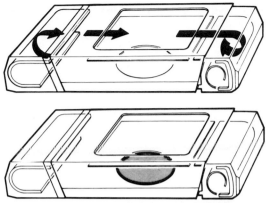

Figure 11-23
See-through Film Changer

(Top) Film is transported from the stack-loading magazine through the film changer, exposed, and collected in the receiving cassette. The compression system consists of a front compression plate of carbon fiber–reinforced plastic, intensifying screens, and a back compression table. This unit allows real-time exposure monitoring as well as video recording. (Bottom) A circular, 200-mm (8 inch) x-ray transparent opening in the center of the exposure field makes it possible to monitor the angiographic exposures (see Fig. 11-24). (Courtesy of Elema-Schonander, Schumburg, IL)

ports closed, is preloaded in the darkroom. It is inserted at the load position of the film changer with the receiving cassette of the unit in place. The tray on which the magazine rests is advanced electrically, automatically opening the lid of the magazine as it moves forward. Two levers enter the open small ports at the bottom of the magazine and flip a single film upward. The film is then conveyed into the opened screens. The screens close, an exposure is made, the film is carried into the receiving magazine, the levers flip another film into place, and the cycle is repeated.

The imaging sequence is controlled by a preprogrammed punch card. Films per second, injector activation, and longitudinal tabletop shift are accomplished with this program.

"See-through" film changers used with an image intensifier make it possible to leave the patient on the angiographic table for the fluoroscopic placement of a catheter (Figs. 11-23 and 11-24). The see-through film changer has an 8-inch center opening, which facilitates patient positioning, collimation of the primary beam, and observation on the television monitor of the injection of the contrast material. A videotape or video disc recorder can be used to immediately replay and evaluate the study.

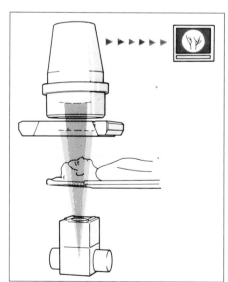
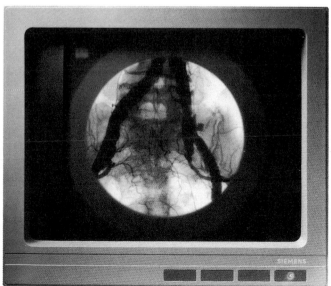

Figure 11-24
Real-time Angiographic Monitoring

A see-through film changer allows real-time monitoring of angiographic exposures. (Left) The film changer is aligned with the central x-ray beam. The video image shown is a 200-mm (8 inch) circular area. A 35 × 35 cm x-ray film is used in the changer (see Fig. 11-23). (Right) The correct position of the catheter and contrast medium flow can be observed during the exposure sequence. (Courtesy of Elema-Schonander, Shumburg, IL)

Roll Film Changer

In a roll film changer, a roll of x-ray film, usually 14 inches wide (and about 60 feet in length), is pulled through a pair of intensifying screens. Before each exposure, the screens open and the exposed film advances into a receiving magazine. The screens then close to maintain screen film contact and an exposure is made. The process is repeated as often as is necessary, up to six frames per second. The exposed films are taken to the darkroom in a take-up magazine (see Fig. 11-22). Fifty or more 11 × 14 inch images are possible per roll, although there is a loss of film when a new leader must be applied to the receiving magazine when scout films or short serial runs are exposed.

A biplane roll film changer is available that has an 8- or 12-frame-per-second capability. However, a distinct disadvantage of this system is that both units are permanently linked in an L-shaped form. The individual units cannot be separated or moved in any direction for tube angled techniques. Film loading must be performed in the x-ray room with the room lights off.

Full-Length Cassette Changer

Cassette changers holding four (14 × 51 inch) cassettes can be used to sequentially image the abdominal aorta and peripheral artery runoff. Traditionally, different speed-intensifying screens have been used in these cassettes to overcome differences in body part thickness. For example, if a 400-speed system were used to image the abdomen and a 100-speed system were used to image the distal extremities, the system would vary in speed from top to bottom by a factor of 4:1. This type of gradient compensatory screen has limited application because as portions of the system are reduced in speed, the patient receives more x-ray than is needed for adequate imaging of a specific part. The distal extremities in the aforementioned example receive approximately four times more radiation than is needed for proper imaging.

The use of a compensatory wedge filter, combined with up to a 1200-speed, rare-earth screen film combination is recommended for this procedure in place of compensatory screens (Figs. 11-25 and 11-26).

High-speed, rare-earth imaging systems provide additional benefits when used for angiography. The increased film blackening produced by these screens permits the use of smaller focal spots. Patient and vessel motion is minimized by

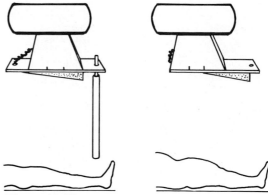

Figure 11-25
Compensatory Filter for Full-Length Arteriography
An aluminum wedge filter attached to a sheet of aluminum or plastic can be used during full-length arteriography to overcome tissue differences. (Left) The wedge filter can be moved within the track of a cone or collimator by using a dowel inserted in an opening in the filter base. A cord or some type of security device is required to keep the filter from sliding out of the track. (Right) With a larger patient, the wedge filter can be moved toward the feet to allow the unattenuated beam to expose a thicker abdomen or thighs. (Courtesy of Eastman Kodak Company)

the use of shorter exposure times, and more frames per second may be possible.

Many new angiographic tables have a stepped moving top that allows the table to be moved in longitudinal increments during a runoff study.

The movement of the table and appropriate changes in exposure factors are controlled by a preprogrammed punch card. Films per second, injector activation, and tabletop shift are automatically accomplished.

Some Technical Considerations

Some difficulties are common to all serial film or cassette changers.

THE CAPACITY OF THE X-RAY TUBE. This can be a limitation when serial angiographic studies are performed. The selection of an appropriate focal spot to improve radiographic detail as well as a short exposure time should be made only after tube ratings have been considered. Also, some generators are inadequate for serial changer use in terms of the maximal exposure length per cycle. The output of new equipment must be determined and then weighed against the maximal exposure length per cycle of a new or existing film or cassette changer.

CONTROL OF SCATTER RADIATION. This is the most significant technical difficulty encountered with simultaneous biplane angiographic techniques. The relation of the internal collimator shutters to a keyhole diaphragm or an extension cone attached to the collimator must also be considered (Fig. 11-27).

GRID SELECTION FOR ANGIOGRAPHY. The selection of a proper grid for a serial changer should be discussed with a manufacturer's representative. When working in a single plane and using a perpendicular x-ray beam, a cross-hatch grid may be advantageous over a linear grid. For example, many changers are equipped with a 12:1 ratio linear grid with a focal range of 36 to 40 inches. This means that in any study attempted with this unit, the radiographer must use the 12:1 ratio focused grid, whether the study is a pediatric angiogram or an adult abdominal aortogram in the lateral position. The result: too much grid for the infant, perhaps not enough grid for a large adult. If an 8:1 ratio aluminum interspaced grid is used as the basic grid in the serial changer, then a second

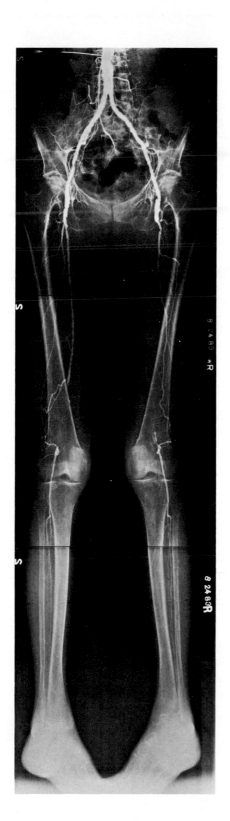

◀ **Figure 11-26**
Full-Length Arteriography

Sequential imaging of the abdominal aorta and the arteries of the lower extremities is possible with a cassette changer that holds four 14 × 51 inch cassettes. Because of the differences in tissue thickness from the abdomen to the ankles, a variety of techniques have been developed to balance the densities.

Different speed intensifying screens (e.g., from speed 400 to 100) can be used to overcome differences in patient thickness. High-speed, rare-earth screens are used for the dense abdominal area and a slower speed screen for the ankles. The distal extremities receive up to four times more x-radiation than needed for adequate film blackening.

Better than gradient screens is a compensatory filter (see Fig. 11-25). The vascular study shown in this illustration was made with a single exposure using a leaded-acrylic compensatory filter mounted in the external tracks of a collimator. A technique adequate for abdominal radiography was used. The design of the wedge filter determines the amount of x-radiation permitted to proportionally expose the lower extremities. With this technique, each segment of anatomy received the amount of x-ray needed for proper exposure. (Courtesy of Nuclear Associates, division of Victoreen, Carle Place, NY)

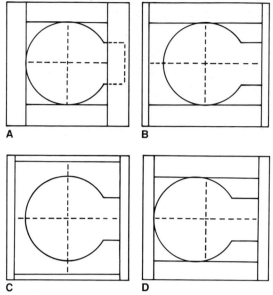

A   B

C   D

Figure 11-27
Collimator Shutter Adjustment to Keyhole Aperture

The relation of the shutters of the collimator to a keyhole aperture mounted in the external tracks of the collimator can contribute to increased scatter radiation on the image. A dashed line *cross hair is used to indicate the position of the central ray for a lateral cerebral angiographic image with the patient in the supine position. The keyhole is configured to image the vault of the skull and the neck. The central ray is directed to the area of the sella turcica on A, B, and C. When the shutters are restricted to the circle opening in the keyhole, the cervical area is not imaged (A). If the shutters are opened to include the neck, the opposing shutter is also open, since they work in synchrony (B). Since the keyhole functions as the final shutter in the collimator, the internal shutters could be completely open with only the keyhole being used to restrict the beam (C).*

If the central ray is directed 1 to 1 1/2 inches inferior to the sella turcica, all shutters are optimally used (D). Before an exposure is made the shutters should be adjusted so that they are visible at the edges of the illuminated circle of the keyhole diaphragm.

overlay grid such as a 5:1 ratio or 6:1 ratio grid could be used for a cross-hatch effect. Fiber interspaced grids are usually acceptable in the cross-hatch mode, since defects in one grid are often obliterated in the weave pattern created by the other grid. The combination of 8:1 ratio and 5:1 ratio is equal to, or better than, the scatter cleanup capability of a 12:1 ratio linear grid.

Some benefits of a cross-hatch combination include:

1. The linear 8:1 grid can be used without the overlay grid at moderate kilovoltage levels for tube angle techniques.
2. The increased focal film range helps the radiographer overcome the FFD variations associated with tube angle techniques required for patients with short necks or a severe kyphosis (see Table 5-1).
3. An 8:1 grid permits reduced exposures for pediatric angiography.
4. The cross-hatch combination can be used to clean up the increased scatter generated by larger patients.
5. The lower ratio linear grid can be used with smaller field sizes in selective and subselective studies.

Simultaneous Biplane Techniques

Regardless of the type of collimator or grid used, there is a considerable increase in film density due to the scatter radiation generated with biplane procedures (Figs. 11-28 and 11-29). In general, if an adequate biplane study has been made and a single repeat examination is needed, an increase in technical factors may be required to overcome the density effect generated by biplane cross-fogging. Occasionally, a biplane examination will be made of the abdominal aorta, and the lateral projection will be used only during the aortic opacification stage. The images in the biplane mode are technically adequate until the study reverts to single plane operation. If the anteroposterior single plane is adequately exposed, the anteroposterior images made in a biplane mode will frequently be overexposed owing to the increase in scatter radiation from the lateral exposure.

Cross-fogging of film with simultaneous biplane angiography also results in more scatter per image when compared with a single plane study. Each film in each frame is exposed to the scatter radiation from both exposures. Even when every effort is made to use a moderate kilovoltage range, tight collimation of the primary beam, and high ratio grids, the cross-fogging still occurs. The scatter radiation generated in the anteroposterior and lateral planes is easily absorbed by the cross-hatch grid in the lateral plane. In the lateral position there is an air gap, which provides additional scatter cleanup. Unfortunately, the linear grid in the anteroposterior plane is often unable to absorb the

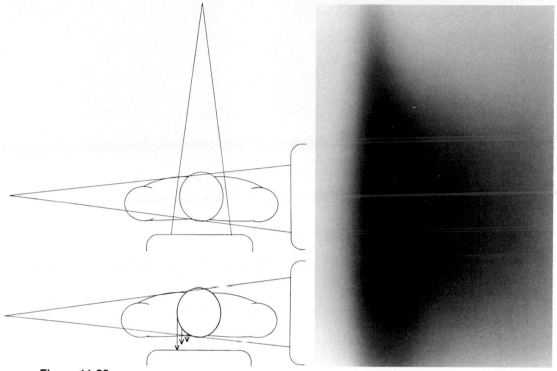

Figure 11-28
Biplane Angiographic Studies

(Top left) When a simultaneous biplane angiographic study is performed, an increase in density may be noted on the anteroposterior radiograph. The density decreases in intensity from the entrance beam side of the lateral tube. (Bottom left) To determine the amount of scatter generated on the anteroposterior image by the lateral beam, a simple test can be performed. A phantom is positioned for simultaneous anteroposterior and lateral projections. With both serial changers running simultaneously, only a lateral exposure is made. (Right) Note the wedgelike scatter on the anteroposterior frame, wider at the entrance point of the lateral beam but diminished in intensity towards the center of the frame. The radiographic density that appears on the anteroposterior image is due to scatter from the lateral exposure (see Fig. 11-29).

With a biplane cut film changer study, an alternate load–alternate exposure biplane technique will avoid cross-fogging of the radiographic films. The frontal magazine should be loaded with film in frames 1, 3, 5, 7, and so on; the lateral magazine is programmed with film in frames 2, 4, 6, 8, and so on. When the study is performed, film 1 is exposed in the anteroposterior frame; no film is in the lateral changer at this point. Film 2 is then exposed in the lateral changer, with no film in the anteroposterior frame, and so on. Alternate loading will eliminate biplane scatter problems.

scatter generated in both planes. Particularly disturbing is the density increase across the anteroposterior plane created by scatter from the lateral beam. With the left lateral study, the x-ray beam enters the right side of the patient's head and exits from the left side to expose the film in the lateral changer. The anteroposterior radiograph will exhibit a decreasing wedge of density from the right to the left side of the image. The placement of a primary beam attenuator on the outer aspect of

the frontal changer can help to minimize this density effect (Fig. 11-30).

One example of the effect of scatter generated by the lateral beam can be seen in Figure 11-28. The single frame was taken from the anteroposterior changer, which was run simultaneously in the biplane mode with the lateral changer. Only the lateral x-ray tube was energized for a conventional scout image. The wedge density pattern, wide at the beam entrance and diminishing across the

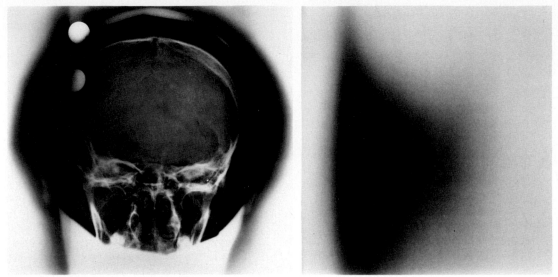

Figure 11-29
Biplane Leak

Scatter can be generated in the anteroposterior plane by the lateral beam. (Right) Note the wedgelike scatter, wide at the entrance point of the lateral x-ray beam and diminished toward the center of the frame. Both changers were energized simultaneously in the biplane mode, but only the lateral tube was used to make an exposure. (Left) A simultaneous biplane exposure demonstrates a density increase on the right side of the skull.

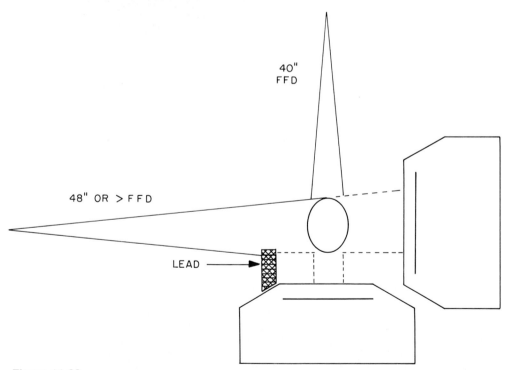

Figure 11-30
Difficulties with Scatter During Biplane Serial Cerebral Angiography

Although cross-hatch grids may be used with the lateral projection during cerebral angiography, a linear grid is required for the anteroposterior tube-angled projection. There is often an increase in density across the anteroposterior image, decreasing from the tube side to the lateral changer (see Fig. 11-29). Placing a primary beam attenuator on the tube side of the frontal changer restricts the inferior portion of the lateral primary beam. The lead must be carefully placed to avoid cutting off the posterior segment of the skull in the lateral view. Elevating the head on a radiolucent sponge reduces the effect of scatter (see Fig. 11-31).

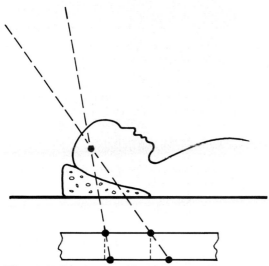

Figure 11-31
The Towne Projection and the Parallax Effect

The parallax effect can be lessened considerably by reducing the caudad angulation of the x-ray tube. The black dot *represents a radiographic detail within the skull. Note the separation of the image when an increased tube angle is used. If a fractional focal spot (0.3 mm) or small focal spot (0.6 mm or less) is available, the patient's skull can be elevated on a 15-degree radiolucent sponge and the tube angle decreased. A larger focal spot cannot be used with this technique.*

frame, was formed by the scatter generated from the lateral x-ray beam. Scatter from the anteroposterior skull study produced by both the lateral and anteroposterior beams can be reduced by elevating the head on a radiolucent sponge to form an air gap (Fig. 11-31). The lateral beam must also be adjusted to a higher level. To overcome magnification in the lateral position, the lateral tube can be moved to a 48- or 72-inch FFD, with an appropriate increase in technical factors.

During operation of cut film changers, cross-fogging can be eliminated by alternate loading of the film magazines. The magazine frames 1,3,5,7, and so on can be loaded in the frontal unit and frames 2, 4, 6, 8, and so on in the lateral unit. When the film changer is activated, film 1 is exposed in the anteroposterior unit, film 2 is then exposed in the lateral unit, and so on, thereby eliminating the cross-fogging effect. With some newer cut film changers, full magazine loading is permitted for alternate biplane angiography. When using roll film changers the alternate exposure technique wastes every other frame in both projections.

Although the use of a cross-hatch grid is rec-

ommended for perpendicular beam biplane studies, it is impossible to use a cross-hatch grid in the frontal plane during a cerebral angiographic procedure because of the tube angulation needed for this position. A linear grid is used for the anteroposterior projection of the skull, and a cross-hatch grid is often used for the lateral projection. Although an increase in kVp can be tolerated by the cross-hatch grid, the corresponding increase in scatter radiation, unfortunately, cannot be overcome by the linear grid in the anteroposterior plane (see Fig. 11-29).

An externally mounted grid can overcome another major technical problem when using biplane 14 × 14 inch serial changers. It is extremely difficult to maintain good object film contact in the lateral position of a cerebral angiogram, since the skull must be centered to the 14 × 14 inch grid. A 10 × 12 inch grid placed on the side of the anteroposterior changer, nearest the lateral film changer, decreases the OFD in the lateral plane (Fig. 11-32).

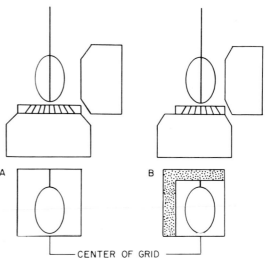

Figure 11-32
Cerebral Angiography with a Large-Frame Serial Film or Cassette Changer

(A) When the skull or another small body part must be centered to the grid in the anteroposterior position on a large-frame (14 × 14 inch) film or cassette changer, an increase in OFD occurs in the lateral position. (B) By using a smaller grid (10 × 12 inch) the center of the grid can be moved closer to the lateral film changer. The patient can then be positioned closer to the lateral film changer, with a reduction in the OFD. Alternate film loading of the changers, if possible, completely avoids biplane scatter.

BIPLANE OPERATION WITH A SINGLE GENERATOR. A problem can occur if both x-ray tubes are energized from a single generator. Although sharing the energy of a single generator may be acceptable for some biplane procedures, in general it should be avoided.

With both x-ray tubes made to operate at the same kvP and exposure times, a biplane split while examining an abdomen would make it difficult to balance exposures, since the lateral projection of the abdomen requires considerably more exposure than the anteroposterior projection. High-speed intensifying screens are often needed in the lateral changer to achieve adequate film blackening.

X-RAY ABSORPTIVE ACCESSORIES. Attenuation of the x-ray beam can be caused by an x-ray absorptive head support or tabletop.

A simple test to demonstrate beam attenuation by a headboard can be performed using a skull phantom positioned halfway off the headboard. The attenuated portion of the skull phantom image will be underexposed when compared with the unattenuated segment (Fig. 11-33).

IMPORTANT

Some head support or tabletop materials can absorb as much as 50% of the remnant beam.

CONTROL OF PRIMARY BEAM LEAKAGE. When a body part is so configured that the rectangular or square shutter pattern of a collimator is not able to conform to the body outline, an unattenuated primary beam may strike the film screen detector, resulting in undercutting of the radiographic image. An example of this is the use of the anteroposterior Towne projection of the skull for cerebral angiography (Figs. 11-34 and 11-35). When the unattenuated primary beam strikes the headboard, scatter is generated and undercutting of the radiographic image occurs. Lead shielding is often placed on a serial film or cassette changer in an attempt to reduce scatter. Since the scatter arises from the tabletop or headboard, the lead shielding (see Fig. 11-34) does not significantly improve image quality. The use of a filter material on the tabletop or headboard, however, will attenuate the primary beam, minimizing undercutting. Sand,

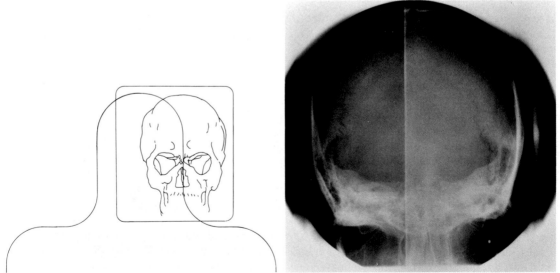

Figure 11-33
Absorption Effect of the Headboard or Tabletop

A simple test can be made to determine the absorption effect of a headboard or tabletop. (Left) A skull phantom is placed halfway off a headboard extension. With the skull centered to the film changer, an exposure is made. The radiograph should show acceptable detail and contrast unless there is significant absorption of the remnant beam by the headboard. (Right) In this example approximately 50% of the remnant beam was absorbed by the headboard. The high absorptive nature of this headboard requires a doubling of exposure factors for adequate radiographic density. Low absorption-plastic or carbon-fiber headboards an be used to avoid this problem.

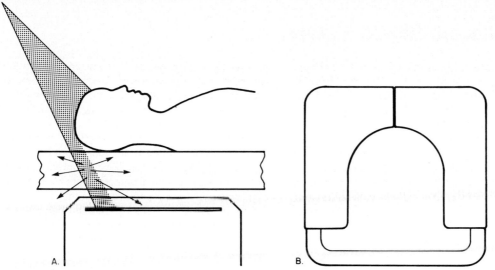

Figure 11-34
Undercutting of the Radiographic Image by a Primary Beam Leak

(A) *An undercutting effect of the image will result if a primary beam leak occurs. The* shaded area *represents the primary beam striking the headboard. (B) Lead shielding often is erroneously placed on the surface of the film changer or cassette changer in an attempt to reduce scatter. Since a significant amount of scatter radiation originates from the headboard, the lead shielding placed on the film changer or cassette changer will have little or no effect on the radiographic image. Although the unexposed borders of the radiographic film shielded from x-rays give the illusion of scatter control, the edges of the radiographic image will be degraded by the undercutting effect of the primary beam leak. The use of primary beam attenuators on the tabletop can lessen the undercutting effect.*

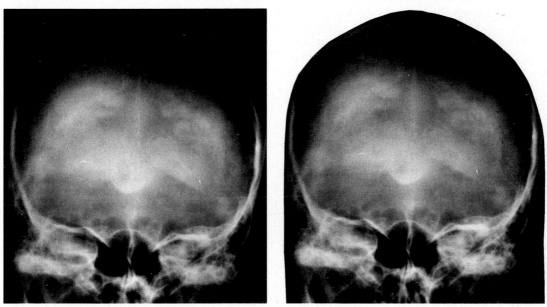

Figure 11-35
The Effect of a Primary Beam Leak on a Skull Radiograph

The rectangular shutters of the collimator do not conform to the contours of the skull, which can cause an undercutting effect. (Left) The right side and the top of the skull are shown, with a primary beam leak of about 1 inch striking the headboard. Note the loss of detail in the skull vault as the scatter from the headboard undercuts the image. A primary beam attenuator on a headboard or tabletop will absorb much of the primary beam and lessen the undercutting effect. A primary beam attenuator on the film changer (see Fig. 11-34) does not eliminate undercutting of the image. (Right) Trimming the extraneous density on a duplicate image with a scissors simulates the effect of lead shielding on the film changer, but it does not improve the image. The loss of detail due to undercutting and extrafocal radiation still exists on the image. (See Chapter 5, Fig. 5-12.)

cornmeal, water, rice, or flour bags or lead-rubber shielding can be used to attenuate the primary ray.

SCREEN FILM CONTACT. With the exception of the vacuum cassette changer, no unit achieves the screen film contact of conventional cassettes.

DETERIORATING INTENSIFYING SCREENS. Intensifying screens are often used for a long period of time without concern for phosphor damage or intensification fall-off. Obvious screen artifacts and poor screen contact are usually seen. Screen speed, however, can deteriorate in a gradual manner. Compensation is often made for this loss in light output by an increase in x-ray factors, which means an increase in exposure to the patient.

IMAGE BLUR. Objects of low contrast such as extremely small blood vessels are difficult to image. High-speed, rare-earth imaging systems are recommended for angiography since their increased film blackening effect permits the use of smaller focal spots and helps to overcome patient or vessel motion. More frames per second are possible with rare-earth systems owing to shorter exposure time potential per frame. Early roll film changers were limited to exposures of 1/30th of a second at four frames per second. Their actual "dwell" time per cycle was quite short, forcing the radiographer to use extremely short exposure times. On larger patients, when exposure length exceeds 1/30th of a second, a two-frame-per-second rate may be required with a roll film changer. Even a larger patient can receive the benefit of more frames per second with reduced image blur in each frame as the result of shorter exposure times associated with rare-earth imaging.

Tube angle techniques can increase the image blur associated with parallax (see Fig. 11-31).

Inherent vibration in the film or cassette changer can create a motion effect with a corresponding increase in image blur.

TRANSPORT CYCLE VS. PHASE-IN TIME. It is important that a service engineer check serial film or cassette changers to ensure proper synchronization of excursion and exposure. In any given cycle of frames per second of a serial film changer there are two distinct segments: the transportation phase, when the film is transported into position, and the compression phase, in which the intensifying screens are closed for optimal screen film contact. During the compression phase of the cut film changer, an exposure is made prior to the opening of the intensifying screens. This reinitiates the transport cycle. A delay can occur in the cycle after the start of compression and prior to the x-ray exposure. Even when compensation is made

for this delay, a second delay from zero to 16 milliseconds—the "phase-in time"—can occur before exposure, depending on the type of x-ray equipment used. Phase-in time can reduce the useful exposure time per cycle (Fig. 11-36).

Without proper synchronization, excursion could begin or end before the making of or termination of an exposure, resulting in underexposed radiographs. If a synchronization problem exists and the survey film for the study is made without the serial film or cassette mechanism being energized, even though the scout film in the actual study may be perfect, the serial run may be underexposed. Cassette or film changers often have an abort mechanism that will shorten or terminate the predetermined exposure if the unit is out of synchronization.

JAMMING POSSIBILITIES. Roll film changers generally jam because of poor film mounting on the receiving or loading spools.

With a cut film changer, adjustment of the levers that flip the film upward must be precise. A special measuring tool is needed for this adjustment.

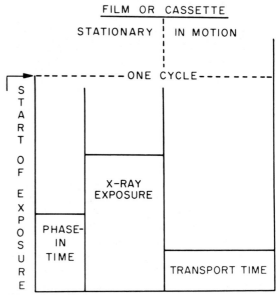

Figure 11-36
Transport Cycle

Closing the relays to produce an exposure robs the radiographer of usable exposure time. Relays can be adjusted to minimize delay. There is, however, a delay prior to exposure known as "phase-in time." This delay can vary with different types of generators from zero to 16 milliseconds.

IMPORTANT

Antistatic agents should be used on the intensifying screens in serial film changers to prevent static artifacts. Silicon coatings applied directly to the intensifying screens must not be allowed to strike the rubber film transportation rollers of cut film changers, since the silicon spray may affect traction of the film.

FILM IDENTIFICATION. With the exception of the roll film changer, films are often not in order when delivered from the automatic processor. Consecutive numbering of the films during a serial angiographic study should be performed with a device that optically transfers pertinent information such as patient name, type of examination, and date directly onto the radiographic film.

FILM PROCESSING AND STORAGE. Manufacturers' recommendations regarding the daily minimal number of films that need to be processed in order to prevent self-exhaustion of the solutions in the automatic processor should be followed. A busy angiographic laboratory should have its own automatic processor.

Roll film must be cut to field size to be stored in conventional radiographic film envelopes. There is considerable waste with almost all film sizes, particularly if small field, tight collimation is used.

A representative angiographic image is shown in Figure 11-37.

Supplementary Serial Studies

Special techniques used to supplement conventional angiography include the following:

1. Stereoangiography. Single-plane stereoangiography can be accomplished using two x-ray tubes mounted side-by-side with an approximately 8-degree angle separation. During a stereo study every other film frame is exposed by the alternate tube. Electrical switching mechanisms alternately activate each tube to produce three-dimensional angiography. The image pairs are viewed simultaneously in a stereo viewer. (See *Stereoradiography.*)
2. Angiotomography. A linear body section device with an exposure angle of 10 to 20 degrees uses a book cassette with up to four pairs of screens to produce multilayered angiotomographic studies. A motor-driven drum

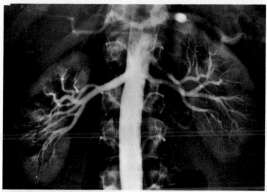

Figure 11-37
Abdominal Aortogram
Careful attention to radiographic technique will result in an optimal study. This abdominal aortogram of a large patient was made with an 800-speed, rare-earth screen film system. The use of a modest kilovoltage value combined with a 12:1 ratio grid produced a relatively high-contrast image. Despite the size and absorptive nature of this patient, careful attention to radiographic technique produced a quality angiographic study. (Reprinted courtesy Eastman Kodak Company)

holds four book cassettes for exposures made at under ¼ of a second each.*

3. Direct roentgen enlargement angiography. A changer used for direct roentgen enlargement angiography should be movable and of adjustable height. The grid should be easily removable for the air-gap technique. Whenever positioning the unit or removing the grid takes an appreciable amount of time, there is a tendency to avoid direct roentgen enlargement angiography as a supplementary procedure (Fig. 11-38).

Direct Roentgen Enlargement

Direct roentgen enlargement (magnification) refers to any radiographic image that is projected to an image receptor some distance from the part under study (Figs. 11-39 and 11-40).

Radiographic enlargement should not be confused with photographic enlargement, which refers to optically enlarging a photographic negative of a radiographic image. For a conventional

*Nadjimi M: Intercranial tumours in the angiogram. Medicamundi 23:13–22, 1978.

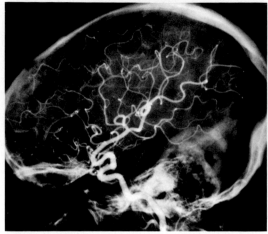

Figure 11-38
Cerebral Angiogram

This lateral projection of a cerebral angiographic study used an alternate-load biplane, direct enlargement technique. A fractional focal spot was combined with a 20-inch air gap to produce a 2× linear (4× area) enlargement. A 1200-speed, rare-earth screen film combination was used without apparent loss of resolution owing to quantum mottle. (Reprinted courtesy Eastman Kodak Company)

2× linear, 4× area magnification study, the part must be equidistant between the tube and the detector. For 3× linear, 9× area magnification, the part is approximately one third the distance (FOD) from the tube and two thirds the distance (OFD) from the detector (Fig. 11-41; Table 11-1).

Different parts of the human body are at various distances from the screen film combination, even when a fixed FFD or OFD is used (Figs. 11-40 and 11-41; Table 11-1). For example, when the patient is placed in the lateral position with the skull equidistant from the focal spot, between the tube and the detector, the vessels to be studied on the right or left side will not be magnified equally. With the patient in the left lateral position, the left middle cerebral artery imaged with a left-sided injection is closer to the detector. Conversely, the right middle cerebral artery imaged with a right-sided injection is farther from the detector and closer to the x-ray source. The right middle cerebral artery will therefore appear larger in size with increased image blur than the left middle cerebral artery. The anterior cerebral arteries are midline and will be magnified approximately to the same degree, regardless of the side that is injected with contrast media (see Fig. 11-40, *right*).

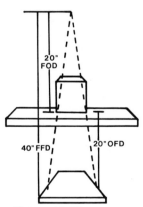

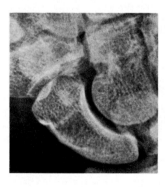

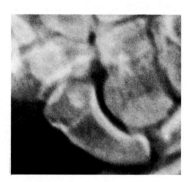

Figure 11-39
Direct Roentgen Enlargement: Focal Spot Comparison

A fractional focal spot tube (0.3 mm or less) is a prerequisite for this technique. (Left) A typical arrangement for direct roentgen enlargement is shown. The part is positioned approximately midway between tube and image detector (20-in FOD; 20-in OFD). This results in a 2× linear, 4× area enlargement. If the part to be examined is positioned 13 inches from the tube with a 26-inch air gap (OFD), the result is a 3× linear, 9× area enlargement (see Fig. 11-41). (Center) 0.3-mm focal spot was used for the enlargement of the scaphoid of the wrist. Note the excellent osseous details. (Right) A 1.0-mm focal spot was used for an exact duplication of the roentgen enlargement technique shown in the center illustration. Radiographic detail is greatly diminished and the image is completely out of focus.

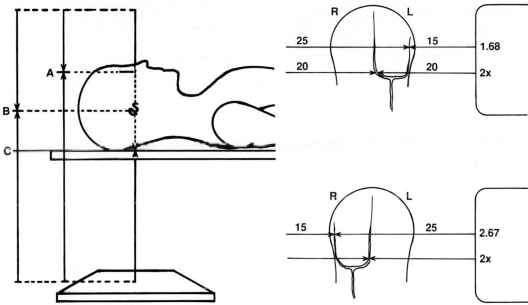

Figure 11-40
Relation of Anatomy to Tube and Detector

Different segments of anatomy enlarge to different degrees, depending on their position within the body (see Table 11-1). (Left) The posterior portion of the skull (C) is equidistant between tube and detector, and a 2× linear, 4× area enlargement will result. When different parts of the skull are to be enlarged, such as the sella turcica (B), the relations between the focal spot, object, and film change dramatically. There will be an increase in the size of the sella turcica greater then 2× linear. If the orbits (A) are to be examined, a severely decreased FOD causes significant enlargement of the orbits. Magnification could be up to 4× linear, 16× area, but the orbits would be out of focus. The FFD is often changed to compensate for this difficulty and the cassette raised closer to the part under study. This is an error, since a 20-inch air gap is required to adequately clean up scatter when a grid or Bucky is not being used. If the orbits are to be enlarged, placing the patient prone will help to maintain a better FOD/OFD relation.

(Right) The side opacified and the vessel to be studied can influence the degree of magnification. For example, with the patient in the left lateral position, the left middle cerebral artery imaged with a left-sided injection is closer to the detector and farther from the x-ray source than the right middle cererbral artery imaged with a right-sided injection. The degree of magnification in this example varies from 1.68 to 2.67 linear. Since the anterior cerebral arteries are midline they are magnified to the same degree, approximately 2× linear, regardless of the side that is injected with contrast media.

When a 2× linear enlargement is exceeded, image blur is increased. When performing direct enlargement studies, not only should geometric relations be a concern but also focal spot size must be considered. (See Table 11-1 for specific linear and area enlargement factors.)

Dosage to the lens of the eyes is a concern. (See *Tomography, Basic Technical Considerations*.)

Basic Technical Considerations

Focal Spot Size

X-ray tubes with "fractional" focal spots (0.3 mm or less) have been used for direct roentgen en-largement techniques for more than four decades. Early fractional focus x-ray tubes had severe rating restrictions, and their use was limited to enlargement of thin body parts. New steep-angle targets have made magnification studies of thicker body parts possible.

A minute radiographic detail present on a conventional radiograph may not be seen on the enlarged study if the structural detail to be enlarged is smaller than the focal spot (see Fig. 11-39).

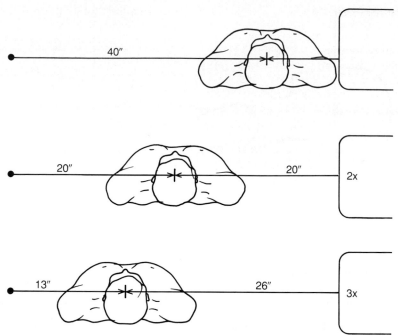

Figure 11-41
Direct Roentgen Enlargement Comparison

(Top) *A patient is positioned for conventional radiography using a 40-inch FFD. (Center) For a 2× linear, 4× area enlargement, the patient is equidistant between tube and detector. (Bottom) A 3× linear, 9× area study has a 13-inch FOD and a 26-inch OFD.*

By separating the image detector from the object under study, a grid-type scatter cleanup occurs. When the radiographic film is in direct contact with the part (top), most of the scatter radiation will strike the film. When an air gap is used (center and bottom) a high percentage of the scatter radiation completely misses the film. (See Appendix 11 for magnification formulas.)

Table 11-1. Distances in Relation to Degrees of Enlargement

40-Inch FFD		Magnification	
FOD	OFD	Linear	Area
25 in	15 in	1.6×	2.56×
20 in	20 in	2.0×	4.0×*
15 in	25 in	2.67×	7.0×
14 in	26 in	2.85×	8.0×†
13 in	26 in	3.0×	9.0×

*A 0.3-mm fractional focal spot is a prerequisite for direct roentgen enlargement up to 2× linear, 4× area.

†A 0.1-mm microfocal spot allows up to an 8× area magnification.

Note: *To minimize the possibility of blooming, the focal spot should not be used at maximum mA. See Figures 11-40 and 11-41 for typical x-ray tube–receptor configurations.*

IMPORTANT

Small focal spots (e.g., 0.5 mm or 0.6 mm) are not acceptable for direct roentgen enlargement studies.

The 0.3-mm focal spot, usually rated less than 200 mA, is universally accepted as the minimal focal spot permissible for direct roentgen enlargement studies. Some radiographic tubes have a 0.1-mm capability with ratings of less than 75 mA. A stationary anode microfocus tube is available with a focal spot corresponding to a nominal diameter of 0.09 mm; its rating is less than 10 mA.

Every effort must be made to ensure the integrity of the focal spot size. Technical factors such as low kVp with maximal permissible mA may contribute to focal spot blooming.

Control of Scatter Radiation

If the image detector is not in close contact with the part under study, most of the scatter radiation generated during an exposure will not reach the film. By using an air gap to separate the image detector from the object under study, instead of a grid, scatter cleanup can be achieved. Increasing the OFD will ensure that a high percentage of scatter, because of its oblique nature, misses the detector.

The primary beam should be restricted to the part under study. If a primary beam leak occurs, undercutting of the image can result.

Screen Film Selection

The use of detail screens is acceptable for high-detail, direct roentgen enlargement of small body parts such as extremities.

The effect of quantum mottle sometimes seen on high-speed, rare-earth images is minimized by the enlargement process. The quantum mottle, still visible on the processed radiograph, does not increase in size since the mottle is generated within the screen. As the degree of enlargement increases, the effect of noise on the image is diminished. Anatomic details increase in size but the quantum mottle remains the same size, making the detector more efficient (Fig. 11-42).

Six hundred to 1200-speed, rare-earth technology permits an increased number of images per second for direct roentgen enlargement angiography without compromising the instantaneous loading capacity of a fractional focal spot tube.

Mammography

One in nine American women will develop breast cancer. The smaller the cancer when found, the greater the likelihood that it will be localized to the breast. The importance of early detection of breast cancer is supported by the recommendations of the American Cancer Society and American Medical Association for periodic breast examination.

A mammogram provides information about normal anatomy as well as pathology. Because of low subject contrast, the types of tissue structures within the breast, represented by muscles, glands, blood vessels, and fatty tissue, differ little in radiodensity. Subject contrast is related to the ratio of the x-ray intensity transmitted through one part of the breast to the intensity transmitted through a more absorbing adjacent area of the breast. Absorption differences in the breast related to thickness and density as well as the radiation quality affect subject contrast.

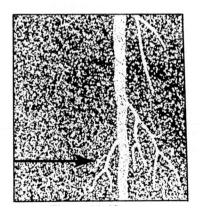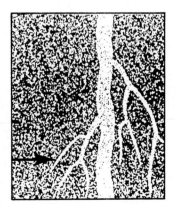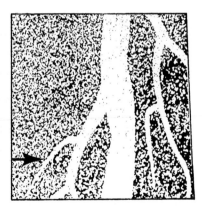

Figure 11-42
The Effect of Quantum Mottle on Enlargement Studies

Occasionally quantum mottle is seen when a high-speed screen film combination is used. (Left) Quantum mottle occurs in the intensifying screen and can damage resolution in the radiographic image. (Center) The effect of quantum mottle on the image can be minimized by the direct roentgen enlargement process, as shown in this 2× linear, 4× area enlargement. (Right) With a greater degree of enlargement, such as a 3× linear, 9× area study, the effect of quantum mottle on resolution is even further diminished. The anatomic details increase in size, but quantum mottle remains the same size because it occurs in the screen, thus making the image detector more efficient. (Reprinted courtesy Eastman Kodak Company)

Special dedicated mammographic equipment and techniques are needed to demonstrate these subtle differences in tissue density (Fig. 11-43). Microcalcifications, if present, and fine parenchymal breast patterns must be clearly demonstrated. Sufficient radiographic contrast is not possible with conventional x-ray equipment. In the kilovoltage range needed for mammography, a molybdenum target tube produces a higher-contrast, almost homogeneous x-ray beam, which improves radiographic contrast and the visualization of minute radiographic details. The use of a beryllium window x-ray tube with minimal filtration is recommended.

Radiographic contrast is essential to image breast microcalcifications. Screen film mammographic techniques require short-scale, high-contrast imaging to demonstrate subtle density differences between waterlike and fatty soft tissues. Optimal kilovoltage settings for short-scale contrast range from 22 to 28 kVp for screen film mammography with a molybdenum target tube and from 45 to 55 kVp for xeroradiography with a tungsten target tube.

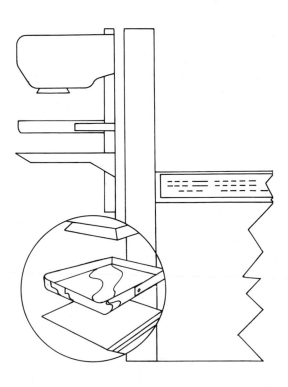

Figure 11-43
Dedicated Mammographic Unit

Conventional radiographic equipment should not be used for mammography. Early mammograms were made with existing conventional radiographic equipment. The collimator was removed from the unit and replaced with special mammographic cones. Filtration was also removed because of the low kilovoltage required for breast examinations. Early direct-exposure films required 22 to 35 kVp at up to 1800 mAs (300 mA at 6 sec) per exposure. These exposure factors were necessary to expose the fine-grain industrial film used for mammography. The patient had to be seated against the side of a table or a special tray for a craniocaudal projection and placed recumbent for a lateral or oblique projection.

In the late 1960s, a dedicated mammographic unit using a molybdenum target with a 30μ molybdenum filter was made commercially available. This unit permitted vigorous compression techniques. The patient was able to be positioned while erect for both the craniocaudal and lateral projections. These units had the compression paddle attached to the bottom of the cone. As the breast was compressed, the FFD decreased, resulting in geometric difficulties.

Newer dedicated mammographic units have a straight-edge compression device (circular insert), independent of the cone or collimator. Some dedicated units have a built-in Bucky for high-contrast mammography. This is particularly helpful when evaluating the dense breast. An automatic exposure device combined with a small focal spot tube ensures high-resolution images.

Magnification techniques can be performed with units that have a microfocus tube, some as small as 0.1 mm. The breast is placed at an increased distance from the detector, approximately midway between the focal spot and the cassette, to produce an enlargement mammogram. Attachments are available to aid in localization techniques prior to biopsy.

Basic Technical Considerations

Filter Concepts

Molybdenum filters are used with molybdenum target tubes for screen film mammography, whereas tungsten target tubes and aluminum filters are recommended for electrostatic imaging.

Image Geometry

The size of the x-ray focal spot and related image geometry must be considered. Selection of a small focal spot (0.6 mm or less) is recommended for screen film mammography. High mA values may result in focal spot blooming. Focal film distance must also be considered. Early dedicated mammographic units used a very short FFD, often less than 13 inches. If the compression plate of a dedicated unit is attached to the bottom of the cone, image geometry may be compromised because FFD decreases as compression is applied.

"Long cone" units have a 60-cm or greater FFD, which improves image geometry.

X-ray Tube Orientation

When conventional radiographic equipment was used for mammography, it was common practice to position the cathode side of the x-ray tube to the base or thicker portion of the breast to take advantage of the anode heel effect. Also, before the use of aggressive compression techniques, the increase in exposure to the thicker portion of the breast at the chest wall was thought to be of value. This position had a distinct disadvantage, however, because although beam intensity increases at the cathode side of the tube, resolution decreases. The effective focal spot widens toward the cathode side of the tube and narrows toward the anode side. This loss in resolution could influence the imaging of minute calcifications, particularly those not in intimate contact with the detector (Fig 11-44).

Compression

As in all medical radiography, it is important that the area to be examined be as close to the image detector as possible. The female breast is conical in shape, thicker at the chest wall than at the nipple. Vigorous compression of the breast brings the breast tissue closer to the image detector (Fig. 11-45). A compression device should immobilize the

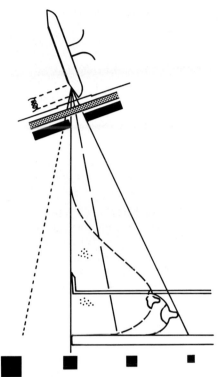

Figure 11-44
Line Focus Effect: Positioning Approach
With conventional radiography, because the cathode (−) portion of the x-ray beam is more intense than the anode (+) portion, the thicker segment of the body is positioned beneath the cathode end of the x-ray tube. There is also an increase in image blur toward the cathode side. Early noncompression mammographic techniques used the increased output of the cathode to overcome the thickness of the breast at the chest wall. Unfortunately, this technique resulted in increased image blur, particularly of anatomic details in the superior portion of the breast (increased OFD).

With modern mammographic units, the x-ray tube is oriented so that the effective focal spot is centered at the chest wall to avoid projection of superior structures into the chest wall, away from the cassette. The anode portion of the beam is used to image the structures near the nipple. In effect, only about one half of the actual beam is used for mammograpy to take advantage of the improved resolution from the line focus effect. The calcifications shown in this illustration would be projected into the chest with a conventional x-ray beam.

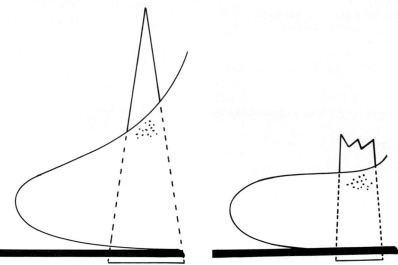

Figure 11-45
The Effect of Compression on Mammography

Most patients are surprised by vigorous compression and may inadvertently fail to cooperate. To ensure patient cooperation, the mammographer must explain to the patient the purpose of compression and the degree of compression needed. It is difficult to adequately image the breast without using breast compression, because the breast is thicker at the chest wall than at the nipple area. Vigorous compression of the breast brings the breast tissue closer to the image detector while lessening the production of scatter. (Left) The conical-shaped breast presents several imaging difficulties. If the proper exposure were used to image the breast tissue near the chest wall, the nipple area would be overexposed. Note the presence of calcifications in the superior portion of the breast and the distance of the calcific flecks from the detector. A widening and therefore a blurring of these structures may occur when they are imaged. The use of a small focal spot helps to overcome this difficulty. (Right) When the breast is compressed to an even overall thickness, calcifications are brought closer to the detector. This change in OFD will help to minimize image blur. When compression is combined with a microfocal spot, image resolution improves dramatically. The decrease in the tissue thickness results in the production of less scatter. Since less radiation is required for the compressed tissue, lower exposure factors can be used.

breast while minimizing its conical shape so that overall breast tissue approaches an even thickness.

Every effort should be made to gain the patient's confidence and cooperation when using a compression device. Compression should be applied slowly and carefully so as not to bruise the skin.

IMPORTANT

Seeing the rib cage on the lateral view of the breast does not necessarily ensure that the entire posterior portion of the breast has been imaged (Fig. 11-46). The radiographer must gently pull the breast tissue away from the chest wall while applying compression so that the posterior segment of the breast will be imaged.

Vigorous breast compression has the following advantages:

1. The structures of the breast are in closer contact with the image receptor, therefore geometric blurring is reduced.
2. There is more uniform tissue thickness, resulting in overall even radiographic density.

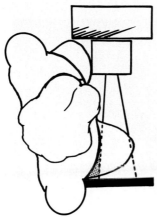

Figure 11-46
Visualization of the Chest Wall

When the rib cage is seen on the lateral projection of the breast, it does not necessarily indicate that the entire posterior breast (shaded area) has been imaged. The mammographer must gently pull the breast tissue forward from the chest wall while lifting the breast tissue into contact with the support tray and gently applying vigorous compression. If the patient's arm is hyperextended, it is difficult to pull the breast tissue forward. The arm should be relaxed, which in turn will relax the muscles along the chest wall.

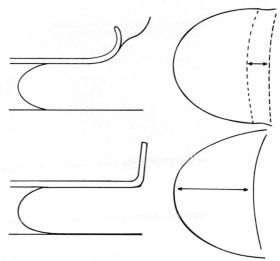

Figure 11-47
Compression Concepts for Mammography

(Top left) When a compression device with an exaggerated curved paddle is used to flatten the breast, tissue can move backward and upward off the curved surface of the compression paddle. The dashed lines (top right) mark the "whiteout" often seen with poor compression. (Bottom left) The use of a straight-edge compression paddle will result in an overall even tissue thickness. (Bottom right) Breast tissue from nipple to chest wall is visible (see Fig. 11-48).

3. Less scatter is produced because of the compression effect.
4. There is a reduction in exposure factors needed to image the breast.
5. Patient motion is minimized.

Occasionally the mammographic image near the chest wall may lack radiographic detail or density, or both, owing to "whiteout" of the tissue near the chest wall as the result of improper compression. When a curved-edge compression device is used, breast tissue can be forced backward and upward along the chest wall, producing a "stepwedge-like" difference in breast thickness, with the tissue at the chest wall considerably thicker than the compressed tissue. The possibility of whiteout of the image is minimized by using straight-edge compression (Figs. 11-47 and 11-48).

Control of Scatter Radiation

Much of the scatter radiation associated with dense glandular breast architecture can be eliminated with a grid (Fig. 11-49). High-quality, fine-line grids, up to 200 lines per inch, or moving grids (Bucky) have been developed for use in mammography. Stationary mammographic grids, usually 3.5:1 in ratio, can be installed within a cassette or can be used on top of a cassette or vacuum bag. Most mammographic units contain moving grids that are either 4:1 or 5:1 in ratio.

If the kilovoltage value of a non-grid technique is to be maintained, an approximate two to two-and-one-half times increase in mAs is needed to overcome the absorptive quality of the mammographic grid. When using the same mAs value, an increase in 3 kVp should be adequate to duplicate non-grid exposures.

Automatic Exposure Control

Modern dedicated mammographic units use an automatic exposure device (AED) to control exposure time. As in conventional radiography, the body part must be positioned carefully over the

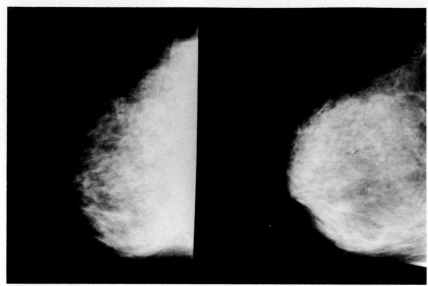

Figure 11-48
Clinical Application of Straight-Edge vs. Curved-Edge Compression
(Left) "Whiteout," a lack of radiographic detail adjacent to the chest wall, is partially due to a portion of the breast tissue being pushed upward and backward along the chest wall by the curved edge of a plastic compression device (see Fig. 11-47). (Right) When vigorous straight-edge compression is used, more uniform compression of the breast tissue adjacent to the chest wall lessens the whiteout effect. The mammographer must gently pull the breast forward while lifting the breast onto the support tray to maximize tissue visualization. (Courtesy W. W. Logan-Young, M.D., Rochester, NY)

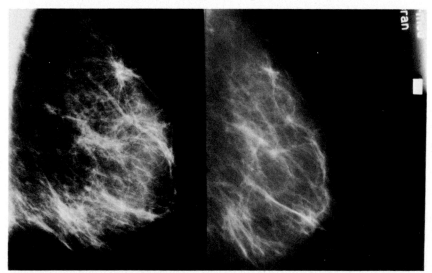

Figure 11-49
Screen Film Grid vs. Direct-Exposure Non-Grid Study
The moving grid (4:1 or 5:1 ratio) was introduced in 1978 as part of a dedicated mammographic unit. It replaced stationary 3.5:1 ratio grids designed to fit inside mammographic cassettes. Radiographic contrast is considerably improved on the grid or Bucky radiograph (left) compared with a direct-exposure industrial film mammogram (right). Direct-exposure industrial film is no longer used for mammography. (Courtesy W. W. Logan-Young, M. D., Rochester, NY)

sensor. A significant difference in the length of the exposures between the breasts should be brought to the attention of the radiologist since radiographic densities can be balanced by the AED, even when significant absorption differences occur.

Mammographic Screen Film Combinations

Two types of screen film combinations are used for mammography: conventional phosphors (emitting primarily a blue light) and rare-earth phosphors (emitting primarily a green light). Appropriate blue- or green-sensitive films are matched to the light output of the screens.

IMPORTANT

Green-sensitive film requires a special safelight filter such as the Eastman Kodak GBX-2 filter. Either blue- or green-sensitive film can be used with the GBX-2 safelight filter. The use of an improper safelight with a green-sensitive film will produce a foglike supplemental density on the radiograph.

Image sharpness is improved with a single intensifying screen and a single-emulsion film designed with an antihalation backing to help prevent crossover of the light within the cassette.

Recent improvements in screen film design permit the use of two intensifying screens with a dual-emulsion, tabular grain, zero-crossover mammographic film.

Intensifying screens should be cleaned at least weekly. With a high patient load, daily cleaning may be necessary.

Film Holders

Maintaining screen film contact is an ongoing concern, regardless of the type of system used. Several types of mammographic film holders are available:

A polyvinyl chloride vacuum bag that produces screen film contact by using an external vacuum source to exhaust air from the bag
A polyethylene bag, air evacuated and heat sealed in the darkroom to achieve screen film contact

A screen film cassette. Because of the low kilovoltage range needed for mammography, the front of a mammographic cassette must be made of a low x-ray–absorbing plastic.

Specific information regarding film holders for mammography can be found in Chapter 6 in the section Specialty Cassettes.

Processing

Processing conditions must be carefully monitored when performing mammography. With an automatic processor, the manufacturer's recommendations for film processing of mammographic film regarding time, temperature, and processor maintenance must be followed.

Mammographic Enlargement Technique

Although a 0.3-mm or less fractional focal spot is a prerequisite for any enlargement technique, it cannot be used for enlargement mammography. For enlargement mammography, a microfocus focal spot is required: a 0.1-mm for $2\times$ linear ($4\times$ area) enlargement and 0.2-mm for $1.3\times$ linear ($1.7\times$ area) to $1.5\times$ linear ($2.25\times$ area) enlargement. A stationary anode tube with a 90μ focal spot is also available for this procedure.

To perform magnification mammography, the image detector is placed at an increased distance from the breast (resulting in an increased OFD and a decreased FOD). The breast, placed approximately midway between the tube and the image receptor, is recorded on an enlarged radiograph, which makes subtle details easier to detect. Because of the increased OFD (air gap), a Bucky is not required for scatter cleanup.

Xeromammography

Xeroradiography uses an electrostatic imaging process. A charged photoconductive plate made of selenium, held in a lightproof container, is used as a substitute for a screen film combination. The xeroradiographic process is described in Chapter 13.

Approximately 45 to 55 kVp is required for xeromammography. Because of this higher kilovoltage level, aluminum filtration is required.

Quality Assurance

The technical parameters for mammography are so specialized that quality assurance (QA) is of utmost importance. As with all radiographic equipment, scheduled periodic checks of peak tube voltage, half value layer, timer accuracy, and focal spot size should be performed.

Radiation Dosage Consideration

The dose levels of a single-screen, single-emulsion mammographic film combination are up to 50 times lower than the dose levels of the direct-exposure film methods used in the 1960s. Patients then were examined using a fine-grain industrial film with 25 to 35 kVp at 1800 mAs (300 mA at 6 seconds) per exposure. Mammographers should be aware of the reduction in dosage made possible by screen film and xeroradiographic techniques.

Feig states that an examination with low-dosage techniques (single-emulsion) would carry a theoretical risk of about one excess cancer case per year for every 2 million women examined.*

The level of risk, one death in 4 million women per year, is extremely small and can be equated with the following: 100 miles traveled by air, 15 miles traveled by car, smoking one fourth of one cigarette, one third of a minute of mountain climbing, and 5 minutes of being a man 60 years of age.

A dual-screen, dual-emulsion (T-grain), zero-crossover film mammographic system is available and is approximately two and one half times faster than single-screen, single-emulsion mammographic imaging products. This system is often used for screening purposes, particularly when examining young women.

*Feig SA: Low Dose Mammography: Assessment of Theoretical Risks in Breast Carcinoma; Current Diagnosis and Treatment. *New York: Masson Publishing, 1983, pp 69–76.*

Chapter 12

Electronic Imaging Equipment and Techniques

Some newer electronic imaging technologies are presented in this chapter. Recording media used with these technologies are addressed in Chapter 13. Information on conventional fluoroscopy is presented in Chapter 4.

The Image Intensifier

The image intensifier is probably the best known medical electronic imaging device. Image intensifiers produce significantly brighter images than conventional fluoroscopes, and because they facilitate viewing and interpretation, they cut down the time of fluoroscopic exposure.

The rods and cones of the eye are visual receptors that are highly sensitive to light stimulation. Rod vision is most sensitive to low light levels. With conventional fluoroscopy, operators must wear adaptation goggles with dark red lenses for up to 20 minutes before a fluoroscopic examination to accommodate their eyes to the low light level of the fluoroscopic image. However, since the advent of television fluoroscopic viewing systems, a darkened room is no longer required for fluoroscopic procedures. Cone vision of the eyes can be used to advantage. The use of partial or total room illumination has several advantages:

1. The ability to perform fluoroscopic vascular opacification procedures in less time
2. Greater patient security, especially for the seriously ill, emotionally disturbed, or uncooperative patient
3. Elimination of the need to adapt the eyes to darkness

As with conventional fluoroscopy, the image intensifier has a shorter distance between the x-ray tube and the patient than the FFD used with conventional radiography (Fig. 12-1). Image blur can be reduced by using a 0.3-mm or 0.6-mm focal spot for fluoroscopic spot film imaging.

Angeline M. Cullinan and John E. Cullinan:
PRODUCING QUALITY RADIOGRAPHS, 2ND ED.
© 1987, 1994 J. B. Lippincott Company.

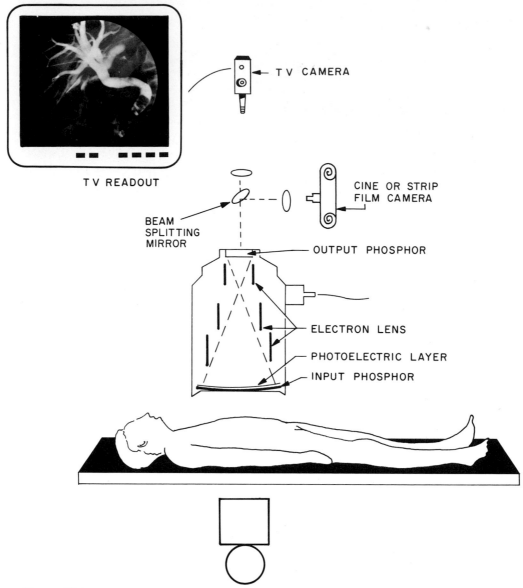

Figure 12-1
The Image Intensifier System

The image intensifier is an electronically enhanced fluoroscope. As with conventional fluoroscopy, the patient is placed between the x-ray tube and the fluoroscopic screen (input phosphor) of the image intensifier. The FOD is approximately 20 inches (a 40-inch FFD is used in radiography), causing anatomic details to be magnified.

Remnant radiation as well as scatter radiation strikes the input phosphor. A fluorescent image is generated and converted into an electronic pattern on the photoelectric layer of the intensifier. Electrons are accelerated to the output phosphor of the intensifier by the application of high kilovoltage. The electron pattern is focused by electron lenses to conform to the smaller size of the output phosphor. A beam splitter (see Fig. 12-5) is used to transmit some of the light to a television camera. The remaining light can be used for motion picture strip film, or cut film imaging. The size of the input phosphor (6–15 inches) determines the viewing field.

A television readout is not essential for image-intensified viewing. A mirror optic system can be substituted for the television.

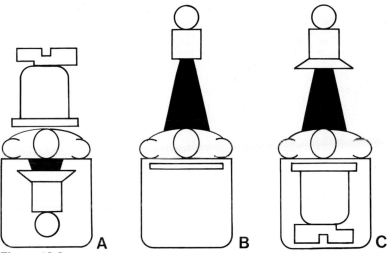

Figure 12-2
Over-table vs. Under-table Image Intensifier

(A) *A conventional fluoroscopic configuration is compared to* (B) *a standard 40-inch FFD table Bucky imaging arrangement. Note the decreased FOD, approximately 20 inches, associated with the fluoroscope.*

(C) *Substantial x-ray exposure to the operator is a concern in connection with the under-table image intensifier when used with an over-table tube for fluoroscopy. With the operator wearing a protective apron and standing beside the patient, the dose from an over-table tube compared with that from an under-table tube can be higher to the hands, the eyes, and the whole body.*

Lead shielding extended from the collimator to the patient can reduce scatter (see Fig. 12-3). A surface shield taped to the side of the patient during an intraventional procedure can reduce scatter radiation up to 75% (Amplatz K et al.: Surface shield: Device to reduce personnel radiation exposure. Radiology 159:3, June 1986).

IMPORTANT

If an under-table image intensifier is used with an over-table x-ray tube, there can be a significant increase in radiation dosage to the fluoroscopist and attending radiographer. Lead shielding should be extended from the over-table tube to the tabletop to minimize exposure to the upper portion of the operator's body (Figs. 12-2 and 12-3).

Remote-Control Fluoroscopy

Remote-control fluoroscopic units have been in use for almost 50 years. A remote-control installation includes a table with an image intensifier and a control booth. An additional video camera is sometimes used for observation of the patient by the fluoroscopist or radiographer (Fig. 12-4). At the control panel a television monitor displays the image from the image intensifier. An audio system is used for communication with the patient. Remote-control units can be installed for use at distant locations.

The image intensifier can be used as a positioning aid by the radiographer. As early as 1973, Dr. Manuel Viamonte stressed that it is feasible for radiographers to operate remote units, because the positioning of the patient under fluoroscopy can be done in such an automatic way.*

Components and Principles of Operation

The image intensifier consists of a large vacuum tube with an input phosphor fluoroscopic screen, which is generally composed of cesium iodide

*Reported in Simkins T: Remote control diagnostic units. Appl Radiol 48:17–22, 1973.

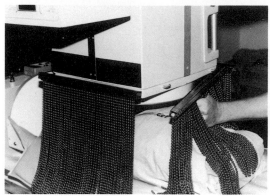

Figure 12-3
The Winkler Radiation Shielding Curtain

The shield consists of a two-layer curtain made of nickle-plated, brass bead chains. The beads in one layer fill the voids between the beads in the other layer. If patient contact is required, the bead chains can drape over the fluoroscopist's wrists and arms, maintaining radiation protection. The bead-chain shield can be mounted directly to the housing of an image intensifier or spot film device. (Courtesy of Nuclear Associates, division of Victoreen, Carle Place, NY)

(CsI) crystals that are laminated to a thin, transparent photoemissive surface called a *photocathode.* CsI crystals, which are hygroscopic (i.e., they absorb water), can be used within the vacuum of

an image intensifier but are not suitable for use in intensifying screens.

The CsI input screen contains more crystals packed together (increased packing density) than in the zinc cadmium sulfide phosphors (ZnCdS) used in early image intensifiers. Over twice the x-ray quanta for the same amount of x-ray exposure is absorbed by the CsI phosphor compared with the ZnCdS phosphor. This improves the quantum detection efficiency (QDE) of the intensifier, which is a measurement of how well x-radiation is detected. Since CsI has about double the packing density of ZnCdS, only about one half as many CsI crystals are needed. The thinner coating of the input phosphor improves spatial resolution and reduces patient dosage, since less x-radiation can be used without a loss of image quality.

As x-radiation from the fluoroscopic tube passes through the patient, representative tissue attenuation is displayed as a fluoroscopic image. The fluoroscopic image is simultaneously converted to an electron pattern on the photocathode. The electrons given off in any segment of the photocathode approximate the amount of light from the same segment of the fluoroscopic image. This process is known as *photoemission.*

The input phosphor is usually 6 or 9 inches in diameter. Some newer image intensifiers have an input phosphor as large as 15 inches in diameter.

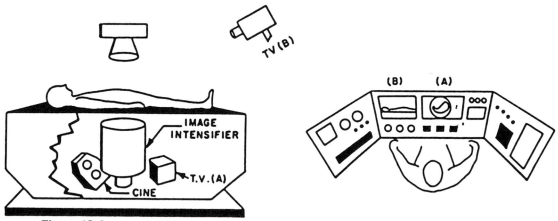

Figure 12-4
Remote-Control Fluoroscopy

(Left) A typical remote-control table consists of an image intensifier with a television camera (A) as well as a cineradiographic camera or a strip or cut film camera. (Right) Although many remote-control consoles are housed in a control booth adjacent to the x-ray table, the workstation could be operated at a remote location in a different room or facility. The radiologist or radiologic assistant sits at the control console and has direct audio communication with the patient. A television camera in the radiographic room (left, B) monitors the patient, who can be observed on the control console (right, B). The fluoroscopic image is viewed on the monitor (right, A).

In theory, the smaller the input phosphor, the finer the spatial resolution. Some intensifiers have multiple scanning fields. The electronically controlled switching mechanism of the dual-mode system gives the viewer the option of scanning 9 inches of a patient for a large field study or 6 inches for a maximal resolution study such as a cine coronary angiogram. When the center portion of an input phosphor, which is almost distortion-free, is used, not only is resolution improved but also the vignetting often associated with the peripheral portions of the fluoroscopic image is minimized.

Electrostatic lenses within the intensifier focus the electron pattern and reduce it in size to the configuration of the output phosphor. The output phosphor, made of fine-grain ZnCdS crystals and situated at the opposite end of the vacuum tube, is smaller in size than the input phosphor. A high-voltage power supply, coupled with a high-voltage cable, causes the electrons to travel at an accelerated speed from the photocathode to the output phosphor of the intensifier. As the electrons strike the output phosphor at an extremely high velocity, they are converted to light energy. Since the output phosphor is 1/2 or 1 inch in diameter on most image intensifiers, even if the electrons were not accelerated by high kilovoltage, there would still be a gain in intensification owing to the minification of the image. The electronic gain resulting from the high kilovoltage adds to the total light gain of the system. The first image intensifiers had a brightness gain of approximately 100 times more than conventional fluoroscopic screens, which originally were the Patterson type B-2 screen. More precise light gain measurement techniques have been developed, and intensifier gain is now evaluated in terms of light output per unit area per given amount of x-ray.

The *minification factor* is the reduction in size of the output phosphor from the input phosphor size. The concentration of the light from the smaller output phosphor also has an intensifying effect. Minification gain (MG) is achieved by electronically focusing the light from the input phosphor to the smaller area of the output phosphor.

$$MG = \left(\frac{\text{diameter of input phosphor}}{\text{diameter of output phosphor}} \right)^2$$

The brightness gain is equal to minification × flux. Flux gain occurs from the acceleration of the electrons striking the output phosphor. The electrons do not strike the output phosphor in a random fashion but are focused by a system of electronic lenses.

The entire system is housed in a glass tube and operates in a vacuum. The image from the output phosphor is transmitted to a mirror viewer or some type of television readout (see Fig. 12-1 and later, Television Viewing and Recording Systems).

As with all radiographic images, one must be concerned about quantum mottle, contrast, resolution, and distortion. Many factors impair resolution in an image intensifier. Some of the more obvious causes for image blur include geometric blurring, which can be due to the size of the focal spot, and phosphor graininess. Quantum fluctuation can be caused by scintillation (known as x-ray noise or quantum noise), which also occurs with low-dosage fluoroscopy.

Image intensifier resolution is measured by a line-pairs-per-millimeter (lp/mm) test object. Most CsI tubes will resolve between 4 and 6 lp/mm, depending on the size of the input screen.

Small image intensifiers with a 6-inch-diameter input phosphor can be mounted directly on a conventional fluoroscopic spot film tunnel. The larger intensifiers, particularly those that have dual- or tri-mode viewing fields, require counterbalanced ceiling mounts.

Newer image intensifiers, with input phosphors of 15 inches or greater, have metal as opposed to glass housings. A metal housing is essential because as the intensifier field gets larger, the glass tube becomes thicker and heavier. The photographic images made from the large output phosphor are of similar quality to full-field radiographs.

Automatic Brightness Control

An automatic brightness control (ABC) is a type of automatic exposure device (AED). An ABC senses the light output of the image intensifier and adjusts kVp or mA, or both, to produce a predetermined fluoroscopic density. The introduction of a contrast agent, differences in patient thickness, or any abrupt density change in the area under study (e.g., from the radiolucent right lung to the radiodense liver) is compensated for by the ABC.

The ABC helps to obtain optimal brightness of the image intensifier as well as good contrast during cineradiography or strip film imaging as patient thickness or density varies.

The Image Distributor

Mirror viewers, television monitors, cine cameras, and single- or multiframe photographic cameras can be linked to an image intensifier. A beam splitter, placed in close proximity to the output phosphor of an image intensifier, provides optical channels for multiple imaging techniques (Fig. 12-5). Some image distributors have up to three ports. One port can be used for mirror or television viewing, a second for cineradiography, and a third for strip or cut film techniques.

The image distributor reflects a predominant percentage of the light from the output phosphor in one direction for photographic recording while transmitting a lesser percentage of light to the mir-

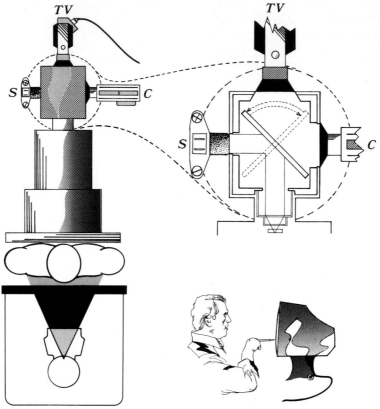

Figure 12-5
Image-Distributor

The image distributor (beam splitter) is placed in close proximity to the output phosphor of the image intensifier (top, left). Several channels are available for diverse imaging techniques (top, right). The image distributor reflects a predominant percentage of the light from the output phosphor in one direction for photographic recording, and transmits a lesser percentage to a television viewing or mirror optic system. A series of lenses and mirrors within the beam distributor are used to channel light to the appropriate camera. A 16- or 35-mm cine camera (C) can be linked to the beam distributor for cineradiography. Seventy-millimeter to 105-mm roll film cameras (S) can be used for either single-spot filming or multiframe imaging. A 4 × 4 inch (100-mm) cut film is also available for single or multiframe imaging. The light image from the output phosphor is displayed on a television monitor (bottom, right). The television monitor is an ideal teaching tool compared with a mirror optic system, which allows only one person at a time to view the fluoroscopic image. Some mirror optic units have dual mirror viewing capability. The fluoroscopist can remain in a fixed position while moving the image intensifier and observing the image on the television screen.

ror or television viewing system. Fiberoptics are sometimes used to couple the output phosphor to an optical system.

The collimating lens is set in relation to the output phosphor and must be focused at infinity. The beam splitting mirror must be in proper alignment (see Fig. 12-5). Contrast and brightness adjustments can be made on the television monitor.

Even if television viewing is preferred by the fluoroscopist, a mirror viewer should be available in the event that the television system fails.

Television Viewing and Recording Systems

The goal of radiography is to produce sufficient diagnostic information with minimal radiation dosage to the patient. The radiographer has some choices that allow dose reduction:

High-speed screen film systems
Strip film or cut film imaging as a substitute for conventional screen film radiography
High-speed cine film
The slowest possible cine frame rate
Video disk–pulsed fluoroscopy
An image intensifier–television system, which can increase light levels as much as 10,000 times when compared with conventional fluoroscopy.

Images viewed on a conventional or image intensified fluoroscopic screen are the reverse of a radiographic image; that is, bone and barium appear black instead of white. The television image can be reversed electronically to resemble a conventional radiographic image.

Three types of television cameras—the vidicon, plumicon, and orthicon—can be used with image intensifiers. The vidicon camera tube is relatively inexpensive but requires a large amount of light from the output phosphor for its operation. The plumicon camera tube is somewhat more light sensitive; the orthicon camera tube is the most sensitive to light.

A video signal is usually transmitted from the television camera to a television monitor through a closed circuit (see Figs. 12-1 and 12-5). The camera tube converts the light image from the output phosphor into a series of electrical impulses in the form of a video signal and usually transmits the image as a 525-scan-line pattern on a television monitor. Although high-resolution monitors of

1024 or 2048 lines are available, they are very expensive and not in common use. Television monitors permit more than one person to view the fluoroscopic image at a time. A disadvantage of the television system is the scan-line-type image that it produces and the potential for electronic noise.

The transmitted signal can be transferred directly to videotape by a videotape recorder. This system has several advantages:

Lower radiation dosage
Instant playback
Stop motion capability
No need for processing
Reuse of tapes

There are also disadvantages to videotape recording:

Poorer image resolution
Potential loss of the image caused by damage to the tape as the result of continual viewing of a single area
Lesser quality slow motion effect
Slower frame rate compared with that of high-speed cineradiography

Video disk scanners use a rigid magnetic or optical disk recording medium rather than a flexible tape. Video disks, used to store thousands of individual images, will be a major part of the electronic file room of the future. The major advantage of the disk recorder over the videotape recorder is that the image is not worn away by viewing individual frames. The video disk scanner has other advantages:

Displays an image at normal, slow, or reverse speeds
Provides stop-motion studies
Freezes a single television frame for image comparison or subtraction techniques

This stop-action storage feature uses short bursts of radiation during fluoroscopy to lower the radiation dosage to the patient. The fluoroscopist can study the stored image on a television screen without additional radiation exposure to the patient. For example, a short burst of x-ray can be used to freeze a projection of the hip during a hip pinning. After a guidewire or pin is inserted, a second pulsed image can be made and compared with the guidewire image. Both images can then be superimposed on a television monitor to compare placement of the metallic orthopedic device and the position of the fracture fragments.

Multiple television monitors are required when more than one video image must be simultaneously compared.

Interventional Radiography

With the introduction of interventional radiography, radiologists are performing outpatient therapeutic procedures in the radiology department. For example, percutaneous transluminal angioplasty (PTA) uses an angiographic catheter with an inflatable balloon to reopen an obstructed artery. Arteriosclerotic narrowing or occlusion results in fatty deposits that may harden and calcify within the arterial walls; arterial blood flow can be obstructed. The balloon tip catheter is guided fluoroscopically to the area of pathology, where it is inflated to compress and laterally displace the plaque formation within the intraluminal layer of the artery. Coronary angioplasty is being used when possible to avoid coronary bypass surgery.

The need for general anesthesia and time in the recovery room have been minimized. These procedures are easier on the patient, lessen the need for surgical intervention, and are relatively inexpensive when compared with most surgical procedures.

Cineradiography

Principles of Cineradiography

Physiologic events that occur too rapidly for normal fluoroscopic viewing can be recorded by cineradiography.

Most cineradiographic units use grid-controlled x-ray tubes that have a third electrode in the cathode assembly. This third electrode controls the flow of electrons across the x-ray tube, permitting extremely short yet accurate exposure times. The cathode focusing cup acts as a grid. This grid is not related in any way to the basic x-ray grid described in the control of scattered x-radiation.

A "bias" voltage applied to the cathode stops the continuous flow of electrons across the x-ray tube from cathode to anode. This occurs even though the filament is heated to thermionic emission levels. When the voltage level at the cathode is dropped to zero, electrons flow across the tube. The current that ordinarily would be flowing through the x-ray tube is stopped by an on-and-off process called *pulsing*. This "gating" effect makes it possible to synchronize the x-ray exposure with the shutters of a motion picture camera.

Sixteen-millimeter or 35-mm motion picture cameras are used for cineradiography. Motion picture cameras typically operate as slow as 8 frames/second (F/s) or as fast as 60 F/s. When slow-motion studies are required, the frame per second rate of the camera is increased. If 24 F/s are made and projected at 24 F/s, a normal rate of motion would be seen. If higher frame rates such as 60 F/s are taken but projected at 24 F/s, it will take approximately 2 1/2 times longer to view the study, resulting in a slow-motion effect. If only 12 F/s were made and shown at 24 F/s, motion would seem to occur twice as fast.

High-speed frame rates can be used to advantage to evaluate swallowing function, cardiac pulsation, or any arterial opacification procedure. Slow frame rates are helpful whenever motion is somewhat limited, for example, to evaluate the stomach with its slow emptying time.

Two different sizes of motion picture film are available for cineradiography: 16-mm film (40 frames/foot) or 35-mm film (16 frames/foot). Cineradiographic framing concepts vary from exact framing of the image to total overframing and are discussed in Chapter 13.

Comparison of Motion Recording Techniques

Multiple methods of recording are available to the radiologist. No one method of image recording, whether a conventional radiograph or a high-frame-rate cineradiographic study, can be used in every diagnostic situation. If dynamic function studies are required, motion picture studies or videotape or video disk recordings are helpful; however, the best recorded detail is still seen on conventional radiographs.

Special cineradiographic tube rating charts, designed for individual imaging systems, must be consulted to prevent tube damage.

Cineradiographic film, accessories, and related equipment are discussed in Chapter 13.

Electronic Radiography

An electronic radiograph has many of the characteristics of a conventional radiograph, with some additional benefits. The electronic image can be manipulated by a computer for the following purposes:

To enhance contrast

To extend image latitude

To electronically reverse the image

To be conveniently stored and easily retrieved from a laser disk. This information can be stored as numbers and will not gradually fade over time as does a silver-containing film.

To be printed as hard copy on film or paper

To be telecommunicated for reconstruction at a remote imaging station

A radiograph is an analog image. This image has high spatial resolution and can be handled and stored easily. To store individual radiographs requires a centralized file and considerable manpower and carries the potential risk for misplacing film jackets.

A digital radiographic system detects x-ray photons; this signal can be converted into digital or numeric values. As numeric values, the image-forming pattern can be manipulated by a computer in real time or at a later time. With a digital image, spatial resolution is poorer than that of an analog system but image contrast is improved.

Images are easily accessed simultaneously at multiple workstations. Multiple modalities can be included in the same patient file, along with patient information and report data.

Digital Subtraction Angiography

An electronic contrast enhancement system with subtraction capability can be linked to an image intensifier. Images can be quickly, easily, and cost-effectively subtracted electronically with a digital subtraction unit. Images can be viewed and recorded in their normal mode or can be reversed electronically. Electronic subtraction eliminates the need for time-consuming frame-by-frame screen film subtraction. The contrast-enhancement capability of the computer permits the visualization of small amounts of diluted contrast material, which would be barely visible on screen film radiographs.

One of the benefits of digital angiographic procedures was avoidance of arterial intervention. With the wider use of digital subtraction angiography (DSA), selective arterial injections are replacing the intravenous injection method, in which all the vessels under study are simultaneously filled with an iodinated contrast material.

Although the resolution on image-intensified studies does not equal that of screen film imaging, it is possible to obtain excellent-quality digital subtraction images (Fig. 12-6).

Although DSA images can be used in place of conventional screen film angiography, subselective and magnification angiography is still used for the demonstration of small vessels before some types of surgery.

Computed Radiography

Two types of electronic enhancement techniques use a laser scanner for their operation. The first uses a pair of conventional intensifying screens in a cassette and an "extended" latitude radiographic film. The radiograph exhibits an extended long-scale contrast with subtle differences in density. This film is scanned by a laser, and data are displayed on a video monitor for computer manipulation and interpretation. Multiformat cameras or laser printers can be used to produce hard copy.

A second, more widely accepted method of electronic radiography requires a reusable photostimulable phosphor-coated plate.* This plate, doped with europium to help with energy retention, is housed in a conventional cassette. Intensifying screens are not needed. After exposure to x-radiation, changes in the phosphors are read by a laser scanner. By scanning a laser light across the plate, energy is released as light. This analog signal, which is digitized and transferred by a digital image processor, can be computer manipulated (enhanced) for interpretation, stored, or reproduced as hard copy.

A distinct advantage of both electronic radiographic systems is that a wide variation in technical factors can produce acceptable images. The image can be manipulated to change density, contrast, and latitude. Underexposed radiographs can be enhanced to an acceptable density level; overexposed images can be reduced in density. In theory, repeat examinations as a result of over- or underexposure should no longer be required. Portions of the image can be selectively adjusted to better portray an area of interest. For example, an anteroposterior radiograph of the thoracic spine can be manipulated to view the ribs or the lung fields. These images can be reversed electronically

---

*Long BW: Computed radiography: Photostimulable phosphor image plate technology. Radiol Technol 61(2):107–111, 1989.

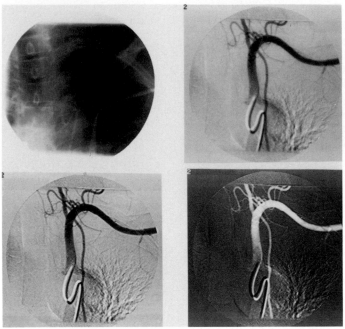

Figure 12-6
Digital Subtraction Angiography

Conventional angiographic subtraction techniques can be time consuming. With a digital subtraction angiographic (DSA) unit, multiple images can be rapidly subtracted electronically, frame to frame, if needed, and recorded with a multiformat camera or laser printer. Although the resolution of the image intensifier does not equal conventional screen film imaging, excellent quality subtraction studies are possible. The computer-enhanced DSA unit permits intravenous injection of contrast material for certain procedures, and the image contrast is superb. Conventional angiographic studies usually require arterial injections, whereas that remains an operator option with the DSA unit.

Register difficulties can be caused by patient or vessel motion during the procedure. Some DSA units use "gated" techniques, so that individual fluoroscopic frames are exposed when vascular pulsation is at a minimum. The patient is linked to cardiographic leads to determine when vascular relaxation occurs, and at that point the exposure is made. Electronic filtering systems can also be used to "smooth" the DSA image, minimizing the blur often associated with conventional subtraction register difficulties.

Images of the left subclavian artery can be compared by technique: (top left) an electronic digital mask image; (top right) an electronically subtracted image; (bottom left) an electronically subtracted image using a filter program to smooth the image; (bottom right) an electronic reversal of the subtracted image.

The catheter is not subtracted because of misregistration caused by a slight movement of the catheter during the injection. (Courtesy of The Genesee Hospital, Department of Diagnostic Radiology, Rochester, NY)

so that white areas appear black. An edge enhancement effect is also possible with this system.

Digitized information can be stored on videotapes, magnetic disks, or optical disks and transmitted by means of television for interpretation or consultation. Optical disk technology has an archival life of more than 30 years.

Other Medical Imaging Procedures

Other types of diagnostic medical imaging procedures are listed in the order of their development. A detailed description of these modalities is beyond the intent of this text; however, because many of these procedures are performed in departments of diagnostic medical imaging, an introduction is appropriate.

Several imaging modalities may be used to demonstrate a single area of anatomy, such as the kidney (Fig. 12-7). The size, shape, and configuration of the kidney is familiar even when presented in various positions or anatomic planes.

Nuclear Medicine Imaging

Radioactive substances have an affinity to specific areas within the body. After an injection or oral administration of a radioactive compound, organs or osseous structures can be evaluated with a gamma camera or other nuclear scanning devices. The absorbed radionuclides are detected by the scanning equipment and are imaged directly on film or a CRT from which hard copy can be made (Figs. 12-7 to 12-9).

Depending on the type of radioactive substance administered and the body part being evaluated, the study can be used to locate a disease process, plan chemotherapy treatment, or indicate normal activity, hypoactivity, or hyperactivity of an organ.

Medical Thermography

All objects having a temperature above absolute zero emit infrared radiation, which can be detected by heat-sensing equipment.

The naturally emitted heat patterns of the body can be detected and displayed on a CRT (Fig. 12-10). No ionizing radiation is required for or produced by this technique, which evolved from heat-sensing detectors used by the military in World War II. Because of its lack of specificity, medical thermography has not been well accepted as a primary diagnostic tool and is often used in conjunction with another imaging modality or physical examination, or both.

Although medical thermography is most commonly used for evaluation of the breasts in conjunction with mammography, it has also been used to detect inflammatory or compromised vascular conditions. Changes in vascular patterns in gangrenous extremities and evaluation of graft sites in severely burned patients are some of the other uses for medical thermography.

Ultrasound

Sound wave technology (ultrasound) evolved from sonar equipment used during World War II to locate naval vessels. Ultrasonography is a nonionizing form of diagnostic imaging. It is especially useful for obstetric and gynecologic evaluations, in which the use of x-radiation is not advisable.

Ultrasound equipment uses a transducer, which emits short pulses of ultrasonic waves in a forward direction. The sound waves continue within the body until they reach a boundary where the density of a structure changes. When boundaries of different densities are encountered, some of the sound waves are reflected backward to the transducer, which is also used to receive the reflected echoes. The images are viewed "live" on a CRT and recorded on single-emulsion film with a multiformat camera or laser printer (Figs. 12-7 and 12-11). Instant photography—a reflective image—is sometimes used, particularly with mobile ultrasonographic units.

Computed Tomography

Computed tomography (CT) is used to image cross-sectional anatomy, which, when displayed on a CRT, can be reconstructed in the transverse, coronal, or lateral plane. In patients with multiple injuries, a single CT examination may demonstrate unsuspected pathology, lessening the need for other imaging procedures. The tomographic feature helps to overcome the superimposition of organs or structures associated with conventional radiography. Multiple thin-section scans are required to image an anatomic area in its entirety.

These studies differ from screen film radiography in that density and contrast can be computer

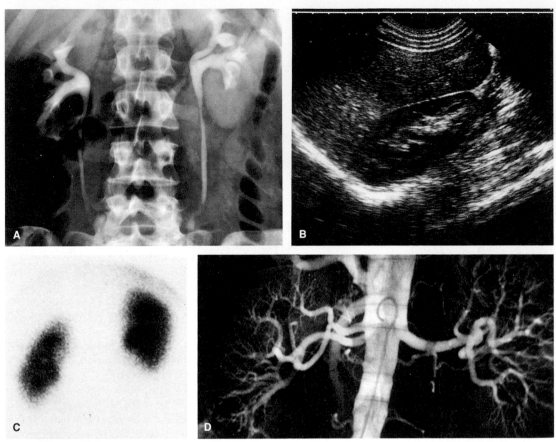

Figure 12-7
Multimodality Image Comparison

The kidneys are shown using several imaging modalities. Interestingly there are similarities between the images even though each modality offers its own information. (A) An intravenous urogram (IVU) represents conventional radiography. (B) The size and shape of the right kidney are easily identified on a sagittal ultrasonic section. (C) The kidneys are again easily recognizable in the radionuclide image. (D) A DSA study of the arterial phase of both kidneys is compared with (E) a conventional renal arteriogram. The DSA image has been cropped to a rectangular shape from the circular image obtained from the output phosphor of an image intensifier.

manipulated to distinguish minute differences between and within tissues. For example, gray- and white-matter densities within the brain can be imaged. The equipment used for CT differs from conventional tomographic equipment in that after the x-ray beam traverses the body, the remnant x-ray beam strikes multiple detectors that sense degrees of x-ray attenuation. This information is sent to a computer, which rapidly evaluates the data. Digital information is then reconstructed by complex computer algorithms and displayed as an image on a CRT monitor. The information is stored electronically and can be retrieved for review as

needed. Hard copies are usually made for diagnostic interpretation (see Fig. 12-7).

Magnetic Resonance Imaging

Magnetic resonance imaging (MRI) equipment generates images based on the electromagnetic properties of certain nuclei of body tissues, most commonly hydrogen. Although the mass of a structure (mass per tissue volume) is a primary consideration in conventional imaging, MRI detects small changes in radiofrequency-perturbed

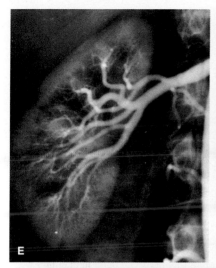

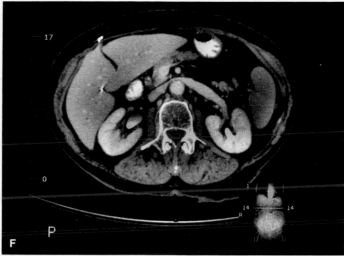

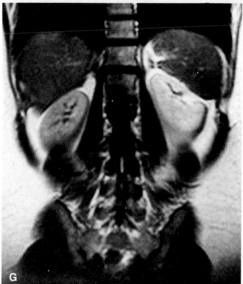

Figure 12-7 continued

(F) Computed tomography is used for an axial contrast-enhanced image of the abdomen at the level of the kidneys. Since only transverse or axial sections could be made with early computed tomographic units, this imaging technology was introduced as computerized axial tomography *(CAT). Complex computer algorithms can now be used to reconstruct transverse anatomy in additional planes.* Computed tomography *(CT) is now the accepted designation for this procedure. (G) A coronal magnetic resonance (MR) image of the abdomen was taken at the level of the kidneys. The size and shape of the kidneys in this image resemble the renal anatomy seen in the IVU (A), the nuclear scan (C), and the renal arteriograms (D and E). At first glance, MR images seem to resemble CT images; however, no bone is seen, which would be well demonstrated on CT images. (A and E, courtesy Eastman Kodak Company; B, C, and D, courtesy of the Vanderbilt University Medical Center, Department of Radiology and Radiological Sciences, Nashville, TN; F and G, courtesy of Picker International, Cleveland, OH)*

hydrogen nuclei within the magnetized tissue samples. Signal strength, therefore, is particularly dependent on hydrogen density. A comprehensive description of the physics associated with MRI is beyond the intent of this book.

Patients are placed on an examining table that slides into and out of the magnet within the gantry. MRI equipment containing powerful magnets is used to alter the normal spinning action of the hydrogen nuclei within the atoms of tissue. In a nonmagnetized state, the spinning action (precession) of the nuclei is random. Within the magnetized field, the nuclei will attempt to align themselves with or against the applied magnetic force field. By introducing a radiofrequency pulse, the spinning nuclei within the tissues absorb energy and change their angle of rotation to the main magnetic field. When the radiofrequency waves are turned off, the excited nuclei produce radiofrequency energy that can be detected, measured, and computer manipulated to produce an image that is displayed on a CRT (see Fig. 12-7).

By varying the MRI pulsing sequence and slice orientation, it is possible to produce clear details of soft tissue structures and obtain useful information about these tissues.

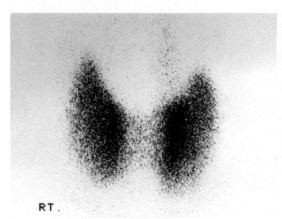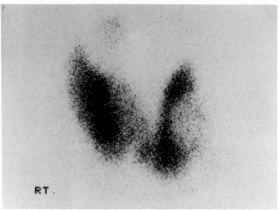

Figure 12-8
Nuclear Medicine Imaging of the Thyroid Gland

In nuclear medicine imaging, a radioactive compound is administered to evaluate organs or osseous structures. When the patient is scanned with a gamma camera or other type of radionuclide scanning device, radioactive substances that have an affinity to specific body parts can be detected and imaged. (Left) After the injection of a radionuclide, the thyroid gland demonstrates the classic, thinning "butterfly" appearance of a normal thyroid gland. Note the pyramidal lobe arising from the left side. (Right) A single cold nodule is noted in the left lobe of a diseased thyroid gland. (Courtesy of The Genesee Hospital, Department of Nuclear Medicine Imaging, Rochester, NY)

Since bone emits little or no magnetic resonance signals, structures obscured by bony tissue on other imaging modalities can be well demonstrated by MRI (see Fig. 12-7). For example, the brain, nervous system, and spinal cord can be evaluated; cardiac muscles, valves, and blood chambers can be easily demonstrated.

A patient with a pacemaker, ferromagnetic aneurysm clips, or a metallic foreign body in the eye should not be scanned with MRI equipment. A large metal prosthesis can create image artifacts if it is in the field. Small metal objects and tools can be strongly attracted to the gantry by the force field, and injury to patients or personnel can occur if safety precautions are not followed.

Three-Dimensional Computerized Reconstruction

Three-dimensional computerized reconstructions are possible from CT, MRI, and DSA images. High-resolution three-dimensional images are used as an aid in surgical planning. A simultaneous display of three-dimensional bone and soft tissue planes of the body and skull can be made from multiple angles.

Picture Archiving and Communication Systems

Picture archiving and communication systems (PACS) can image conventional radiographs or other medical images on a CRT or television moni-

Figure 12-9
Whole Body Scintigraphy

In a nuclear scan of the entire body, note the increased uptake of the radionuclide in the right shoulder. Nuclear bone scans can detect early pathologic changes in bone.

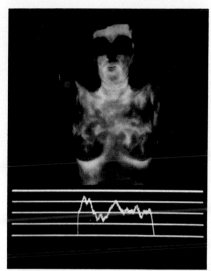

Figure 12-10
Thermographic Representation of the Breasts

A pictorial representation of the infrared heat patterns of the skin is the basis for medical thermography. Medical thermograpy, rarely a primary diagnostic tool, is usually used in conjunction with some other imaging modality or physical examination, or both. Infrared rays lying just beyond the visible spectrum are converted into visible light on a cathode ray tube. Liquid nitrogen, an odorless, colorless, tasteless gas (temperature of −320°F) is used to cool the detector cell in a thermographic unit. The patient should be cooled and examined in a room maintained at 68° to 70° F. Drafts, which cause uneven cooling resulting in artifacts, must be avoided. Before the breast examination shown here, the patient was disrobed to the waist. The arms were elevated for at least 5 minutes to dissipate the heat trapped in the axillae.

The heat pattern can be electronically reversed on a CRT. In this image, heat is represented as white; cooler structures are black. Note the white halo effect (a normal heat accumulation) beneath the folds of the breasts at the chest wall. The patient is wearing glasses, which register as having a lower temperature than the adjacent skin surfaces. The surface temperature of the nose is also lower than that of the face and is seen as a darkened area on the image. Venous patterns are seen as prominent vascular structures distributed throughout the breasts. A "hot" thermographic pattern can represent benign as well as malignant diseases. For example, an abscess may cause a thermogram to appear hot.

The fluctuating scale beneath the breast image is used to measure and compare temperatures from one side of the image to the other. Thermographic equipment can also detect and measure temperature changes within specific areas of the breast. (Courtesy of Wende Logan-Young, M.D., Rochester, NY)

tor. These images can be digitized, manipulated, and transmitted to remote locations by telephone, fiberoptics, coaxial cable, or microwave systems with no degradation in image quality. PACS can include an image distribution capability, a computed radiographic system, an archival system, and teleradiography potential.

Video monitors, as opposed to radiographic viewboxes, are used for viewing and interpretation. Images can be displayed on a high-resolution display system or a three-dimensional display workstation or can be printed on photographic film or paper.

In a large medical institution, diagnostic images may be reviewed many times for teaching purposes. The images can be manipulated by the viewer, similar to CT or MRI image manipulation. With an electronic storage capability, the images are never removed from storage. A PACS can serve as a physician extender; radiologists can consult with each other by way of the television

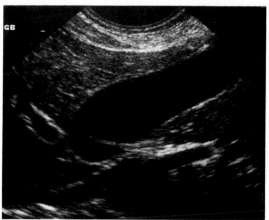

Figure 12-11
Ultrasonographic Images

Medical sonographic equipment emits short pulses of ultrasonic waves from a transducer. These sound waves are used to demonstrate boundaries of tissue where the density of a structure changes. The transducer also receives the backward-reflected sound waves, which are converted to ultrasonic images on a CRT and are usually recorded on single-emulsion photographic film with a multiformat camera or laser printer. Instant photography (reflective paper prints) can also be used to make hard copies. Since ionizing radiation is not required for ultrasound studies, this procedure is routinely used for obstetric and gynecologic studies. A representative image through the liver at the level of the gallbladder is shown. (Courtesy of the Vanderbilt University Medical Center, Department of Radiology and Radiological Sciences, Nashville, TN)

system when necessary. A physician can gain access to images and diagnostic reports from multiple modalities.

Radiographs or multiformat studies imaged from cathode ray tubes or laser printers are currently stored and filed in paper envelopes. This manual filing process is labor intensive and requires considerable filing space. Image archiving and retrieval may eliminate conventional storage and retrieval practices, as well as reduce the number of misplaced films and the time spent locating them.

Recording Media for Specialized Imaging

This chapter describes the recording media often used with specialized equipment for the following procedures:

Cineradiography
Photofluorography
Multiformat cathode ray tube and laser camera imaging
Dental radiographic and pantomographic studies
Intraoperative films for kidney radiography
Radiation therapy treatment localization and verification
 imaging
Duplication and subtraction techniques

Polaroid and xeroradiographic processes are also described.

Cineradiographic Film

Often during conventional fluoroscopic viewing, a physiologic event occurs so rapidly that it cannot be evaluated. Motion picture film is used to record the fluoroscopic image in real time or in slow motion. A specific requirement in a cardiac catheterization laboratory is that the x-ray tube used for cineradiography should have a high continuous load capability, owing to the lengthy fluoroscopic procedures associated with cardiac imaging. Because of the high frame rate per second used, the x-ray tube must also have an extended series length (frames per second; F/s) capability. In addition, since multiple cine runs may be made in rapid succession, there should be maximal dissipation of heat from the anode.

Cineradiographic units that use a grid-pulsed system to control the x-ray tube produce exposures as rapidly as 1 msec (1/1000th of a second) and are synchronized with the open shutter of the motion picture camera. An automatic exposure control known as an automatic brightness control (ABC) can automatically increase kVp, mA, or both, when considerable

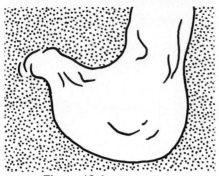 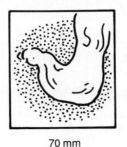

70 mm

35 mm

16 mm

Figure 13-1
Frame Size Comparisons
Four individual frame sizes are represented. (Far left) A 4 × 5 inch spot segment was one of four exposures made on an 8 × 10 inch fluoroscopic spot film. Next to it are a cut or strip film image (70 mm) and two cine film frame sizes (35 mm and 16 mm).

differences in body part thickness or density are encountered. (Cineradiographic equipment is described in Chapter 12.)

Cineradiographic films can be exposed at a rate of from 8 to 60 F/s or greater. Conventional motion picture sound projectors operate at 24 F/s. If only 12 F/s are exposed, a speeded-up impression of the physiologic event occurs when viewed at 24 F/s. If 60 F/s are made and projected at 24 F/s, it takes two and one half times longer to project the study, resulting in a slow-motion effect.

Two sizes of cineradiographic film, 16-mm and 35-mm, are commercially available. Sixteen-millimeter film records 40 individual frames per foot, whereas 35-mm film records 16 frames per foot. The dimensions of each 16-mm frame are 10.5 mm × 7.5 mm, whereas 35-mm film has a frame size of 20 mm × 18 mm, or approximately four times more surface area of increased silver

halide grains than the 16-mm film (Fig. 13-1). Since a greater surface area of silver halide grains must be exposed with the 35-mm cineradiographic film, more radiation is required to achieve the same degree of film blackening.

The size of the framing mode (framing technique) determines the amount of the area blackened on each individual cineradiographic frame (Fig. 13-2).

Special radiographic accessories, such as projectors, film splicers, and film editing equipment, are required for cineradiography. These accessories are more readily available in the 16-mm size. Although devices of this nature are available in the 35-mm size, they are considerably more expensive than their 16-mm counterparts.

The storage of processed cine studies presents a problem, which is compounded by the use of 35-mm film. Not only is 35-mm film two and one half

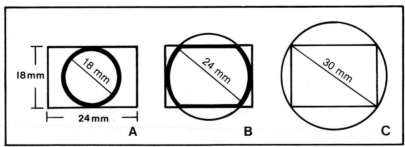

Figure 13-2
Cineradiographic Framing Concepts
Cineradiographic framing can include (A) exact framing, (B) maximal horizontal framing, or (C) total overframing. In A, approximately 50% of the film area is used, whereas in C 100% of the film area is used.

times longer, it is twice as wide, taking up more storage space.

Advantages Over Serial Film or Cassette Changers

A small, difficult-to-perceive change on a conventional radiograph may be more obvious on a motion picture study. Motion recording systems are often used to supplement full-size radiographs. If a comparison is made of the frame speed of a motion picture camera and the frame speed of a serial film changer—for example, 60 F/s vs. 6 radiographs/second—there will be 10 individual cine frames for each serial radiograph. The individual frames of the cine will be of poorer quality than those of the serial film angiograms, but the time interval between frames must be considered.

Disadvantages of Cineradiographic Recording

The loss of detail per individual frame is one disadvantage of cineradiography. Another is the need to restrict the cine field size to the typical 9-inch input phosphor, as opposed to the 14 × 14 inch serial film frame. Serial radiography made with a full-size film changer produces better quality individual images, because the serial images are about 1500 times larger than the cineradiographic frames.

Cineradiography involves cumbersome, time-consuming processing and editing techniques. Careful attention must be given to the processing technique used for cinefluorographic or strip films. A dedicated processor, properly maintained and scrupulously cleaned, is an absolute necessity. The processor selected must guarantee image reproducibility and uniform quality throughout the entire length and width of the film. Temperature control must be automatically regulated. Film surfaces should be continually bathed with recirculated, replenished, and temperature-controlled developer. An efficient replenisher system is a prerequisite for quality cine images because of the rapid solution exhaustion and solution carryover associated with cine processors. Specific instructions regarding chemistry, developer temperature, and other processing parameters must be obtained from the manufacturer of the unit.

Slow-motion cine projection is necessary, including frame-by-frame viewing. A single frame of film must be able to be projected for an extended period of time without damage to the film.

Single-Emulsion Photographic Film

Photofluorographic Film

The photofluorographic unit was designed in the early 1940s for mass screening of the chest to detect pulmonary tuberculosis. A photofluorographic unit contains a single fluoroscopic screen in a lightproof hood and a camera positioned at the back end of the hood. It is used to photograph an image from a full-size fluoroscopic screen on strip film or cut film. Single-emulsion photographic-type film is used to take a miniature photograph of the fluorescing screen (Fig. 13-3). The fluoroscopic image, when recorded on photographic film, resembles a radiographic image. It is an economical and efficient method for mass survey chest radiography.

A magnifying lens or a slide projector is required to view the processed miniature representation of the chest. Although most modern photofluorographic units use considerably less radiation than the original equipment, conventional screen film chest studies require much less radiation for adequate film blackening.

Strip or Cut Film

Seventy-millimeter to 105-mm roll film cameras or a 4 × 4 inch (100-mm) cut film camera can be used for single- or multiframe imaging from the output phosphor of the image intensifier. These cameras require special magazines that can be preloaded with strip or cut film. Self-threading take-up magazines permit the processing of individual strip film studies between examinations. The 100-mm system uses sheet film supplied in a room-light loading package of 100 sheets. This film can be used with either standard (2 F/s) or high-speed cameras (up to 12 F/s). The physical properties of this film, such as stiffness and flatness, are the same as conventional radiographic film.

When a conventional 9-inch input phosphor is used, strip or cut film techniques require considerably less exposure than that needed for a full-

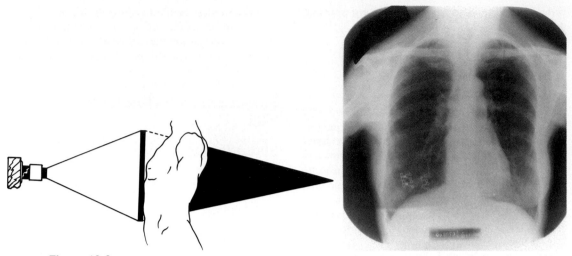

Figure 13-3
Photofluorography

(Left) *Photofluorographic units consist of a fluoroscopic screen in a lightproof hood. A strip or cut film camera mounted at the back end of the hood is used to record the fluoroscopic image of the chest. (Right) A 70-mm photofluorographic study of an adult female in the posteroanterior position was made from a full-size fluoroscopic screen. A single-emulsion photographic film was used for this study.*

size radiograph, because of the increased gain of the image intensifier. Lower radiation exposure, less cost per frame, and relatively easy film handling and storage are advantages of strip or cut film imaging. A disadvantage is that the size of the area to be examined is restricted to the size of the input phosphor of the intensifier (Figs. 13-1 and 13-4). Because of their small size, the strip or

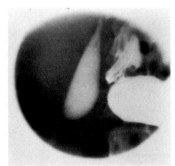

Figure 13-4
Kinescopic Spot Film

Extremely high resolution is possible with fine-line television kinescopic techniques. This image of an opacified gallbladder was made from a 1000-line television monitor on 70-mm strip film. Photographic imaging from the television monitor is not in common use. Most cut or strip film images are made directly from the output phosphor of the image intensifier.

cut film images are usually mounted in clear plastic frames for viewing and storage.

Cathode Ray Tube Film

Single-emulsion photographic films with antihalation backings are used for television monitor (CRT) imaging.

Multiformat cameras require an interface to the imaging device and a television monitor to display a visible image. One or more images are recorded on single-emulsion film. Multiformat cameras can be used to photograph images generated by digital subtraction angiography, ultrasonography, computed tomography, or magnetic resonance. (For representative images see Chapter 12.)

Laser Imaging Film

The raster lines of the television screen, electronic noise, and other types of interference are often simultaneously recorded when photographic techniques are used to transfer an image from a television monitor to single-emulsion film. An extremely fine-grain single-emulsion laser recording film, sensitive to laser light, has been developed to record data "written" directly on the film by a laser beam, thus eliminating raster lines on the processed image.

Dental Radiographic Film

Dental radiographic film is used in direct exposure techniques. This film has emulsion on both sides and is prepackaged in a light-tight, usually waterproof, envelope containing one or two films. Since it is impossible to identify each dental film with a label or lead marker during the procedure, the film manufacturer impresses a small raised dot on the film and packet to determine film placement relationships within the mouth. A manual from the Eastman Kodak Company gives specific dental film usage recommendations.*

The commonly used dental films include the following:

PERIAPICAL FILM. Periapical film is a direct-exposure, dual-emulsion dental film used for routine dental radiography to include the roots of the teeth (Fig. 13-5, *right).*

BITE-WING FILM. Bite-wing film is also a direct-exposure, dual-emulsion film, similar in appearance to periapical film except with a paper "bite-wing" extending at a right angle from the center of the front surface or tube side of the film packet. The bite-wing is held between the teeth to image the occlusal surfaces of the teeth (Fig. 13-5, *center).*

OCCLUSAL FILM. Occlusal film is a direct-exposure, dual-emulsion film, 2 1/4 × 3 inches in size, which is used when larger segments of the maxilla, mandible, or teeth are to be examined (Fig. 13-5, *left).* An occlusal film can also be used to localize calculi in the salivary ducts.

PANTOMOGRAPHIC FILM. A special body section device with the x-ray tube and cassette moving in opposing directions during an exposure can be used to simultaneously image the entire maxilla and mandible (Fig. 13-6). A narrow-slit primary beam is used with a long exposure time to produce a linear tomographic image of the upper and lower teeth. The anatomic area seen with this technique is referred to as a *plane* or *focal trough.* The pantomographic cassette uses intensifying screens with dual-emulsion screen-type radiographic film.

Intraoperative Film

Dual-emulsion x-ray film in a disposable plastic holder that can be sterilized and placed within the abdomen during kidney surgery is used with a direct exposure technique to determine whether calculi or calculi fragments are present. One study reports the use of a miniature vacuum cassette with a single high-definition intensifying screen and a single-emulsion film.* The cassette is gas ster-

---

*X-Rays in Dentistry. *Publication Number D1-5. Rochester, NY: Eastman Kodak Company.*

*Pochaczevsky R: Kidney cassettes for intraoperative radiography. *Radiology 123:237–238, 1977.*

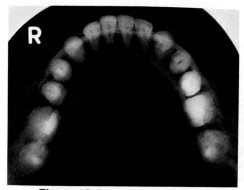
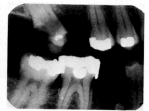
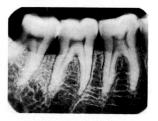

Figure 13-5
Dental Radiographic Images
Typical radiographic images are produced by direct exposure dental techniques. (Left) An occlusal film demonstrates almost all of the teeth of the mandible. Large segments of the maxilla, mandible, or teeth can be examined with occlusal films. (Center) A bite-wing film is used to evaluate the occlusal surfaces of the teeth. (Right) A periapical film used for routine radiography includes the roots of the teeth. (Reprinted courtesy Eastman Kodak Company)

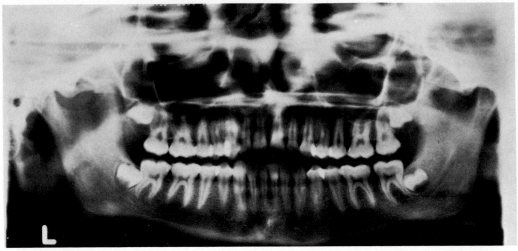

Figure 13-6
Pantomographic Study

Pantomographic units use split-scan tomographic techniques, with the tube and film moving in opposite directions to each other. This study includes the entire maxilla and mandible from one temporomandibular joint to the other. Note the horizontal parasitic streaks above the inferior orbital ridges caused by the horizontal linear movement of the tube and film. (Reprinted courtesy Eastman Kodak Company)

ilized and can be easily positioned beneath the kidney, within the abdomen. Both the prepacked direct exposure holder and the vacuum cassette have a notch or concavity to accommodate the renal pedicle (Fig. 13-7).

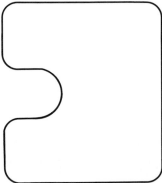

Figure 13-7
Intraoperative Kidney Film

A dual-emulsion, direct-exposure x-ray film in a plastic holder (shown), or a single high-definition intensifying screen that requires a single-emulsion film, can be used during kidney surgery to determine whether calculi or calculi fragments are present. The notch or concavity of the film or cassette is designed to accommodate the renal pedicle.

Radiation Therapy Imaging

Portal Localization Film

Portal radiographs are often made as part of radiation treatment planning to ascertain the position of the radiation beam and the shielding blocks. This beam–block relation to patient anatomy is an important part of the treatment. When portal localization radiographs are needed, a single exposure is often made with the radiation shielding blocks in position; a second exposure of the adjacent anatomy is then made on the same film with the blocks removed (Fig. 13-8).

Although medical screen film as well as fine-grain industrial-type films are used for radiation therapy imaging, the cassettes used for these techniques are quite different from medical radiographic cassettes. Therapy imaging cassettes do not contain conventional intensifying screens. The cassette used for portal imaging has a 1-mm-thick copper front screen in combination with a posterior lead screen. The copper screen intensifies the primary radiation and blocks electrons generated within the patient, keeping them from the film. The lead back screen also serves as an intensifier, providing additional exposure to the film, mostly as a result of backscattering of electrons.

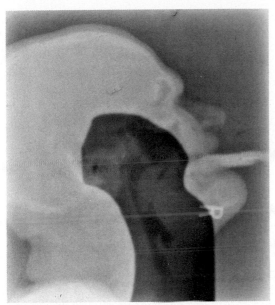

Figure 13-8
Radiation Therapy: Portal Localization Image

A portal localization radiograph of the soft tissue structures of the mouth and neck was obtained before radiation therapy. A double-exposure technique was used. The first exposure was made with shielding blocks in place to outline the field size. A second exposure was made with the blocks removed to demonstrate anatomy adjacent to the treatment area. Note the unusual shape of the actual treatment field, which was designed to minimize exposure to adjacent tissue. (Reprinted courtesy Eastman Kodak Company)

Portal Verification Film

Verification cassettes have anterior and posterior lead screens. A newer version uses a copper front and a posterior plastic screen. The plastic screen does not intensify the radiation but is used as a spacer to ensure contact of the x-ray film with the anterior copper screen. Blur is reduced and resolution is improved, because the image-forming electrons from the copper front screen are in better contact with the radiographic film.

The techniques and films used for treatment localization and verification differ in the following ways:

Film in a prepacked envelope is used with the portal localization or verification cassettes. Each sheet of film is prepackaged in a light-proof envelope by the manufacturer, and the cassettes can be loaded and unloaded in room light.

The radiographic film used for portal verification is a screen-type film used to minimize radiation to the patient during the pretreatment localization process (see Fig. 13-8).

The x-ray film used with the verification system is a slow, fine-grain, direct exposure film, since the actual radiation used for the treatment exposes the film. The verification film is left in position beneath the patient throughout the entire treatment (Fig. 13-9).

Sophisticated electronic and computed radiographic systems that allow manipulation and enhancement of portal and verification images are available.

Duplication and Subtraction

Duplication Film

Duplication images are made for teaching files, legal records, and as a courtesy to referring physicians. Original images can be retained while duplicates are forwarded to interested parties.

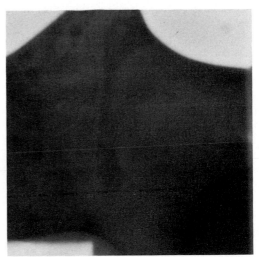

Figure 13-9
Radiation Therapy: Portal Verification Image

A portal verification radiograph with treatment shielding blocks in place records the radiation exit dose from the patient for the entire treatment. This radiograph documents the actual radiation treatment and can be used to evaluate localization errors that may have occurred during treatment. (Reprinted courtesy Eastman Kodak Company)

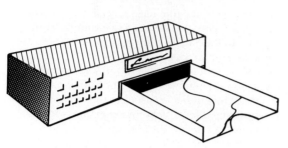
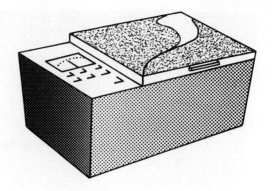

Figure 13-10
Duplication and Subtraction Printers

(Left) Duplicating film and a superimposed radiograph are fed into a roller-operated duplication printer in a darkroom. After exposure of the duplication film by the printer, the film is processed in an automatic processor and an exact duplication of the original radiograph is obtained. Subtraction techniques are also possible with some units of this type. (Right) A duplication/subtraction printer contains three light sources: a bright light for registration of superimposed images, a white light for exposing the subtraction mask and print, and an ultraviolet light for exposing duplicating film. This type of printer provides good contact because of equalized pressure over the large surfaces of the film. A timer permits variations in exposure lengths for better control of subtraction densities.

This process, photographic in nature, requires a duplicating printer or copier that uses ultraviolet light to make a contact print of a radiographic image (Fig. 13-10, *left*). The image is transferred to a sheet of single-emulsion duplicating film of the same dimensions.

The printing of any photographic film from a negative results in a positive. Duplication film, however, is sensitometrically designed to produce an exact duplicate of the original image. Since duplication film is single emulsion, the emulsion side must be placed against the radiograph to minimize lack of sharpness in the printing process. The back of the film is covered with an antihalation coating to stop light from passing through the film and scattering. The procedure must be performed under safelight conditions.

Subtraction Film

Radiographs are summation images, with considerable superimposition of structures. The subtraction process is used primarily for vessel evaluation in angiography to erase overlying structures that can mask diagnostic information.

Subtraction techniques are photographic in nature and usually use the same equipment as duplication techniques (see Fig. 13-10, *right*) Subtraction techniques, however, are considerably more complex to perform than are duplication procedures. Although there may be minor differences in duplication/subtraction equipment design, they all operate in essentially the same manner.

The tasks required for subtraction techniques include:

1. An angiographic scout image devoid of contrast material is used to produce a reverse image on subtraction film. This reverse tone image is known as a *mask.*
2. An angiographic image is selected from a serial study after the injection of a contrast medium.
3. The processed mask (step 1) must be superimposed, that is, "registered," on the selected angiographic image (step 2).
4. A copy of the superimposed mask and angiographic images, in register, is made on subtraction film.

In theory, the mask should subtract the structures common to the mask and the angiographic image. Osseous structures and soft tissues should be subtracted while the image of the opacified vessels remains, since it is unique to the angiogram (Fig. 13-11). It is almost impossible to produce a perfect subtraction image because slight movement by the patient between exposures can cause registration problems. When subtracting thoracic or abdominal angiographic images, cardiac motion, breath-

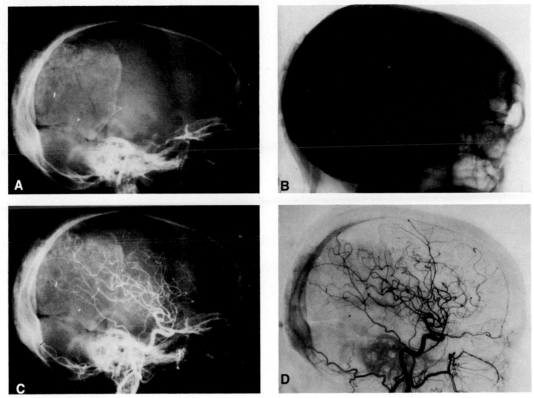

Figure 13-11
Subtraction Technique

Radiographs are summation images with considerable superimposition of anatomic structures. Subtraction is used to "cancel out" overlying structures in a radiograph. (A) A radiographic image devoid of contrast medium is selected to produce a subtraction mask (a reverse-tone image). (B) The mask is then registered on (C) an angiographic image. (D) A copy of the superimposed images produces a subtraction image. The mask serves to subtract out structures common to both the mask and the angiographic image. Osseous structures are subtracted but the contrast medium remains, since it is unique to the angiographic study. The mask is usually made from a scout film taken just before the injection of the contrast material. (Courtesy of The Genesee Hospital, Department of Diagnostic Radiology, Rochester, NY)

ing, vessel pulsations, or changes in position of gas or fecal shadows can cause register problems.

Boundary edges on the subtracted image will occur if any of the images—mask, scout, and so on—are not properly registered. These edges can interfere with visualization of vascular structures on the final subtracted image.

IMPORTANT

If it is not possible to register all radiographic details because of voluntary or involuntary motion, an effort should be made to register the area of interest.

Some radiographers prefer to place the subtracted mask against the angiogram with the emulsion side away from the radiograph. Although this produces a slightly unsharp image, they believe that this slight defocusing effect makes register misalignment less obvious.

If a higher level of subtraction is indicated, a second-order subtraction technique using two masks is suggested. The first-order mask is placed over the scout (base or zero) radiograph, and a second mask is made using subtraction film. The processed second-order mask is carefully superimposed on the first subtraction mask and then taped to the radiograph to be subtracted. The use of the bright light in the duplication/subtraction unit helps in the registering of the two masks to the radiograph when performing this multi-mask technique.

Most duplication/subtraction printers use the following types of light:

Conventional white light for exposing the subtraction mask and print
A bright white light for image registration purposes
Ultraviolet light to expose the duplicating film

All duplication and subtraction films can be processed in 90-second automatic processors.

Two television cameras can be used to simultaneously record an electronically reversed scout image and the angiographic image. The images can be electronically superimposed for a subtraction effect and hard-copy images recorded from the CRT. Digital subtraction techniques use computer technology to electronically produce subtracted angiographic images. The use of a computer to enhance the image permits the injection of smaller amounts of contrast medium. (See Chapter 12 for additional digital subtraction information.)

Instant Photography

Instant Photographic Film

Instant photography has been commercially available for more than 40 years. Instant photographic media contain their own processing systems. A

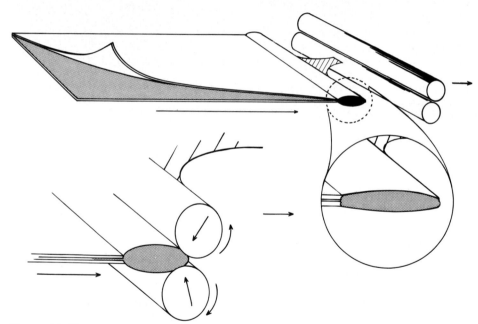

Figure 13-12
Polaroid Radiographic Process

The Polaroid radiographic system is a type of instant photography. The Polaroid radiographic packet consists of three major segments: a photosensitive emulsion; a metallic foil envelope, which contains a gel-like processing solution; and a receiving sheet, which accepts the image from the exposed negative.

Under room-light conditions, a Polaroid film is placed in a special cassette using a single-intensifying screen. After an exposure is made, a special unit is required to process the film. A paper tab is used to pull the exposed photosensitive film and the receiving paper through metallic rollers that rupture the envelope (insert) and spread the processing agent evenly over the surfaces of the film and paper. The developing gel functions as both developer and fixer. When the process has been completed, the receiving paper is separated from the photosensitive paper and a reverse image results. In the Polaroid image, dense structures such as bone and barium appear black.

foil pod containing a special processing gel is ruptured as the exposed film is pulled through a pair of rollers for processing. Instant black and white photography can be used to record medical images from CRT monitors.

The Polaroid X-ray System

The Polaroid x-ray system works in a manner similar to the Polaroid photographic process. Polaroid radiographic film can be loaded in room light into a special radiographic cassette containing a single intensifying screen. After a radiographic exposure, the Polaroid film packet is placed in a special roller processor. The film is pulled through the rollers, and a processing gel is spread over the exposed film (Fig. 13-12). A reverse-image paper print results. Bone appears black instead of white, as seen on conventional radiographs. This paper print requires reflective light for viewing.

Since the Polaroid x-ray system was available before the introduction of the automatic processor, it was immediately accepted by orthopedic surgeons for operative x-ray procedures as a method of reducing operating and anesthesia time. Although this system is no longer in common use, veterinarians find it useful when examining the extremities of large animals at remote locations.

The Polaroid Dry Imaging System

A dry processing technology that uses carbon-based film and a laser imager eliminates the need for a darkroom, wet chemical processing, and wet chemical waste. This unit can be used with nuclear medicine and ultrasound scanners to produce 8 × 10 inch images in about 90 seconds. The images resemble conventional black-and-white silver halide films with comparable stability and archival qualities.

Xeroradiography

The xeroradiographic process and its recording media differ from screen film imaging. An electrically charged selenium-coated plate is used in place of x-ray film in a special lightproof cassette. The xeroradiographic cassette must be handled carefully to avoid discharging of the plate, which can result in image artifacts. Special conditioning

and processing units are required for this procedure (Figs. 13-13 and 13-14).

The selenium plate must be electrically charged in a special conditioning unit. When an exposure is made, the x-ray beam forms a latent image within the electrical charge. X-rays passing through the body electrically discharge the plate in direct proportion to the density or mass of the overlying tissue (Fig. 13-15). The surface of the exposed plate is dusted with a thermoplastic powder known as toner in a processing unit designed for this purpose. The toner adheres to the exposed plate in amounts proportional to the charge remaining on the plate after exposure. The powder

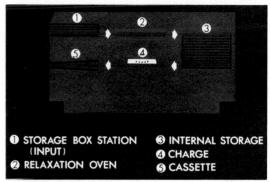

Figure 13-13
Xeroradiographic Conditioner
The xeroradiographic process requires special image receptors, processors, and conditioning equipment. A reusable selenium-coated photoreceptor plate is used in place of intensifying screens and x-ray film.

A xeroradiographic plate conditioner functions as follows: The storage box station (1), which holds up to six reusable selenium-coated plates in a standby position, is taken from the processing unit (see Fig. 13-14) and inserted into the conditioner. The plates are transported within the conditioner to the relaxation oven (2) and heated (relaxed) to remove any residual electrical charge remaining from a previous exposure. The plates are then placed in internal storage (3) where they cool to room temperature in a storage magazine, which can accommodate up to 16 plates.

When an empty cassette is inserted into the conditioner, a plate is moved from the storage magazine to be sensitized, that is, given a uniform electrostatic charge (4). The plate is now sensitive to x-radiation and light. The charged plate is automatically loaded into a light-tight cassette (5) and released from the conditioner. When the sealed cassette with its charged plate is removed from the conditioner, it is ready for an x-ray exposure. (Courtesy Xerox Corporation, Xerox Medical Systems, Pasadena, CA)

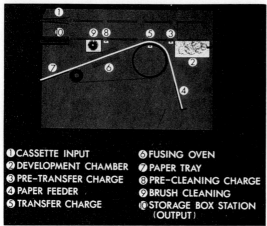

Figure 13-14
Xeroradiographic Processing Unit

A xeroradiographic processing unit functions as follows: The cassette (1) holding an exposed plate is inserted into the processor. Improperly oriented cassettes will not be accepted by the processor. The exposed plate is automatically removed from its cassette and transferred to the development chamber (2) where a charged developing powder, known as toner, is sprayed on the surface of the selenium-coated plate. More toner is attracted to areas that have a remaining high charge; less toner is attracted to less charged regions (see Fig. 13-15). Pre-transfer charging (3) neutralizes the remaining charge on the plate, and the layer of developing powder is charged negatively to increase the efficiency of the transfer process.

A sheet of paper moves from the paper feeder (4) into the transfer position (5) for contact with the plate. At a registration point, the plate and paper meet. A transfer charge is passed over the back side of the paper, drawing developer powder to the paper. The paper is then withdrawn from the plate and carried to the fixing station. In the fusing oven (6) the paper surface is heated to permanently fix developer particles to the paper. The finished xeroradiograph exits into the paper tray (7) ready for immediate viewing.

Residual powder that may remain on the plate following the transfer is removed by a neutralizing charge (8). This pre-cleaning charge helps to free residual powder from the plate surface. A rotating fine soft brush (9) removes the developer from the plate. The plate is then deposited into the storage box (10), which must accumulate six plates before the storage box can be released to be taken to the conditioner unit (see Fig. 13-13). (Courtesy Xerox Corporation, Xerox Medical Systems, Pasadena, CA)

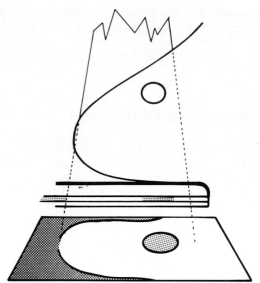

Figure 13-15
Exposure of a Charged Selenium Plate

A dense circular mass in a breast is depicted. The shaded area *represents unexposed regions of the xeroradiographic plate. The x-ray beam used for this representation was collimated to the shape of the breast. In this illustration, the dense circular lesion absorbs most of the x-rays, so that the discharge of the selenium-coated plate surface is minimal. There is little effect on the original surface charge of the selenium plate in the area of the lesion or in the unexposed portions of the plate outside the tightly collimated x-ray beam. The x-ray beam passing through the radiolucent breast "erases" much of the charge.*

Xeroradiographic systems have a wide exposure latitude because the development process is particularly responsive to charge differences. In an actual xeroradiograph, density changes would vary throughout the entire image, ranging from soft tissue densities to dense bone structures (see Figs. 13-16 and 13-17).

image is then transferred to a copy paper (9.5 × 13.5 inches) and heat-sealed in the processing unit. The selenium plate can then be returned to the conditioning unit to relax the plate image, after which the cleaned, relaxed plate is recharged for reuse.

Xeroradiography has a wide recording latitude with an edge enhancement effect. In xeroradiography, sharp structural edges are enhanced by the attraction of the toner material on the plate. Immediately adjacent to sharp-edged structures,

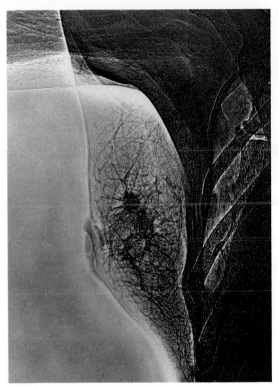

Figure 13-16
Xeroradiographic Image of the Breast
(Positive Mode)

This image exhibits wide exposure latitude. A stellate carcinoma of the breast is shown, with skin thickening and nipple retraction. The chest wall, including the osseous details of the ribs, can be seen. The black densities in this illustration would be blue in an actual xeromammographic study. See Figure 13-17 for an example of reversal (negative mode image). (Courtesy Xerox Corporation, Xerox Medical Systems, Pasadena, CA)

little or no toner is deposited. This effect is known as *deletion*. Sharply delineated edges of vessels, osseous structures, and calcifications benefit from the deletion effect (Fig. 13-16).

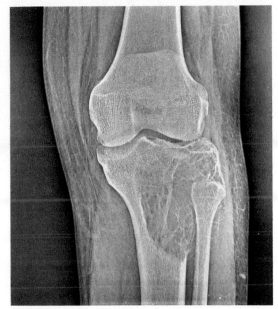

Figure 13-17
Xeroradiographic Image (Negative Mode)

A negative mode xeroradiographic image is obtained by altering conditioning and processing parameters on the xeroradiographic equipment. This anteroposterior image of the knee demonstrates a destructive lesion that encompasses the lateral aspect of the upper tibia. Note the soft tissue visualization throughout the entire image. (Courtesy Xerox Corporation, Xerox Medical Systems, Pasadena, CA)

Xeroradiographic images are blue and white as opposed to black and white radiographs. In positive-mode xeroradiographic studies, blue represents the dense areas and white represents the radiolucent areas. When conditioning the plate, this process can be reversed to a negative mode, with white made to represent the more dense areas and blue the more radiolucent areas (Fig. 13-17).

Chapter 14

Quality Assurance Guidelines

A radiographic study that is of high quality may sometimes contribute more to patient care than some of the newer imaging modalities.

At a conference of the World Health Organization in 1980 in Germany, the following definition was developed: "Quality assurance is the organized efforts by staff to insure the consistent production of adequate diagnostic information at the lowest possible cost with minimum exposure to both patients and personnel to radiation."*

Some Radiation Protection Considerations

Most radiation received during one's lifetime will be manmade.

Health care workers are issued radiation safety monitoring badges or dosimeters if they are employed in areas where studies using radiation for diagnosis or treatment are performed. If it is necessary to work near an x-ray source, radiation protection and monitoring devices must be provided. A film badge, thermoluminescent dosimeter (TLD), or ionization chamber can be use to monitor radiation exposure to personnel.

Personnel can be protected from x-radiation by the use of lead barriers in walls, windows, doors, movable lead shields, and lead sheeting. Radiation dosage to personnel can also be reduced by increasing the distance between the operator and the x-ray source. Exposure control cords should be up to 12 feet in length on mobile equipment to permit the operator to stand at a greater distance from the x-ray source. Exposure control cords on permanently installed units should be very short to ensure that an exposure cannot be made from out-

World Health Organization: Quality Assurance in Diagnostic Radiology. Geneva: WHO, 1982.

Angeline M. Cullinan and John E. Cullinan:
PRODUCING QUALITY RADIOGRAPHS, 2ND ED.
© 1987, 1994 J. B. Lippincott Company.

side of the control booth. Concern for a patient should not be an excuse to expose another radiographer or other professionals to x-radiation. Patient holding devices should be available, especially for pediatric studies. X-ray personnel should wear lead aprons and gloves whenever they may be exposed to primary or scatter radiation. Fluoroscopists should consider using protective eyeglasses and thyroid shields in addition to a lead apron and gloves.

Direct reading ionization chambers and TLDs, placed in the path of the primary beam, can be used to monitor entrance skin exposure (ESE) from medical and dental x-rays to patients. Patients can be protected from excess radiation in several ways:

Filtration of the x-ray beam. Filters remove soft radiation that would be absorbed by the patient but do not produce useful information on the radiograph.

Beam-limiting devices. These restrict the x-ray beam to the area of interest.

Shielding. Like beam restriction, shielding restricts the field size and can selectively protect radiosensitive areas. All patients with reproductive potential are entitled to gonadal shielding. Many accessories can be used for protective purposes, including pelvic lead sheeting or a lead shield attached to the collimator for positioning in the x-ray beam (see Chapter 5, Fig. 5-6). At a bedside examination, the patient lying adjacent to a patient being examined should be considered. People accompanying a patient are also at risk; for example, the mother of a child who is being examined may be pregnant.

Occasionally, special coverage of the thyroid gland or lenses of the eyes is indicated.

Leakage radiation from the x-ray tube is a another concern. The x-ray tube shielding should not permit leakage radiation to exceed 100 mR/hr/meter/ from the source when the machine is operating at maximal output. A Victoreen R-meter or TLD can be used to test for leakage radiation.

Selective positioning. Some patient positioning techniques reduce dosage to radiosensitive areas. For example, in the anteroposterior position for skull tomography, the unattenuated primary beam enters through the lens of the eyes. With the patient in the posteroanterior position, attenuated remnant radiation exits through the lens of the eyes (see Chapter 11, Fig. 11-18). The posteroanterior position can also be used for studies of the full vertebral column of young females to minimize dosage to the breasts.

Adherence to the 10-day rule. Attention to the menstrual cycle in women of child-bearing age can reduce the possibility of radiation exposure to a fetus.

Exposure factor selection. The use of proper technical factors, such as an optimal kilovoltage technique, ensures adequate penetration of the part under study with decreased absorbed dosage.

Use of high-speed screen film combinations whenever possible. Rare-earth technology significantly lowers radiation dosage without compromising the image.

The National Council on Radiation Protection estimated that more than 40% of the annual collective effective dose equivalent from medical x-ray examinations results from two fluoroscopic examinations, the upper gastrointestinal study and the barium enema.* Since approximately 50% of patient exposure with these studies is the result of fluoroscopic screen film imaging, the substitution of a 1200-speed for a 400-speed screen film system would reduce patient exposure by approximately 17%. Further reduction in dosage could be accomplished with a high-ratio grid in the spot device linked to a 0.6-mm focal spot. Bucky-like radiographs can be obtained with this arrangement, thereby eliminating the need for some overhead Bucky images.

Avoiding repeat radiographs. Careful attention to technical details and positioning before making an exposure can often eliminate the need for a repeat examination.

Quality Control and Quality Assurance

Even minor variations in equipment standards, each within acceptable tolerances, can collectively degrade a radiographic image. Everything may be within specifications and yet the quality of the medical images may not meet departmental standards. Quality control (QC) techniques ensure standards in a specific piece of equipment; quality assurance (QA) programs ensure standards between x-ray units and the x-ray procedures performed with these units.

FDA Roundup Medical Devices Report, May 18, 1989.

Quality assurance goals mandate technically reproducible follow-up studies over an extended period of time. Documentation of technical factors and related information for each study is important. QA testing procedures are now mandatory in many states.

IMPORTANT

After ascertaining a need to measure a specific function, measurement parameters should be developed. Each test should be reproducible, relevant to patient care, easy to perform, and as low in cost as possible. Testing equipment should comply with all local, state, or federal codes or regulations for electrical and radiologic safety. Agencies such as the American College of Radiology (ACR) and the Joint Commission on Accreditation of Health Organizations (JCAHO) have established regulations for accreditation and certification.

Quality Control Testing of the Automatic Film Processor

Quality control testing and quality assurance programs begin with the automatic processor (Table 14-1). Often radiographic equipment seemingly fails to perform properly, when in reality minor changes in the processor are responsible for the poor-quality images (Table 14-2). Every radiographic room or mobile unit serviced by a faulty processor can be affected by it. A poorly calibrated or malfunctioning automatic processor can undermine a technique chart, accurately calibrated x-ray equipment, and the best efforts of a radiographer

to produce quality radiographs (Fig. 14-1). A processor QC program can help to minimize the repeat rate, patient exposure, and departmental operating costs.

Preventive Maintenance

In order for the processor to operate efficiently, an established preventive maintenance routine should be faithfully followed. Daily and weekly cleanup procedures will result in a well-maintained processor that will require minimal servicing. Some recommended tasks include the following:

1. Daily cleaning with a nonabrasive cleaner. Dried precipitation from evaporated chemicals on the rollers can cause transport problems. A single dirty roller can cause a breakdown in the automatic processor.
2. Developer and fixer tanks must be covered with lids to reduce chemical evaporation, which can cause oxidation of the developer and diminish its chemical activity. If a processor is used in a low-volume area, evaporation covers are very important.
3. The top lid of the processor should be propped open at shutdown. This will help to prevent the precipitation of chemicals on the lid, which may fall back into the solutions and cause contamination.
4. The water tank should be drained when the processor is turned off to minimize the formation of algae.
5. Lubricants should not be used on the roller gears because of possible contamination of the solutions.

Table 14-1. Some Basic Quality Assurance Tests for the Automatic Processor

Test	Test Tools	Comments
Processor function and replenishment; documentation of sensitometric properties of radiographic film	Sensitometer,* densitometer,* stepwedge, graduated beakers, thermometer	Changes may affect density, contrast, and fog level on processed radiograph.
Safelight	Film, stopwatch, mask	Improper filter or wattage can add supplemental density to film (fog).

Electronic sensitometers and densitometers, some with sophisticated software programs, are also available (see Fig. 14-3).

Table 14-2. System Control Trouble-Shooting List

Film Appearance	Fog	Speed Index	Contrast Index	Possible Cause
Image density too high	↑	↑	↑	Developer temperature too high Developing time too long Faulty developer mix Insufficient mixing Slight overreplenishment of developer
Image density too low	↓	↓	↓	Developer temperature too low Developing time too short Exhaustion of developer Insufficient developer replenishment rate Faulty developer mix
Increased fog level, loss of image contrast	↑	↔	↓	Contamination of developer-fixer Insufficient fixer replenishment rate
Increased fog level, increased image density with loss of image contrast	↑	↑	↓	Contamination of fixer-developer Faulty developer mix Insufficient mixing Safelight fogging
Increased fog level, loss of image density and contrast	↑	↓	↓	Insufficient starter Excessive overreplenishment of developer Complete oxidation of developer
Loss of image density and contrast	↔	↓	↓	Developer overdiluted Insufficient replenishment rate of developer
Increased speed and loss of contrast	↔	↑	↓	Slight fixer contamination No splash covers Poor dryer exhaust Fixer percolation

Reprinted courtesy Eastman Kodak Company.

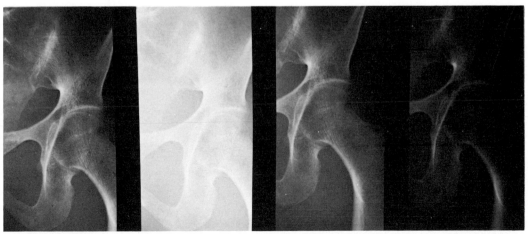

Figure 14-1
Automatic Processor Quality Control

Severe differences can occur in radiographic densities as the result of mechanical or chemical problems in an automatic processor. These four radiographs of a pelvic phantom were all exposed with the same calibrated x-ray unit, cassette, technical factors, and collimator shutter pattern. Immediately processed in four different automatic processors, they exhibit severe variations in density due to processor malfunctions. Since one rarely has the opportunity to compare images from processor to processor, daily quality control testing of all processors is essential.

X-ray Film Processing

The benefits of state-of-the-art x-ray equipment and a high-quality screen film product can be lost if the film is not processed properly.

Care must be taken in the selection of safelight filters. Special filters are required to match the spectral sensitivity of the film in use. For years, the Eastman Kodak Wratten Series 6B safelight filter was in common use. This filter was designed to be used with blue- and ultraviolet-sensitive medical x-ray films. With the introduction of orthochromatic medical x-ray film, a filter was designed that could be used with blue-, ultraviolet-, and green-sensitive film products. This filter is the Kodak safelight filter type GBX-2.

A dark green filter is available for photofluorographic and cinefluorographic panchromatic films; however, these films should be handled in total darkness until at least one half of the development time has expired.

If a safelight designed for blue-sensitive film is used with orthochromatic x-ray film, which is primarily green-sensitive, there will be fogging of the film. A number of other potential sources of fog exist:

An improperly attached filter
A faded filter
A crack in the filter or safelight housing
Number and location of safelights
A safelight bulb wattage that exceeds the recommended level. Light bulb wattage level information and a simple safelight test kit are available from most film sales representatives.
Light leaks around doors, passboxes, or the processor
Indicator lights on equipment, such as a humidifier, telephone, silver recovery units, and so on
Phosphorescent clothing or accessories, such as some wristwatch dials

---

IMPORTANT

After exposure to x-radiation, film is usually more sensitive to low-level light.

Automatic Processor QC Tasks

Processing QC should be done in the morning, before processing any films, before and after processor cleaning, and after fresh chemicals have been added to the replenisher storage tanks.

Monitoring Developer Activity

Monitoring of the developer process includes checking the length of development and the developer temperature. The number and size of films fed into an automatic processor and the time of the development can affect developer activity. (See Chapter 7, Flooded Replenishment.) The processor temperature should be compatible with the make and type of film being used.

Automatic film processors should be set according to the manufacturers' recommendation. However, some film products cannot tolerate the 95°F developer temperature recommended by processor manufacturers.

The temperature must be monitored using a digital thermometer (Fig. 14-2).

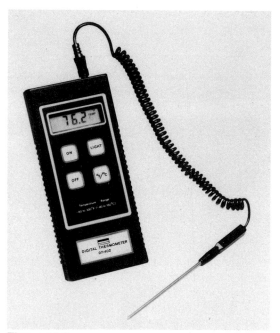

Figure 14-2
Digital Thermometer
A battery-powered, hand-held thermometer with a detachable emersion probe can be used to check film processor solution temperatures. Multiple probes can be used with a single display unit to eliminate possible cross-contamination of chemicals. (Courtesy Nuclear Associates, division of Victoreen, Carle Place, NY)

A mercury thermometer should not be used in the darkroom. If it breaks, mercury in the x-ray developer will contaminate the solution, even at a few parts of mercury per million. It is almost impossible to remove all traces of mercury from a developing tank or darkroom.

Monitoring Chemical Activity

Among the factors that affect chemical activity are replenishment rates and solution contamination. Replenishment rates can be easily measured by disconnecting the replenisher lines so that the replenisher solution that is fed into the processor flows into graduated beakers. The replenishment tanks should contain only as much solution as can be used within 2 weeks.

Care must be taken to avoid contamination of the developer by the fixing solution. It is advisable to change solutions in the automatic processor at least every 6 months. More frequent changes may be required depending on the workload of the department. When the solutions are being changed, a more thorough cleaning and inspection should be made using a maintenance checklist.

Sensitometric Control Film

Processor activity should be evaluated by a sensitometric film strip exposed by a sensitometer. The color of the light source of a sensitometer must match the primary light sensitivity of the film strip, such as a green light source for a primarily green-sensitive film.

New sensitometers are available for simultaneous exposure of both emulsions (Fig. 14-3). This is essential when using dual-emulsion, zero-crossover film.

A densitometer contains a light source and a timing mechanism for precise, repeatable light exposure to x-ray film and is used to evaluate the sensitometric readings from the processed image. Speed, contrast, and fog should be evaluated daily (see Fig. 14-3), and a log should be maintained.

The test strips should be exposed and processed in the same manner every time to reduce variability.

Electronic automatic scanning densitometers that can measure, analyze, and store data and create reports and processor control charts are essential for rapid and accurate QC testing of the automatic processor (see Fig. 14-3). (An introduction to sensitometers and densitometers can be found in Chapter 7.)

With a screen film system, an x-ray machine is sometimes used to expose a stepwedge to monitor the processor. However, a sensitometer is recommended for this task, since the x-ray machine may vary in radiation output.

X-ray Equipment Maintenance

QA techniques help to fine tune imaging equipment and accessories. It is imperative that QA tests be documented, continually updated, and available for reference. Records must also be maintained when modifications are made to the equipment. These records can be used to evaluate room downtime, repair costs per room, and the need to update existing equipment or to purchase new equipment.

Protocol and Recommendations

A regular schedule should be adopted for QA testing on all radiographic and fluoroscopic equipment (Table 14-3). Test tools should be reliable to guarantee accurate, reproducible results. Each component of the radiographic/fluoroscopic system should be subjected to the following guidelines:

1. There should be specific materials and equipment available for each test. It is important that approved QA test tools be used. Instructions for the use of the tools, descriptions of the tests and test results, and suggestions for monitoring test evaluations are included with each test tool.
2. Test procedures should be standardized to ensure reproducible results.
3. Preventive maintenance schedules should be set up to detect variations in equipment function.
4. Protocol should be clearly stated so that corrective procedures can be initiated and carried out whenever test results indicate a deviation from normal.
5. Records and service reports should be main-

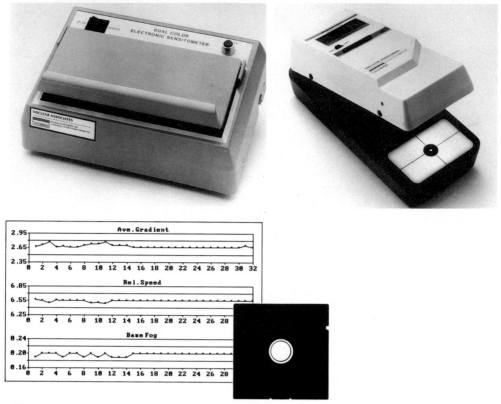

Figure 14-3
Electronic Sensitometers and Densitometers

(Top, left) A microprocessor-based sensitometer is capable of a double-sided simultaneous exposure of a dual-emulsion test film or a single exposure of single-emulsion test film. The double-sided, simultaneous exposure is required for zero-crossover films. The unit contains a real-time clock for automatic time and date stamping of the test film. This unit has a dual-color capability for use with blue-sensitive and green-sensitive sheet film and cine film. (Top, right) A transportable, battery-operated densitometer is convenient to use. The processed film is read on a three-digit liquid crystal display. (Bottom) A computerized quality-control processor program can be used to evaluate an x-ray film processor in seconds. It measures and analyzes data and generates reports, control charts, and corrective action forms. This program can be used with any sensitometer-densitometer combination for multiple-film processors. (Courtesy Nuclear Associates, division of Victoreen, Carle Place, NY)

tained for each piece of equipment for which a problem is indicated and should include the date of testing, corrective action taken, date of action, and so on. This record will help to document recurrent problems and to check variations in equipment that may occur between scheduled tests.

6. If an x-ray unit is altered in a major way, including replacement of parts, quality control testing of the equipment must be done in order to compare image quality to the original parameters.

Documentation

The guidelines for quality assurance are usually set by a radiation safety committee that usually includes a radiologist, a physicist, and a radiation safety officer. A procedure manual should be designed by this committee. It should list the following information necessary for accurate QA testing:

1. Individuals responsible for testing, supervising, and servicing the equipment
2. Types of QA testing

Table 14-3. Some Basic Quality Assurance Tests

Test	Test Tools	Comments
Screen film contact	Wire mesh	Poor screen film contact affects detail (see Figs. 14-19 and 14-21)
Grid uniformity	Cassette/film	Performed to check for damage to grid (see Fig. 5-17)
Grid alignment	Grid phantom	Performed to check for alignment of the grid to the table (can also be a visual check) (see Fig. 14-4)
Focal spot size	Pinhole camera	Demonstrates the intensity distribution of the projected focal spot (see Fig. 14-15)
	Star test pattern test tool, a stand on which to mount test pattern	Central ray alignment is critical for accurate measurements (see Fig. 14-14)
	Slit camera assembly and stand	Recommended device for measuring focal spot size and focal spot blooming (see Fig. 14-16)
Beam alignment	Alignment test tool or four small objects (coins)	Misalignment can cause cutoff on edges of radiograph (see Fig. 14-6)
Timer accuracy	Spinning top (single-phase equipment)	Timer accuracy can be determined by number of dots recorded in a given time (see Fig. 14-9)
	Motor driven Spinning top (three-phase equipment)	If spinning top is used for three-phase equipment an arc (continuous line) results; requires a template for evaluation (see Fig. 14-10)
	Oscilloscope (three-phase equipment)	Requires service personnel for performance of test
AED control (automatic exposure reproducibility)	Stepwedge, ruler, containers, water or tissue-equivalent material, densitometer	Performed to determine if phototimer or ionization exposures are consistent
KV accuracy	Test cassette	Performed to check calibration of kilovoltage (see Fig. 14-12)
mA accuracy	Stepwedge	Performed to check mA linearity
	Oscilloscope	Requires qualified service personnel for performance of test
Beam quality	Al and Cu attenuators	Performed to check for half-value layer
Tomographic accuracy	Aperture plate phantom	Evaluation of fulcrum, stability, exposure uniformity, and cut level accuracy (see Fig. 14-17)
Optical system (fluoro, image intensifier)	Wire mesh segments, phantom	Performed to evaluate resolution or loss of resolving power; exposure rates; and brightness (see Fig. 14-18)
Television (mirror optics; fluoro, image intensifier)	Aluminum blocks, penetrometer	Performed to evaluate low-contrast structures
Automatic brightness control	Aluminum blocks, resolution test pattern	Performed to evaluate ability of brightness control to adjust to patient size or variations in density
Viewbox	Light meter, mask	Performed to check for percentage and uniformity of transmitted light through the glass panels (see Fig. 14-20)

3. Description of test procedures and equipment to be tested
4. Frequency of testing
5. Test forms for specific tests or equipment
6. A log of tests performed and test results
7. Service repair sheets
8. Policies for monitoring and documenting dosage to personnel
9. Well-defined radiation safety policies for the holding of patients, gonadal shielding, pregnant patients, and operator guidelines. Proper technique, careful positioning, and beam collimation should be used with gonadal shielding, not as a substitute for it. Policies and procedures for pregnant patients should include:
   a. Establishing if the patient is pregnant
   b. Selection of x-ray techniques that minimize fetal exposure if an examination is indicated
   c. Determining fetal dosage
   d. Developing departmental policy regarding advising the patient and her physician about the exposure to the fetus before the study
10. Records of dosage to anyone outside of the primary field. Visitors as well as patients and hospital personnel are entitled to radiation protection.
11. Guidelines for posting of technique charts. Technique charts should be mounted in an easily accessible area and should contain all pertinent data, including the filter in use. In addition to technical factor selection, they should refer to placement of gonadal and breast shielding as well as patient positioning techniques to reduce dosage.
12. Guidelines for testing new screen film products. When a new screen film product is introduced, an established testing protocol should be used to evaluate this product as follows:
   a. The room selected for comparison to an existing product should be calibrated.
   b. The same phantom should be used for all exposures. Whereas newer anthropomorphic phantoms simulate anatomy, the chest phantom containing air-dried lungs is not recommended when evaluating a screen film system for mediastinal structures. With this phantom, details behind the heart can be seen at 60 kVp, although modern chest techniques use 100 kVp to 150 kVp for the same effect in an adult pa-

tient. System speed and resolu tion, however, can be checked using this chest phantom.
   c. The only change in technical factors should be the length of the exposure, since time changes are linear on a properly calibrated unit.
   d. The same focal spot should be used for all exposures. Technical factors should be restricted to a single mA station to avoid mA output variability. A modest mA value should be selected to avoid blooming of the focal spot.
   e. A fixed kilovoltage value should be used so that any visible change in radiographic contrast can be attributed to the film being evaluated.
   f. The field size should remain the same regardless of the size of cassette being used. If various cassette sizes are used in conjunction with a positive beam limiting (PBL) device, the PBL must be overridden.
   g. Processing of all films in the comparison test should be limited to the same previously calibrated automatic processor.

Responsibilities of the Staff Radiographer

Quality assurance is an ongoing process. Unfortunately sometimes simple mechanical tests may be overlooked because of the current interest in electronic testing. Radiographers should report any difficulty with x-ray equipment such as missing hardware, improper lubrication, or a need for a component adjustment. When assigned to a radiographic room, a radiographer should make a visual check of the following:

1. Mechanical stability of the x-ray tube. Vibration in the tube crane can produce image blur. Instability in the system is particularly damaging to conventional tomographic images.
2. Bucky stability. If the Bucky vibrates excessively during exposure, the cassette will also vibrate and image sharpness will deteriorate.
3. Equipment locks. Bucky tray locks and tube crane locks should be checked, since a malfunctioning lock may result in vibration in either the crane or Bucky tray.
4. Tube crane–Bucky alignment. Alignment of the x-ray tube to the grid and distance indicator must be accurate. If a tube is rotated from its normal position for a horizontal beam ra-

diograph, misalignment to the grid can occur. When the tube is returned to its conventional position, a minor tilt against the grid may cause grid cutoff. A simple tube realignment adjustment is shown in Figure 14-4.

5. Control panel function. Meters and dials must be observed for fluctuations, since minor changes in radiation output may affect radiographic density. Radiation output changes may reflect tube aging or a need for calibration of the equipment.

6. Condition of the electrical cables. Rotation for horizontal beam studies may cause the tube cables to become entwined, putting stress on tube connections. The retaining rings of the cables at the termination points should be checked for tightness. Breaks in the insulation or shielding should be noted. A hanging cable that rubs against the equipment or a wall may become frayed.

Responsibilities of the QA Technologist

QA specialists should be familiar with test equipment, trained to perform QC tests, and able to evaluate and interpret the results of the tests. Responsibilities of the QA specialist should be well defined. The more clearly the tasks and departmental standards are defined, the closer personnel will come to achieving optimal image quality.

To avoid improper use of equipment, the QA technologist must establish effective communication among radiographers, radiologists, and equipment manufacturers concerning equipment operation and limitations. Additional responsibilities include familiarizing all radiographers with new equipment and its usage and developing in-service classes in conjunction with service or sales representatives to aid in the education of new staff and students.

QA programs are easier to implement with the help of a QA committee consisting of a staff radiologist, physicist, in-house service or engineering specialist, staff technologist, and other departmental employees. Unfortunately, QA specialists are often viewed as obstructionists if they insist that a room be closed until equipment tests are completed. A clearly defined schedule for QA testing avoids this conflict.

Many noninvasive tests can be performed by a radiographer, but invasive tests that require the electrical attachment of test tools to the imaging equipment should be performed by qualified service personnel.

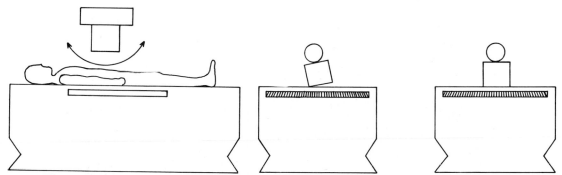

Figure 14-4
X-ray Tube–Bucky Alignment

Birail tube stands or ceiling-mounted tube cranes can be used in many positions, including horizontal cross-table radiography. When the tube is rotated in its housing and then returned to its normal position, misalignment can occur. (Center) A minor tilt (1 or 2 degrees) against the grid can result in grid cutoff. It is good practice to check grid–tube alignment prior to the making of a radiograph. A simple tube realignment adjustment may be required. (Left) By standing at the side of the table, adjacent to the Bucky tray opening, the radiographer can easily see tube angulations to the head or foot of the table. Unfortunately, from this position tube rotation to or away from the radiographer is hard to detect visually. (Right) By standing at the end of the table and lowering the radiographic tube and collimator so that the flat surface of the exit portion of the collimator is flush with the x ray table, one can guarantee proper tube–grid alignment. For precise alignment, a grid alignment QC test tool is recommended.

Retake Analysis Program

A retake analysis program should be used to evaluate all repeat radiographs and to help identify the reasons for additional exposures. In addition to increasing patient dosage, a repeat radiograph costs more than the price of the film used. Time spent by the radiographer and other personnel, room scheduling conflicts, and cost of chemicals and other disposables all add to the expense of a repeat radiograph. A repeat analysis program can help to identify topics that could be addressed in an in-service training program. Film sales organizations are usually helpful in setting up this type of program. To ensure cooperation in a retake analysis program, the technical staff must be assured that the information is not intended to be used for disciplinary purposes.

Studies have shown that the reject rate as the result of equipment problems is quite low. Most of the radiographs are rejected because of patient positioning, patient or equipment motion, or the selection of the wrong exposure factors. When repeating a radiograph, the technical information and the rationale associated with the selection of the original technique help the radiographer make corrective decisions. Understanding the rationale for a specific examination helps the radiographer to help the radiologist. A clinical history may influence the selection of technical factors, since disease or injury can affect the technical options. If a radiographer has no information about a specific disease process before the exposure, an over- or underexposed image due to pathology is not a technical error (Fig. 14-5).

Occasionally, radiographs of marginal quality must be accepted for interpretation. Because of the nature of the examination or the age or condition of a patient, it may not always be advisable to repeat a study.

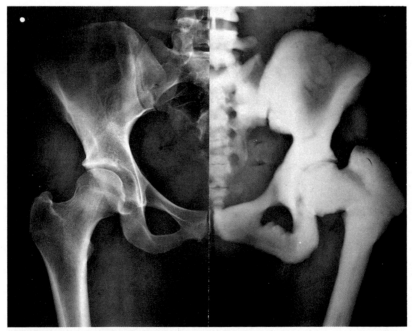

Figure 14-5
The Effect of Pathology on Technique
Normal pelvic bony anatomy (left) *is compared with a pelvis with osteopetrosis* (right). *An increase in bony density requires an increase in x-ray exposure. Conversely, an osteoporotic condition requires a decrease in the exposure needed for normal bone. (Courtesy Cullinan AM: Optimizing Radiographic Positioning. Philadelphia: JB Lippincott, 1992)*

Basic Quality Assurance Test Procedures

The QA tests described in this book are not all-inclusive but serve only as an introduction to the basic QA tests for radiographic/fluoroscopic equipment and accessories (Tables 14-1 and 14-3). Many QA testing reference books and video programs are available, and it is not the purpose of this book to develop an elaborate QA protocol that can be used in every radiology department. X-ray equipment and x-ray accessory manufacturers and medical film sales organizations can provide help in establishing a comprehensive QA program.

General Radiographic Equipment and Accessories

The following test procedures are commonly performed by radiographers to ensure proper equipment performance.

ELECTRICAL AND MECHANICAL SAFETY CHECKS. Electrical, mechanical, and safety guidelines may vary within different areas of the hospital or x-ray facility. An awareness must be developed by the staff as to the potential for accidents and approaches to avoid these problems.

Inspection and maintenance of electrical equipment and related power circuits is an important part of a quality assurance program.

All department personnel should be alerted to potential electrical hazards, particularly with equipment used for patient care or diagnostic imaging. Although the radiographer is responsible for the operation of the radiographic equipment, he or she must also consider other types of electrical equipment in the room, such as electrically operated tables and chairs, illumination devices, dental equipment, and so on. Complex electrical equipment in a special procedures room requires careful electrical monitoring, since many instruments are simultaneously connected to the patient. Very high electrical current can cause physical damage to the patient, such as ventricular fibrillation, paralysis of the respiratory muscles, and burns.

Appropriate equipment grounding is the responsibility of the in-house engineer or x-ray equipment service representative. Responsibility for preventive maintenance for electrically powered equipment and related power circuits belongs to the engineering staff of the facility. Advice is also available from equipment vendors.

In a book of this nature, information cannot be provided to the reader about all electrical and mechanical hazards and their detection and elimination. Power cords and plugs should be periodically checked and should be of a type that will not easily damage. Proper plugging and unplugging of the equipment should be part of the general instructions to radiographers. Strain protection for the cord and plug is essential. Every effort should be made to protect the cord from abnormal wear. Radiographers should examine each cord when used, checking the plug for loose and broken grounding pins, exposed conductors, and so on.

Attention should be paid to replacement of counterbalance cables, x-ray cables, or other accessories. Even a minor incident in which an x-ray table bumps into a tube crane or gets caught on a footstool should be discussed with the service engineers.

PROCESSOR CONTROL TESTS. The use of an x-ray film with QA test tools requires that the x-ray test film used for the testing have the same emulsion number as the film used as a control. When the box of film used for calibration is almost empty, a new box of film should be introduced into the testing procedure. The new and old control films should be compared for matched densities in order to isolate density changes that may have occurred because of a variation in film emulsions. (See Table 14-1 and previous discussion in this chapter.)

BEAM ALIGNMENT AND COLLIMATOR ACCURACY. Alignment tests are made to ensure that the light field and x-ray field are in alignment. The light field of the x-ray collimator should correspond to the predetermined field size of the x-ray beam. Misalignment of the light field can be caused by a change in location of the light bulb filament, the position of the mirror, or change in the position of the collimator housing. This information can be obtained by using a collimator and beam alignment test tool. This tool can also be used to test fluoroscopic alignment and collimation (Fig. 14-6, *left*).

Collimator shutter alignment can also be determined by a simple test using markers such as coins for shutter localization (Fig. 14-6, *right*).

Positive beam-limiting devices must be tested to determine that the PBL automatically adjusts to the cassette size in use.

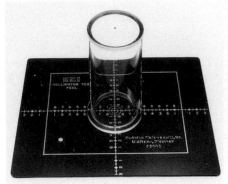
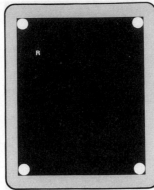
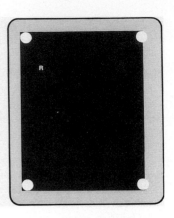

Figure 14-6
Collimator Test Tool

(Left) A collimator test tool is used to verify proper alignment of a collimator light field with the x-ray field. This test tool can indicate a 1% or 2% misalignment at a 40-inch FFD. It can be used at any FFD for conventional radiography and is useful to check fluoroscopic alignment and collimation. This device has a steel ball, mounted in the center of a disc at each end of a 15-cm-high clear plastic cylinder. If the central ray is perpendicular to the detector, the steel balls will be superimposed. (Courtesy Nuclear Associates, division of Victoreen, Carle Place, NY) (Right) An easily performed collimator test uses four coins and a localization marker positioned on a cassette in a pattern corresponding to the pattern of the light field. The radiographic image of the coins should appear within the projected light field. The unilateral cutoff of the coins in the image on the far right indicates misalignment of the light beam and collimator shutters. (Reprinted courtesy Eastman Kodak Company)

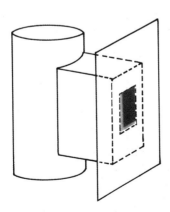

Figure 14-7
Primary Shutter Cutoff Test

A misaligned shutter above the mirror within the collimator may cause a discrepancy between the light field pattern and the x-ray pattern. Although the illuminated field size may appear adequate, a shutter cutoff may occur, particularly with tight beam collimation of an extremity. (See Chapter 5, Fig. 5-7.) (Left) A simple test using a sheet of screen-type film in a direct-exposure holder taped against the exit of the collimator will demonstrate pattern misalignment. The exposure is made after the shutters are adjusted to the desired field size. The proximity of the film to the shutters helps to image the defect. (Right) In this illustration, two shutters are out of alignment in relation to the light field. This test can also be used to determine if a crack exists in the mirror. (See Chapter 5, Fig. 5-5.)

Occasionally one of the upper shutters in a collimator will be out of alignment and will extend into the x-ray field. Since the exit shutters form the light-field pattern as well as the x-ray field pattern, the x-ray field may be smaller than the light field. A segment of the anatomy may not be imaged because of the shutter misalignment. A simple test can be used to determine if this problem exists (Fig. 14-7).

EXTRAFOCAL RADIATION TEST. A simple test to determine the presence of extrafocal radiation can be accomplished without special test tools (Fig. 14-8).

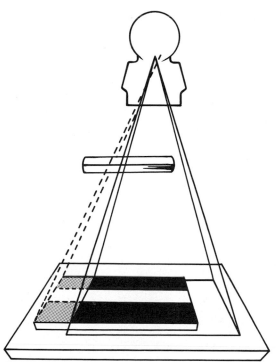

Figure 14-8
Test for Extrafocal Radiation

Extraneous details external to the collimator shutter pattern may be the result of extrafocal radiation. (See Chapter 5, Figs. 5-11 and 5-12.) To test for its presence, a radiograph can be made of a metal bar, suspended midway between the focal spot and cassette, with the x-ray shutters opened as far as possible. The cassette is positioned slightly out of the field to include the portion of the bar that is also out of the x-ray field. The exposure made demonstrates the dense opaque bar as white on a black background. Note the extraneous gray and white densities outside of the collimated field, which are due to exposure of the film by extrafocal radiation (dashed lines).

MANUAL TIMER ACCURACY. Manual timer accuracy can be checked on a single-phase, full-wave or half-wave rectified unit by using the spinning top test (Fig. 14-9).

TIMER ACCURACY AND REPRODUCIBILITY OF mA SETTINGS. X-ray timer accuracy and consistency of radiation output from each mA station should be measured over the life of an x-ray tube. A minor error in exposure times can have a major effect on radiographic density. For example, a 1/120th of a second error in a timer can double radiographic density if it occurs while using a 1/120th of a second exposure. An x-ray timer and mAs test tool can help to provide this information (Fig. 14-10).

AUTOMATIC EXPOSURE CONTROL. The testing of automatic exposure control for reproducibility should include compensation for patients of different thicknesses and kVp variations. A Lucite phantom can be used to check the mR output and to determine if exposure times are reproducible. Another test uses two heavy aluminum plates with a low-contrast resolution test tool.

KILOVOLTAGE ACCURACY. Kilovoltage accuracy and half-value layer (HVL) testing are done to determine beam filtration (Fig. 14-11).

At a given kVp, total filtration in the x-ray beam can be determined by a measurement of the HVL. Exposures are made using increasing thicknesses of aluminum or copper attenuation filters. Aluminum is used for mid-range (80–140 kVp) generators, copper for high-range (140–400 kVp) generators.

Readings are made using a dosimeter and plotted on paper for interpretation. The HVL is determined when the dosimeter readings are reduced to one half of the exposure's initial value.

IMPORTANT

The aluminum attenuation plates should not be made of an alloy of aluminum, since it could affect HVL measurements.

ESTIMATES OF TUBE POTENTIAL AND BEAM FILTRATION. The Wisconsin Test cassette is frequently used to estimate tube potential (kilovoltage) and beam filtration at various exposure levels (Fig. 14-12). These measurements should be made with exposure factors that are typically used in the clinical setting.

For accurate assessment of a generator, waveforms should be evaluated from an oscilloscopic screen.

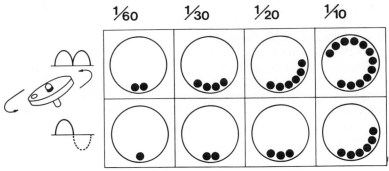

Figure 14-9
Timer Accuracy Test

Timer accuracy can be checked on a single-phase, full-wave or half-wave rectified unit by the use of a spinning top. The spinning top is a circular lead disc, approximately 3 inches in diameter, with a small hole 1/16 of an inch in the outer portion of the disc. The disc is mounted on an axis and made to spin freely with the flat surface of the disc parallel to the cassette. When an x-ray exposure is made with the disc rotating, the peak of each individual pulsation of a waveform is recorded on the radiographic film as a black dot. Each 1/120th of a second exposure will produce a single black dot on the radiograph if the timer is operating accurately. Typical short radiographic exposures (1/60th, 1/30th, 1/20th and 1/10th of a sec) are shown for (top) single-phase, full-wave and (bottom) single-phase, half-wave exposures. If the current is not rectified, only half the number of dots will appear on the processed radiograph.

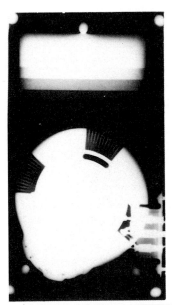
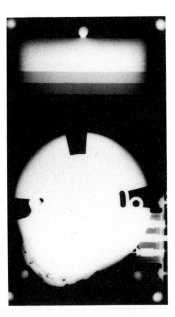
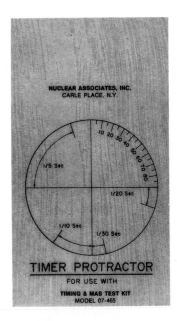

Figure 14-10
Timing and mAs Test Kit

(Left and center) A synchronous rotating slit can be used to check x-ray timer accuracy and mAs uniformity. Accurate timer phasing is ensured by a precision 1-rps motor. (Right) A transparent protractor is used to measure the length of the three-phase exposure. This test can also determine if radiation output is constant for a given mAs when different mA stations are used. (Courtesy Nuclear Associates, division of Victoreen, Carle Place, NY)

Figure 14-11
X-ray Exposure Meter

A variety of devices are available for routine checks of x-ray exposure and exposure rate. This battery-operated x-ray exposure meter can be used for entrance skin exposure measurement, fluoroscopic exposure measurements, radiography output checks (mR/mAs), beam quality/half-value layer, mAs reciprocity, and mA station checks. Remote chambers are available for mammographic and cine imaging systems.

The exposure meter or an optional remote detector is placed on the x-ray table, and the beam is collimated to the detector. An exposure is made and information is presented on a liquid crystal display. (Courtesy Nuclear Associates, division of Victoreen, Carle Place, NY)

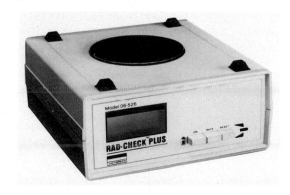

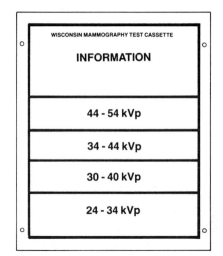

Figure 14-12
Wisconsin kVp Test Cassette

The Wisconsin kVp test cassette can be used for an accurate, simple measurement of the kVp of an x-ray generator. HVL can be estimated by making the test exposure at 60 kVp. Since an x-ray film is required for this procedure, a hard copy record is generated for each test.

(Left) The test cassette, calibrated for blue or green film, measures the overall penetrability of the x-ray beam in the 50 to 150 kVp range. (Right) A Wisconsin Mammographic test cassette, also calibrated for blue or green film, measures the kVp of a mammographic unit in the 24 to 54 kVp range. Both cassettes are accurate within ± 3 kVp. Cassettes should be recalibrated every 2 years, or sooner if the cassette has been dropped or damaged. Calibration can be performed by the National Bureau of Standards or by vendors who have calibrated NBS cassettes. (Courtesy Nuclear Associates, division of Victoreen, Carle Place, NY)

A standard aluminum stepwedge (penetrometer) may be used to establish a baseline image for a quick check of consistency in radiation output.

FOCAL SPOT SIZE MEASUREMENT. The nominal or effective focal spot size is an estimation determined by the manufacturer of the x-ray tube. The filament is wound to certain size specifications and set into the cathode focusing cup at a predetermined distance from the anode. The size of the focal spot has a significant effect on resolution. There are four recommended tests:

1. Focal spot test tool. A simple "pass-fail" test can determine if an x-ray tube focal spot has been damaged (Fig. 14-13).
2. Resolution star pattern test. A resolution star pattern can be used for measuring the resolution properties of focal spots. The star pattern consists of an array of alternating highly absorbing (usually lead) and low-absorbing wedges. This device is a line-pair resolution test pattern. The image obtained with this pat-

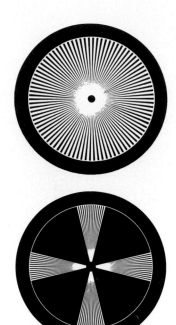

Figure 14-14
Focal Spot Size Measurement

Test patterns consisting of lead-foil screens (rasters) sandwiched between two plastic plates can be used to measure focal spot size. By observing the regions of blurring that occur when a star pattern is imaged by an x-ray source of finite dimension, focal spot size can be determined. Calculation of the focal spot size depends on an awareness of the geometric factors and the distance from the center of the pattern to the region where blurring occurs. (Courtesy Nuclear Associates, division of Victoreen, Carle Place, NY)

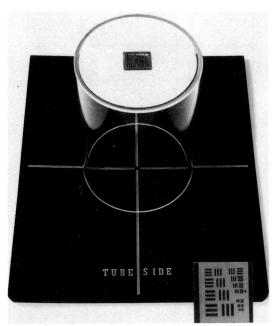

Figure 14-13
Focal Spot Test Tool

A simple pass-fail test is used to determine focal spot damage. A radiograph is made by using a test pattern on a 6-inch-high stand. The resulting image is compared with a chart showing resolution and focal spot size (in millimeters) supplied by the manufacturer. (Courtesy Nuclear Associates, division of Victoreen, Carle Place, NY)

tern does not provide a visual display of intensity distribution but does provide the limit of resolving power of the focal spot. This test can be performed on a wide range of focal spots without removal of the collimator (Fig. 14-14).

3. Pinhole method. A pinhole camera is used, which includes a pinhole diaphragm to produce images of the projected focal spot. The image of the pinhole represents a two-dimensional intensity distribution of the projected focal spot. This tool is used to determine the overall shape, orientation, and the relative location of the small and large focal spots. The image can be helpful when aligning the slit camera. The pinhole technique demonstrates not only focal spot size but also the intensity distribution of radiation from the focal spot (Fig. 14-15).

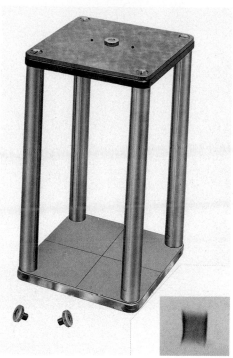

Figure 14-15
X-ray Pinhole Camera

The pinhole camera contains a small and precise pin-hole, which is used to determine the focal spot size of an x-ray tube. Four precision pinhole assemblies are available to measure the dimensions of focal spots. The pinhole camera height is adjustable, up to 24 inches, to maintain a minimum magnification factor of two. An exposure made through the pinhole results in a focalgram (insert). The small screwlike parts lying by the stand are additional pinhole assemblies. (Courtesy Nuclear Associates, division of Victoreen, Carle Place, NY)

4. Slit measurement technique. A slit camera is used to reproduce the intensity distribution in the actual focal spot projected on an x-ray film (Fig. 14-16). The slit measurement technique was recommended in NEMA standard

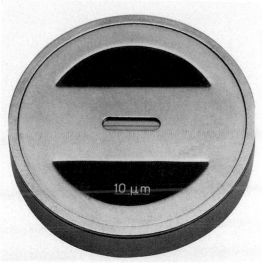

Figure 14-16
Slit Camera

The slit camera method is used with a focal spot stand to measure focal spot size, modulation transfer function, and focal spot blooming. (Courtesy Nuclear Associates, division of Victoreen, Carle Place, NY)

XR5-1992 for measuring focal spot size, focal spot blooming, and modulation transfer function (MTF); MTF can be developed from the slit image, using a microdensitometer scan and computer.

Comparisons between the last three methods show that the star pattern and pinhole images can be used for acceptance testing of x-ray equipment. The star pattern provides a quantitative evaluation of the size of the focal spot, whereas the pinhole image is a qualitative evaluation of the focal spot distribution. The slit measurement technique—the better indicator of focal spot size—can be used to measure the focal spot size, to determine focal spot blooming characteristics, and to measure MTF (Table 14-4). The slit technique requires about one tenth the mAs needed for the

Table 14-4. Focal Spot Evaluation Test Comparisons

Star Pattern Test	*Pinhole Camera Technique*	*Slit Camera Technique*
Limit of resolution	Orientation Intensity distribution	Focal spot size Modulation transfer function Blooming

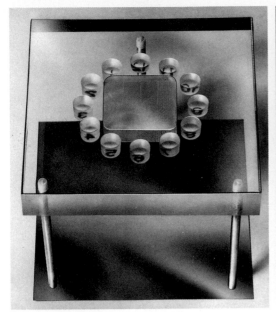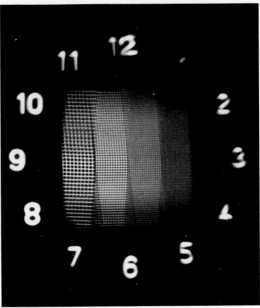

Figure 14-17
Tomographic Phantom

(Left) A tomographic phantom containing lead numbers over a 12-mm depth is used to check the cut level accuracy, evaluation of the fulcrum and bearing conditions, and exposure uniformity. A copper mesh is enclosed in the phantom to measure in-depth resolution. (Right) A tomographic phantom test film. (Courtesy Nuclear Associates, division of Victoreen Carle Place, NY)

pinhole technique for proper exposure. Two exposures are required to measure the focal length and width.

NEMA standards require the use of any fine grain x-ray (nonscreen) film for focal spot imaging. Except for focal spots smaller than 0.3 mm, tube loading is not a problem with the star pattern. Because of the high mAs values required for pinhole imaging, a low-speed detail screen film system is sometimes substituted for nonscreen film, since a reduction in exposure by 50 or more times is possible with the screen film system.*

TOMOGRAPHIC TEST TOOL. The tomographic test tool is used to determine the location of the focal plane, thickness of cut, overall resolution in the plane of the cut, x-ray exposure uniformity, and the beam trajectory during the exposure (Fig. 14-17).

MONITORING OF FLUOROSCOPIC UNITS. Fluo-

roscopic units should be monitored for the following:

Fluoroscopic radiation output per minute. A highly absorptive metal plate is positioned in front of the image intensifier with maximal kVp and mA levels set on the control console. Maximal output readings are determined with an ionization chamber.

Image intensifier automatic brightness adjustment. If an increase in kVp or mA is required to maintain the preselected brightness of the automatic brightness control, the light output of the image intensifier and the TV monitor should be checked.

Image intensifier focusing.

Television and recording camera resolution. Resolution test patterns are available for television and strip film recording cameras (Fig. 14-18).

INTENSIFYING SCREEN CONTROL. Age of intensifying screen, make of screen, speed of screens, and so on should be monitored for consistency.

Everson JD, Gray JE: Comparison of focal spot measurement techniques: The new slit, pinhole, and star resolution pattern techniques and screen film systems as the image receptor. Radiology 165:261–264, 1987.

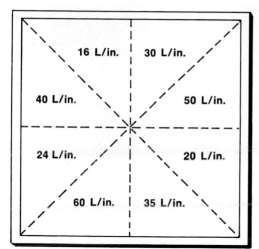

Figure 14-18
Fluoroscopic System Resolution Test Tools
A 7 1/2-inch-square plastic plate that holds eight groups of 7-inch-square copper or brass mesh screening arranged in a pie-shaped configuration can be used to optimize television system focus, mirror optics, and image intensifier settings. The screen mesh shown ranges from 16 to 60 lines per inch. Other resolution test tools are available in ranges from 30–100 mesh and 60–150 mesh. The pie-shaped wire mesh is arranged in an irregular rotation for discrete visualization of screen groupings. (Courtesy Nuclear Associates, division of Victoreen, Carle Place, NY)

Consistency in screen speed can be determined by comparing images with those made with standard quality control tests. Cassettes should be labeled with the type of intensifying screens, date installed, cassette number, and last scheduled cleaning of the screens. An artifact on an image as a result of a dirty or damaged intensifying screen can affect image quality. Careful handling of intensifying screens and film will minimize artifacts.

Intensifying screens should be routinely cleaned with the product recommended by the screen manufacturer. A specific schedule should be designed to include all intensifying screens. Special attention should be paid to the cassettes used at the bedside, in the operating room, or other remote imaging areas. Mammographic screens, in a busy facility, may require daily cleaning.

Common screen defects can usually be detected by visual inspection; however, visual inspection may overlook artifacts. An ultraviolet lamp helps to identify dirt, stains, or screen defects.

INTENSIFYING SCREEN FILM CONTACT TEST. Poor screen film contact contributes greatly to image blur. Screen film contact can be determined with a simple wire mesh test (Fig. 14-19).

FILM INVENTORY CONTROL. Films should be stored in a temperature-controlled environment to avoid fog build-up or deterioration. Film has an expiration date and should be rotated in storage so that the oldest film is used first.

GRID RADIOGRAPHS. The condition of a grid, including the presence of defects, can be determined by simply making a radiograph of the grid. This easily performed test can provide valuable data. (See Chapter 5, Figure 5-17.)

GRID ALIGNMENT TEST. A test tool is suggested for precise alignment of the central ray to the grid. A visual inspection may indicate tube–grid misalignment (see Fig. 14-4).

TEST OF POSITIONING FOAM BLOCKS. Foam-support positioning blocks should be evaluated radiographically for the presence of opaque media or other artifacts. A small amount of opaque material can simulate calcifications. These sponge blocks are easily overexposed.

CARE OF PROTECTIVE DEVICES. Apron racks should be installed in every room and on mobile units so that these garments are hung correctly to avoid damage. Lead aprons, gloves, and other protective devices should be visually checked for defects.

VIEWING CONDITIONS. The light output reading of the viewbox in the processing area should match the light output of the larger banks of lights in the area of interpretation (Fig. 14-20). Many large, multibank viewboxes produce ambient light leaks around the radiographs, which cause the images to appear darker than they appear on a single viewbox. This can be particularly disturbing when interpreting mammograms. Special smaller viewboxes with adjustable internal shutters to block out ambient light should be considered for viewing mammograms.

IMPORTANT

The area near the processor where radiographs are initially checked may have viewboxes with a different degree of brightness or different color fluorescent lights than the viewboxes in the area of interpretation.

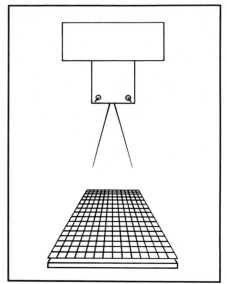

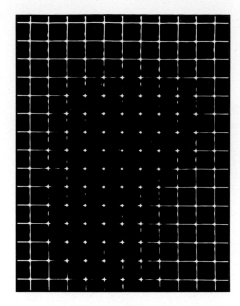

Figure 14-19
Screen Film Contact Test

(Left) A test for screen film contact in a cassette involves placing a wire mesh test tool directly on the cassette and exposing the film. A radiograph of the mesh is made using a background density of approximately 1.0. Wires in an area of poor contact will exhibit image blur. (Right) When evaluated on a viewbox, they will seem to be slightly darker than the wires in surrounding areas. For proper evaluation, the image should be placed on a viewbox and viewed at a distance of between 10 and 12 feet. The diffuse halo-like shadows associated with poor screen film contact are more obvious at these distances. If an extended viewing distance is not practical, the images should be viewed at an oblique angle to avoid the brightness of the direct light emitted by the viewbox. All cassettes should be tested at least annually. Since larger cassettes are more prone to screen film contact difficulties, they should be checked every 6 months or less. New cassettes should be tested before being put into service. (Reprinted courtesy Eastman Kodak Company)

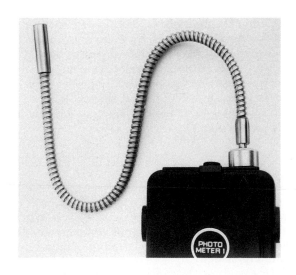

Figure 14-20
Measurement of Light Output

The Precision Photometer can be used to measure the brightness and uniformity of an x-ray viewbox or to verify that an x-ray tube/collimator light or CT system light source used for patient alignment and localization complies with appropriate regulations and guidelines. The fiberoptic probe can be used to measure relative densities of areas on radiographs or the luminance of video screens. (Courtesy Nuclear Associates, division of Victoreen, Carle Place, NY)

ISOLATION PROCEDURES. When appropriate, isolation clothing such as gowns and masks should be used. If necessary, isolation and reverse isolation techniques should be reviewed before performing an examination.

Mammographic Equipment

The QA standards in mammography have not only improved mammographic imaging but also have been the catalyst for interest in quality assurance throughout all phases of radiology. Mammographic QA testing has discouraged the use of conventional radiographic units for screen film mammography, while helping to foster the acceptance of dedicated mammographic equipment.

The American College of Radiology (ACR) accreditation program, a voluntary program for evaluation of mammographic screening sites, requires participants to document information regarding the type of x-ray equipment, image receptor, technical factors, and quality control practices used. Mammograms and ACR mammographic phantom images must be submitted by the mammography facility for evaluation by a panel of radiologists and medical physicists. Radiation dose and equipment output are also evaluated in this program. Since quality assurance is subject to ongoing changes, any facility that is considering applying for ACR mammographic credentialing should check with the ACR for updated information on these guidelines. (See Appendix I for the ACR address.)

The following mammographic QA procedures are generally carried out by physicists:

Entrance exposure and average glandular dose measurements
kVp accuracy reproducibility
Beam quality (half-value layer) evaluation
System performance of the automatic exposure control
Beam restriction accuracy
Focal spot size measurement. This is particularly important if image magnification techniques are to be performed.
Uniformity of image receptor speed

Other mammographic QA tests are performed by radiographers:

Processor quality assurance, which should include replenishment rates, film transport time,

and archival quality of the images. Whenever possible, a screen film mammographic imaging site should have access to a dedicated processor operated and maintained as recommended by the manufacturer. The chemistry chosen for the processor must be compatible with the film in use.
Screen evaluation for cleanliness and screen film contact (Fig. 14-21). Dust or dirt on an intensifying screen blocks the light emitted by the screen during an exposure, producing an artifact that may simulate microcalcifications. In a high-volume facility, screens may require daily cleaning. Screens should be cleaned with a soft, absorbent, lint-free, antistatic wipe and an antistatic cleaner recommended by the manufacturer of the screens.
Exposure of an ACR-approved mammographic phantom (Fig. 14-22).

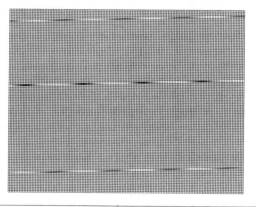

Figure 14-21
Mammography Screen Film Contact Test Tool
The conventional screen film system resolves 4 to 8 cycles/mm, whereas mammographic systems resolve 16 to 20 cycles/mm. Screen film contact is essential for all conventional radiographs, but the loss of contact and resolution is critical in mammograms, which often contain areas of tiny calcifications or very subtle nodules.

A fine-mesh contact tool, consisting of a copper screen with 40 wires per inch, is needed for evaluating high-resolution mammographic screen film systems. With the contact tool placed over the cassette, the compression device is moved as close as possible to the x-ray tube and an exposure is made. Dark areas within the image would indicate poor screen contact. (Courtesy Nuclear Associates, division of Victoreen, Carle Place, NY)

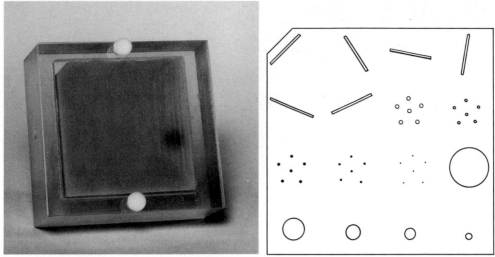

Figure 14-22
Mammographic Accreditation Phantom

(Left) Use of this phantom is an integral part of the ACR mammographic accreditation program. As a quality control tool it can help to evaluate overall imaging. (Right) The phantom is a square wax block containing test objects such as aluminum oxide specks to simulate punctate calcification, thin nylon fibrils to simulate soft tissue fibrillar extensions into adipose tissue, and parts of spheres that mimic tumor-like masses. With the addition of two 2-cm acrylic plates to check the automatic exposure control of the mammographic unit the phantom is equivalent in x-ray attenuation to a 4.5-cm compressed "average" breast. An acrylic disc, 4 mm thick by 1 cm in diameter, can be used to check system contrast. (Courtesy Nuclear Associates, division of Victoreen, Carle Place, NY)

Evaluation of darkroom conditions, including cleanliness, lighting, safelighting, and film handling. Walls, cabinets, floors, countertops, and processor trays should also be cleaned regularly.

A major cause of fogged mammograms is the use of the wrong safelight in the darkroom. A filter such as the Eastman Kodak GBX-2 should be substituted for a Wratten series 6B filter when using orthochromatic films. The GBX-2 filter can be used with most blue-, ultraviolet-, and green-sensitive radiographic films.

Glossary of Related Terminology

Radiologic technology has its own unique language by which members of the profession communicate with each other. Radiographers must be familiar with two forms of terminology. The first, medical terminology, which deals with the terms used to describe the anatomy and pathology of the human body, has been well documented. The second, the terms associated with the principles of radiographic exposure, is not found as readily. Whenever an unfamiliar term or word is encountered by a radiographer, several reference books must often be consulted before an adequate explanation can be found. Many textbooks fail to explain the differences or similarities of the terms used in radiologic technology. For example, *incandescence, fluorescence, luminescence,* and *phosphorescence* are all forms of light, but their meanings are distinctly different. The terms *accommodation* and *adaptation* are not interchangeable, although both refer to the response of the eyes to light. There is a difference in how this response is achieved.

More than 300 terms and items related to radiologic technology are included. The definitions are commonly used but are not necessarily those found in a standard or medical dictionary. For example, when *radius* is listed, no mention is made of its medical use, that of a bone in the forearm.

A list of abbreviations associated with radiographic principles of exposure is presented in Appendix I.

Absorption the process by which an x-ray beam gives off all or some of its energy as it passes through matter. (See *Differential absorption.*)

Absorption blur the blur in an image owing to absorption differences caused by the shape of the structure.

Absorption differences variations in the thickness, density, and atomic composition of the subject being imaged that cause differences in attenuation of the x-ray beam.

Accommodation automatic adjustment of the lenses of the eyes to various distances.

Actual focal spot see *Focal spot.*

Adaptation the process of adjustment of the eyes to various intensities of light in order to increase sensitivity to low light levels; in radiology, dark adaptation of the eyes requires approximately 20 minutes either in a darkened room or the wearing of light adaptation red goggles; adaptation is necessary before the eyes can see a dimly illuminated conventional fluoroscopic image.

Afterglow a persistence of image (lag) after the activating force has ceased; common to low-light-level conventional fluoroscopic screens; not acceptable in intensifying screens or image intensifiers. (See *Phosphorescence.*)

Air-gap technique the separation of the cassette from the subject being examined in order to produce an air gap; a method of reducing scatter radiation.

Alignment the act of arranging the central ray, patient, and image detector in a straight line.

Alternating current see *Current.*

Aluminum equivalent the thickness of any absorbing material that would attenuate the x-ray beam to the same degree as a given thickness of aluminum.

Amp a unit of electrical current.

Angeline M. Cullinan and John E. Cullinan:
PRODUCING QUALITY RADIOGRAPHS, 2ND ED.
© 1987, 1994 J. B. Lippincott Company.

Ampere a rate or measure of electrical current; produced by 1 volt acting on the resistance of 1 ohm.

Amplitude a term related to conventional tomography; defined as the motion of the x-ray tube during an exposure; a pluridirectional tube–cassette motion has approximately a five times increase in amplitude compared with a linear motion.

Angstrom the internationally accepted measurement of wavelength.

Anode the positive electrode or pole of an x-ray tube, valve tube, or any diode tube; when rapidly moving electrons interact with the target of the anode, as in an x-ray tube, x-radiation is produced.

Anode heel effect see *Heel effect.*

Aperture a sheet of lead with an opening that restricts the primary beam; the exit segment of a radiographic collimator.

Automatic brightness control an automatic exposure device that senses the light output from the output phosphor of the image intensifier; the ABC adjusts either kVp and/or mA to produce a predetermined fluoroscopic density.

Automatic exposure device see *Timer.*

Autotransformer an electrical device with a single coil of wire wound around an iron core; part of its turns are common to both the primary and secondary circuit; the primary and secondary windings are connected in series with no electrical insulation between the primary and secondary sides.

Average gradient the slope of the characteristic curve of a radiographic film in the useful density range of diagnostic medical imaging.

Backscatter see *Radiation.*

Back-up time represents the maximal exposure that an automatic exposure device will permit with given mA and kVp values.

Barium an opaque medium (metal) used in the form of barium sulfate; a white, crystalline, water-insoluble powder for fluoroscopic examinations of the gastrointestinal tract.

Base plus fog the density of an unexposed x-ray film that has been processed. Film base opacity and inherent fog due to age or storage conditions compose the base plus fog density.

Beam radiant energy (x-rays) moving in a straight line from a source; since the x-ray beam starts from a small, almost point source, a divergent effect occurs; anatomic structures at the outer edges of this divergent beam can be distorted; the central portion of the beam produces images with minimal distortion; angulation of the path or the beam relative to the object can produce elongation or foreshortening of the image.

Beam splitter an optical system consisting of lenses and mirrors used to reflect a predominant percentage of the light from the output phosphor of an image intensifier toward a photographic recording device.

Blooming a change in values (usually increased) in focal spot dimensions; high mA, low kVp techniques may cause a focal spot to bloom.

Blur used most often to describe lack of image sharpness; see *Detail* and *Resolution.*

Body section common term used for tomography; other synonyms include planigraphy, laminagraphy, ordography, stratigraphy; see *Tomography.*

Bremsstrahlung radiation "braking radiation" is a literal German translation; a heterogeneous beam of radiation created as electrons interact with the target; the attraction between the negatively charged electrons and the positively charged nuclei cause the electrons to be deflected and decelerated from their original path, with some loss of energy.

Bucky diaphragm a grid that is made to move before, during, and after the x-ray exposure to obliterate grid lines and grid artifacts; the grid is suspended beneath the table but above the x-ray cassette; see *Grid.*

Calcium tungstate a type of phosphor that emits primarily blue-violet light when activated by x-radiation; used in the manufacture of intensifying screens; because of its poor absorption/conversion ratio, calcium tungstate is rarely used for intensifying screens greater than 250 speed.

Calibration the determination of accuracy of equipment operation by comparing results to a known standard or value.

Caliper a measuring device, usually divided into centimeters, used to measure part thickness; used in conjunction with a technique chart.

Canting the manufacturing process of inclining grid lines uniformly and bilaterally; the canting process determines the grid focal range.

Capacitor a device able to hold and store an electric charge; often used with a type of mobile radiographic unit.

Capacitor discharge unit a mobile unit using capacitors as a source of electricity during the exposure.

Cassette (1) a light-tight holder for x-ray film; usually contains two intensifying screens; (2) a light-tight take-up container for roll or strip photographic film; (3) a light-tight container for electrostatic imaging plates.

Cathode the negative electrode or pole of an x-ray, valve, or any diode tube; when heated, the filament of the cathode emits electrons; this effect is known as thermionic emission.

Central ray center of the x-ray beam emanating from the focal spot of the x-ray tube.

Characteristic curve see *Sensitometric curve*.

Characteristic ray see *Ray*.

Cineradiography motion picture recording of the fluoroscopic image from the output phosphor of an image intensifier.

Circuit breaker a device used to break or open a comparatively high current; a safety feature.

Collimator a device with a series of lead shutters used to confine a beam of radiation to the field of interest; usually square or rectangular in shape.

Compression a method of reducing the thickness of tissue being imaged to allow a reduction in technical factors and restrict motion.

Compression device (mammography) a rigid, thin, radiolucent plastic paddle used to help eliminate blurring due to motion, to separate structures within the breast, and to decrease breast tissue thickness.

Compton effect when kVp is increased, the incoming x-ray photon has increased energy and can strike an electron in an outer shell and be deviated from its original path with a reduction in energy; commonly referred to as *scatter*.

Condenser another term for capacitor.

Conductance the reciprocal of resistance.

Conductivity the specific electrical conducting ability of a substance; the reciprocal of resistivity.

Conductor a medium that can be used to transmit or carry electricity, heat, or sound.

Cone a beam-restricting device in common use before the design of the collimator; the beam-restricting pattern may be circular, square, or rectangular; occasionally used in conjunction with a collimator.

Constant potential electric current with a constant direct voltage.

Contrast (1) differences between adjacent densities on a radiograph; the number of tonal differences visible on a radiograph determines the scale of contrast; short-scale contrast is demonstrated by abrupt difference in density; longer-scale contrast is presented as a greater range of tones with more shades of gray; contrast is primarily controlled by kilovoltage; (2) radiographic contrast consists of both film contrast and subject contrast; (3) the term *contrast* is also used in reference to opaque or radiolucent media introduced into the body to enhance subject contrast.

Contrast medium radiopaque or radiolucent media used to produce short-scale contrast in an image of an organ or vessel of low contrast. Radiolucent or negative contrast media, such as gas or air, do not absorb x-radiation; radiopaque or positive contrast media, such as barium sulfate or iodine, absorb x-radiation.

Coulomb a quantity of electricity equal to 1 ampere/sec.

Current (1) the movement or flow of electrical charges (electrons) by means of a conductor; (2) alternating—a regular reversal of direction and speed of electrons; (3) direct—a continuous flow of current in one direction; direct current is required for the operation of an x-ray tube.

Cut (tomography) a level or section determined by the focal plane during tomography.

Densitometer a device for determining the degree of blackening of photographic or radiographic film due to the amount of light or x-radiation received; quantitative measurements, known as *sensitometry,* can be made of the response of the film to exposure and development.

Density (1) optical or radiographic density; degree of blackness on a radiographic image; measured by the log of the light incident to the radiograph to the light transmitted through the radiograph (2) the mass/cm³ of a substance or tissue density affects optical density by its absorption of x-radiation.

Detail the sharpness of the structural edges of the radiographic image, often referred to as *recorded detail;* sometimes referred to as *umbra, sharpness, definition,* and *resolution;* usually measured in line pairs per millimeter; affected by focal spot size, intensifying screens, and changes in geometry or patient motion; it is usually referred to as *blur.*

Detent a mechanical or electrical device that is used to limit or prevent motion in an x-ray tube, Bucky tray, spot film device, and so on. A detent is also used for tube–film alignment.

Diaphragm (1) aperture; a primary source beam-restricting device; usually mounted as close to the source of x-radiation as possible; (2) keyhole; a beam-restricting device usually added to the external tracks of a collimator; the opening is often formed to the shape of the part being examined; when used for cerebral angiography, the shape of the skull and cervical area results in a keyhole-like opening.

Differential absorption the relative differences in attenuation of x-radiation by air, fat, water (soft tissue), bone, and metal; the degree of absorption is influenced by the atomic number and thickness of the absorber; equal thickness of dissimilar materials may have different degrees of absorption.

Digital image a computer-based image that converts numeric measurements to densities that can be displayed on a cathode ray tube or television monitor. Computer manipulation of the image is possible.

Digital storage the ability of a unit to store digital information for television readout or hard copy at a later time.

Diode any vacuum tube with two electrodes (positive and negative); such as an x-ray tube, valve tube, or crystal that permits unidirectional electron flow.

Direct current see *Current.*

Direct exposure technique a cardboard or plastic film holder, often with a thin lead foil backing to minimize backscatter; used with x-ray film sensitive to the direct action of x-radiation; screen-type radiographic film when used without intensifying screens in a direct exposure holder requires up to four times more radiation than do direct exposure films for the same examination.

Distortion the size and shape of the radiographic image compared to the size and shape of the object being radiographed; overall equal size distortion is referred to as *magnification;* shape distortion results in elongation or foreshortening; there is some degree of enlargement present in all radiographs.

Divergent see *Beam.*

D-Max the maximal density possible on a radiograph as seen on the shoulder portion of the sensitometric curve.

D-Min the least density on a radiograph, after exposure, usually higher than base plus fog density.

Dose the amount of radiation received as radiation absorbed; expressed in terms of the traditional unit of the rad; the international unit of measure of absorbed dose is the Gray.

Dose equivalent a unit used to express an estimation of biological effects upon people who have been exposed to various qualities of radiation; the traditional unit of DE is the rem; the international unit, the Sievert; in diagnostic radiology, the rad, rem, and roentgen are said to be equivalent.

Dosimeter a direct-reading miniature ionization chamber, usually pencil size; used in personnel monitoring for measuring accumulated dosage of radiation.

Duplication the process of copying a radiograph.

Dye a term erroneously used to describe opaque contrast media.

Dynamic moving; as with fluoroscopy, a dynamic image.

Edge gradient a term sometimes used to define the area of penumbra or lacking sharpness seen on a radiograph caused by the shape of an object and its relation to the central ray.

Electromagnet a magnet produced in a core of iron when an electric current is passed through the coils of wire wound around it; unlike a permanent magnet, an electromagnet can be turned on and off.

Electromagnetic induction with an electromagnet, a magnetic field exists only while the current is flowing; current can be induced in a second wire if the wires cut through the magnetic field lines produced by an electrical current; since both coils are not electrically connected, the first coil induces an electrical current in the second coil by mutual induction; the force in the second wire is directly proportional to the number of turns in the first wire.

Electromagnetic spectrum bundles of electrical and magnetic fields arranged in nature in an orderly fashion according to the wavelength of their energies.

Electron a negative atomic charge that revolves around the nucleus of the atom; in a stable atom, the number of electrons is equal to the number of protons in the nucleus; when there is an excess or deficiency of electrons, the atom is ionized.

Electrostatic imaging a dry imaging process such as used in xeroradiography.

Element the simplest substance composed of atoms of the same atomic number.

Emulsion the radiation-sensitive portion of film that contains the latent image prior to development and the visual image after development of the exposed film; composed of a gelatin mixture containing a silver halide compound; emulsion is coated on one or both sides of the film base.

Energy the ability to perform work; exists in nature in many forms such as kinetic energy, potential energy, magnetic energy, and molecular energy.

Enlargement increase in image size; generally associated with lack of sharpness; affected by FFD, FOD, and OFD; direct roentgen enlargement requires a 0.3-mm focal spot or smaller to minimize loss of sharpness.

Exponent scientific notation used to write very large or small numbers; may be expressed as either a positive or negative number.

Exposure (1) a measure of the ionization produced in air by x-rays or gamma rays; (2) subjection of sensitized film to light or x-rays, either directly or with intensifying screens.

Exposure angle the angle through which the x-ray beam moves during a tomographic exposure; determines the thickness of a tomographic section.

Exposure rate exposure expressed in R (roentgen) divided by T (time in minutes).

Exposure time a measure of time of x-ray exposure expressed in seconds or fractions of a second.

Extended processing see *Processing (extended).*

Field size the area and shape of the segment to be exposed to x-radiation.

Film badge a dental film in a special holder usually worn by personnel who may be exposed to ionizing radiation; the degree of blackening on the processed film is used to determine the amount and quality of radiation exposure received.

Film changer a device used to make serial radiographs at multiple frames per second. A cut film changer moves individual sheets of film through a pair of intensifying screens; a roll film changer transports a continuous roll of film through a pair of intensifying screens.

Film sensitivity the response of x-ray film to a given range of light, such as ultraviolet, blue, or green, or to x-radiation.

Film speed measure of film sensitivity to exposure to produce a specified optical density, usually 1.0 plus base fog.

Filter any obstacle removing low-energy quanta (photons) from the x-ray beam through which x-rays pass from the focal spot to the object under study; total filtration includes added and inherent filtration.

Fluorescence a form of luminescence that emits light only when subjected to an activating force.

Fluoroscope a device used for dynamic evaluation of organs and structures; radiation from an x-ray tube usually mounted beneath an x-ray table passes through the patient to produce a visual image on the fluoroscopic screen; zinc cadmium sulfide is the basic phosphor used for conventional fluoroscopic screens.

Focal plane the layer or level in maximal focus in relation to the x-ray tube and cassette during tomography.

Focal spot (1) actual—the section on which the anode of an x-ray tube intersects with an electron beam emanating from a filament; (2) effective—the size of the projected focal spot in a specified direction; measured with the slit camera method; (3) projected—the projection of the actual focal spot along the central ray, perpendicular to the x-ray port plane and passing through the center of the focal spot; often referred to as the *focal spot.*

Fog additional density on a radiograph due to several conditions such as exposure to scatter radiation, light, chemicals, and so on.

Fulcrum the point selected between the x-ray tube and cassette to determine the focal plane during a tomographic exposure.

Fuse a device used in the electrical circuit to open the circuit as protection against overloading.

Gamma (film) the slope of the straight-line portion of the characteristic curve used to indicate the contrast of the film.

Generator a device that can be used to convert mechanical energy into electrical energy.

Gonad a generic term used to describe male or female reproductive organs.

Gradient the slope of a straight line drawn tangent to the characteristic curve at some point on the curve.

Grid (1) a radiographic accessory designed to minimize the effect of scatter radiation; (2) radius or focus—an imaginary point in space where imaginary lines drawn from the outer aspects of the grid would intersect; (3) ratio—the height of the lead lines of the grid to the width of the interspaces between the lead strips.

Ground an electrical connection of an electrical conductor to the earth.

H & D curve see *Sensitometric curve.*

Half-value layer the amount of any material (e.g., lead, copper, cement, or aluminum) that will reduce the intensity of a beam of radiation by 50%; also known as half-value thickness.

Half-value thickness the thickness of an absorptive material that, when placed in the x-ray beam, will lower the beam intensity by one half its original value; also known as half-value layer.

Heat units a heat unit (HU) is the energy produced in the form of heat by 1 kVp and 1 mA for 1 sec (single-phase, fully rectified radiographic equipment); a multiplication factor

is used to calculate heat units generated by three-phase equipment.

Heel effect a variation in intensity of x-radiation from cathode to anode; sometimes referred to as anode heel effect; the projected focal spot size is also affected by the heel effect.

Helix a cylindrical coil of wire.

Heterogeneous x-ray energies of varying wavelengths and intensities.

Hysteresis loss a form of power loss from the core of a transformer.

Homogeneous x-ray energies of similar wavelengths.

Image detector the term often used for any recording media; used to image radiation for direct viewing or hard copy; also known as *image receptor* in addition to radiographic and photographic film and conventional fluoroscopes, the image may be recorded on Polaroid film; image-intensified fluoroscopic screens; motion picture film; cathode ray tubes; and electrostatic recording media.

Image distributor see *Beam splitter.*

Image intensifier electronic-enhanced fluoroscope with a brightness gain as much as 10,000 times greater than a conventional fluoroscopic screen; makes television viewing, motion picture recording, and strip film recording possible.

Impedance total resistance, in alternating current, which includes inductance, capacitance, and electrical resistance.

Impulse 1/120th second of a commercial 60-cycle alternating current; see *Timer, impulse.*

Incandescent glowing, white hot; usually refers to the illumination of the filament of the x-ray tube: see *Thermionic emission.*

Incident light see *Density.*

Index a factor used to measure a ratio against a given standard.

Induction the generation of an electrical current in a second coil by close subjection to another coil bearing an electrical charge; electrical current can be induced in the second wire if the wires cut through the magnetic field lines produced by the current flowing in the first wire.

Inertia a property of matter that causes a body at

rest or in motion to remain at rest or in motion until an external force changes its state.

Instantaneous load the maximal kVp and mAs values that can be used for a given length of time for a single exposure.

Insulator a material (nonconducting) that resists the conduction of electrical current.

Intensification factor the exposure ratio required to produce a given density without intensifying screens compared to the exposure required for an equivalent image made with intensifying screens.

Intensifying screen fluorescent crystals coated on a paper or plastic base; used in conjunction with single-emulsion film (one screen) or dual-emulsion x-ray film (two screens) to convert x-radiation into light.

Intensity the rate, roentgens per second, at which x-radiation reaches the film; the total energy passing through an area per unit area, per unit time.

Inverse square law a law expressing that the intensity of radiation is inversely proportional to the square of the distance from the source of radiation.

Ionization occurs when an interaction within an atom causes a transfer of energy to an orbital electron sufficient to remove the electron from orbit, thereby converting the atom to ions.

Ionization chamber (1) an automatic exposure timer used to achieve reproducible radiographic densities over a wide range of body sizes and thicknesses; (2) a radiation-sensing device (such as a geiger counter) used to detect and measure ionizing radiation.

Isotope any two atoms of the same element and same atomic number with different mass numbers.

Joule a derived unit of work or energy in the SI system of measure where 1 watt per second is equal to 1 joule.

Jukebox a device that holds a number of optical disks for archival purposes. Specific disks can be retrieved as needed.

keV the effective voltage value; the direct current voltage required to generate the same amount of energy as an alternating current with a given resistance; eV = 0.7 pV; pV = 1.41 eV.

Kilo a prefix for 1000.

Kilovolt 1000 volts.

Kilovoltage (1) optimum—a radiographic technique using a fixed kVp with variable mAs; (2) variable—a radiographic technique using a variable kVp with a fixed mAs.

Kilovolt peak the highest kilovoltage that occurs during an x-ray exposure; the peak voltage is not present throughout the entire exposure with single-phase equipment; the beam contains photons of various energies.

Kilowatt 1000 watts.

Kinetic energy the energy of motion.

Lag afterglow; light from a fluoroscopic screen after the activating force has ceased; see *Phosphorescence.*

Laminagraphy see *Tomography.*

Laser L(ight) A(mplification) by S(timulated) E(mission) of R(adiation); a laser beam is used to "write" directly on photographic film in laser printing devices to eliminate the electronic interference and raster lines associated with cathode ray tube imaging.

Latent image changes in the sensitive film emulsion by which silver ions in the silver halide crystal are converted to neutral silver atoms by the exposure to x-radiation. These changes require development of the x-ray film to produce a visible image.

Latitude this term has several applications in medical radiography: (1) film latitude is a design parameter using sensitometry to define the range of contrast possible in an image, with a given film product; multiple tonal shades (long-scale contrast) represent extended latitude; abrupt black and white changes in density are associated with lower-latitude, high-contrast film products; (2) technical latitude is generally described in terms of the high kVp and lower mAs values that result in a longer scale of contrast on the image; changes at higher kVp are more easily tolerated than changes at lower kVps; slow screen film combination speeds making larger changes more tolerable (increased exposure latitude).

Lead marker a lead number, letter, or word used on a cassette or film changer for identification.

Light adaptation see *Adaptation.*

Linear energy transfer the measurement of the amount of energy transferred from x-radiation to the soft tissues of the body.

Linearity density comparisons between mA stations as determined by an image of a step-wedge. A doubling of an mA setting should produce a doubling in the film blackening effect.

Line pair a quantitative measurement of resolution; one opaque line and one space. The higher the number of line pairs per millimeter, the better the resolving power of the screen film system.

Line spread function a test used to measure the light diffusion (blurred or unsharp edges of the image) associated with intensifying screens; this information is then used as the basis for determining the modulation transfer function of a screen film combination.

Logarithm (log) the exponent or power to which a fixed number (base) must be raised to produce a given number. A logarithmic scale used with a characteristic curve makes it possible to compress a significant amount of data into a small manageable space.

Luminescence the production of energy in the form of light without producing heat.

Magazine a take-up cassette for exposed strip, roll, or cut film.

Magnetic field the area of magnetic influence in space around a current carrying wire; the magnetic force only exists while current is flowing through the wire.

Magnification see *Distortion, size, shape* and *Enlargement.*

Mass the amount of matter in a body as measured by its inertia; the weight and compact nature of a substance.

Matter any substance composed of atoms that occupies space.

Micro a prefix for 1/1,000,000th.

Milli a prefix for 1/1000th.

Milliampere 1/1000 ampere.

Milliampere second product of the milliampere value times the length of exposure expressed in seconds (mA $\times$ T).

Minimal reaction time see *Minimal response time.*

Minimal response time represents the time required for the shortest possible automatic exposure.

Modulation transfer function a mathematic method of measuring image detail (sharpness and resolution) on the radiographic image; calculated from line-spread function data.

Molybdenum an element used for the anode and filters of mammographic x-ray tubes; used as a base for tungsten rhenium anodes in conventional x-ray tubes.

Mottle any disturbance in the signal being recorded; various types of mottle can interfere with diagnosis, including (1) grid mottle—a widening or banding of grid lines "captured" while the grid is in motion; (2) structure mottle—characterized by either film grain or uneven distribution of phosphors in the intensifying screen; structure mottle is rarely seen on a radiograph; (3) quantum mottle—a variation in optical density (on a radiograph) resulting from the random distribution of the x-ray quanta absorbed by the x-ray detector; density fluctuations seen on an exposed processed radiograph can generally be characterized as quantum mottle.

NEMA National Electrical Manufacturers Association.

Neutron an elementary particle of an atom. Equal in mass to the proton but possessing no electrical charge.

Noise any disturbance in the visual signal being recorded; see *Mottle.*

Nonconductor any substance (usually very resistant) that does not readily transmit electricity, heat, or sound.

Nonopaque radiolucent; easy to penetrate with x-radiation.

Nucleus central portion of the atom containing protons and neutrons and, therefore, most of the mass of the atom.

Off-focus radiation see *Radiation.*

Ohm's law V = IR; I = V/R; R = V/I; the relation in an electrical circuit between the potential difference, current, and resistance.

Opaque having the ability to stop light or other forms of radiant energy; blackened (exposed) radiographic film is opaque to light; dense structures such as bone are opaque to radiant energy; contrast media (barium, iodinated oil, or aqueous products) that can absorb some or all the radiant energy are used to make soft tissue or organs visible.

Optical density the measurement of the percentage of incident light passing through a radiograph.

Optical disk a recording device which uses laser energy to store and retrieve digital data.

Optimal kilovoltage technique see *Kilovoltage.*

Oscilloscope an electronic device used to convert electrical current into a visible pattern on a cathode ray tube.

Parallax effect the impression of a change in position of an object as seen on dual-emulsion film when a tube-angled technique is used.

Penetration the ability of x-radiation to pass through an object; influenced by kilovoltage and the density (mass) of the object.

Penetrometer an aluminum stepwedge used to test mA linearity and the penetrating effect of kilovoltage.

Penumbra geometric blurring at the edges of a structure, immediately adjacent to the umbral (distinct) shadow on the image; affected by focal spot size, object film distance, focal film distance, and the shape of the object.

Periodic table an arrangement of the elements shown in related groups in order of their atomic numbers.

Phantom tissue-equivalent materials used to simulate the absorption characteristics of the human body; may be made of aluminum, such as a stepwedge, or materials such as plastic, shaped as a mannequin or model of an individual body part.

Phosphor a substance that can absorb energy in one form (such as x-radiation) and re-emit the energy in another form (such as visible light).

Phosphorescence the giving off of light from a phosphor after the activating force has ceased; lag; afterglow.

Photoelectric effect interaction of a low to moderate single photon with an electron in which the electron is ejected from its orbit in the form of a photoelectron.

Photofluorogram radiograph (usually of the chest) made by photographing an image from a fluoroscopic screen housed in a lightproof hood.

Photographic effect the effect of x-rays or light on x-ray emulsion.

Photon a quantum or unit of radiant energy.

Phototimer see *Timer.*

Pinhole camera an assembly of equipment, including a pinhole diaphragm, which is used to produce images of the projected focal spot. The pinhole image is a display of the two-dimensional intensity distribution of the projected focal spot.

Planigraphy see *Tomography.*

Polarity a positive or negative state of electrical current.

Position a specified body position (e.g., supine, prone, recumbent, erect, Trendelenburg) used to refer to the physical position of the patient.

Potential difference the energy available to move current in an electrical circuit.

Processing (automatic) the chemical development, fixation, washing, and drying of x-ray film in an automatic film processor. Dry-to-dry cycles vary from 30 seconds to more than 3 minutes.

Processing (extended) an increase in developer time or developer temperature, or both, to increase the speed and slope of the characteristic curve of a specific type of film, usually mammographic film. Film contrast is increased and exposure factors reduced.

Projection refers to the path of the central ray of the x-ray beam.

Proton an elementary particle of an atom that possesses a positive charge; the atomic number of the atom indicates the number of protons present in the atom.

Quality (1) quality is often used to describe the penetrating nature of the x-ray beam as influenced by kilovoltage and filtration; increased kVp produces a more penetrating beam; increased filtration removes soft wavelengths from the beam, thus producing a more homogeneous beam; (2) quality is also used to describe the overall technical appearance of a radiograph; the esthetic appearance of a radiograph is referred to as image quality, which can be affected by sufficient radiographic density, adequate contrast, and minimal distortion, rendering radiographic details visible; (3) image quality can be further expanded to include positioning and processing parameters.

Quality assurance (1) according to federal government recommendations (HEW publication-FDA 80-8110), "quality assurance in diagnostic radiology is defined as planned and systematic actions to insure that a diagnostic facility will produce consistently high quality images with minimum exposure of patients and personnel: quality assurance actions include both quality control techniques and quality administration procedures"; (2) according to the World Health Organization, Germany, 1980, "quality assurance is the organized efforts by staff to insure the consistent production of adequate diagnostic information at the lowest possible cost, with minimum exposure to both patients and personnel to radiation"; (3) quality assurance (QA) programs must include ongoing evaluation of processor, generator, scatter control mechanism, recording media, and so on. QA tests must be documented, updated, and continually available for reference and as support for ongoing continuing education.

Quality control according to federal government recommendations (HEW publication-FDA 80-8110), "quality control refers to those procedures and techniques used to monitor or test and maintain the components of a radiation imaging system. Quality control techniques are directly concerned with equipment."

Quantity quantity is a unit of substantive measure of radiation; quantity is often used to describe the amount of milliamperage and time (mAs) used for an exposure or the amount of exposure measured in roentgens (R).

Quantum a unit of radiant energy.

Quantum mottle see *Mottle.*

Rad the traditional unit of measure for radiation-absorbed dose; replaced in SI units by Gray, where 1 rad = 0.01 Gy.

Radiation process of transporting energy through space or matter as with x-ray; (1) backscatter—remnant radiation that has passed through the back of the film holder or cassette and is then scattered back toward the x-ray film; (2) elec-

tromagnetic radiation—radiation having electrical and magnetic properties and traveling at the speed of light; (3) ionizing—an atom in its normal state contains an equal number of protons and electrons; if an electrical change occurs in an atom as the result of a gain or loss of an electron, the atom will become ionized; x-radiation can cause this effect; (4) primary—radiation from within the x-ray tube, arising from the actual focal spot; heterogeneous in nature; (5) extrafocal—(off-focus or stem) radiation arising from metal other than the actual focal spot of the x-ray tube; produces extraneous details outside the collimated shutter patterns on the image; (6) scatter—a form of secondary radiation; a change in direction of the radiation with reduced energy (longer wavelength); (7) secondary—radiation produced by the interaction of x-ray with matter (see *Scatter*); (8) remnant—radiation that has passed through the patient toward the image detector.

Radiation-absorbed dose in diagnostic radiology, the energy transferred per unit mass of matter by ionizing radiation; exposure, absorbed dose (rad), and dose equivalent (rem) are said to be equal.

Radiograph the processed visible image produced by x-radiation and recorded on x-ray film.

Radiolucent permits the passage of x-rays; a structure or object that does not appreciably attenuate the x-ray beam.

Radionuclides atomic structures that emit radiation and, in so doing, disintegrate; radionuclides are used in nuclear medicine for diagnosis and treatment.

Radiopaque stops radiation; dense bone or metal objects absorb x-radiation in the medical diagnostic range; also refers to radiopaque contrast media; see *Contrast.*

Radius (1) a line extending from the middle of a circle to a point on its circumference; one half the diameter of a circle; (2) grid radius—see *Grid.*

Range the difference between the smallest and largest set of variables in a series.

Ray (1) a beam emanating from a focal area such as the actual focal spot in an x-ray tube; (2) cathode ray—negatively charged electrons emanating from the cathode or filament of a vacuum tube; (3) characteristic ray—occurs as electrons collide with the atoms of the target and displace structural electrons from any inner shell of the target atom; can also be produced as a secondary effect when x-rays interact with the subject being radiographed; characteristic radiation produced by the interaction of x-ray with matter is usually referred to as *secondary radiation* and is a form of scatter; (4) hard—x-rays produced by higher kilovoltage values; hard rays are capable of increased penetration and possess shorter wavelengths; filtration can remove softer (often non-image-forming), less-penetrating waves; (5) primary—x-ray beam emanating from the actual focal spot; radiation discharged directly from a radioactive substance; (6) roentgen—as a courtesy to Wilhelm Conrad Roentgen, who discovered x-radiation on November 8, 1895, the term *roentgen ray* is sometimes substituted for x-ray; (7) scatter ray—see *Radiation, scatter;* (8) secondary ray—see *Radiation, secondary.*

Real time the viewing of anatomy in motion at the actual time of movement, such as in fluoroscopy, ultrasound imaging, and so on.

Receptor see *Image detector.*

Reciprocity law the reaction of a photographic emulsion to direct x-ray exposure equal to the product of the x-ray exposure and the duration of the exposure. At screen film exposures of approximately 10 msec or less or with long exposures such as those used for tomographic studies the reciprocity law can fail.

Rectification the changing of alternating electrical current to direct electrical current; early rectification units were mechanical switches that controlled the flow of current in a given direction; inefficient when compared with valve tubes or solid state rectifiers.

Rectifier a valve tube or a solid state device used to transform alternating current into direct current.

Reflection (1) turned back; the term *reflection* is used in intensifying screen design when the posterior surface of a screen is reflective in nature; (2) reflection is also encountered in ultrasonography in which high-frequency sound waves are emitted from a transducer; when the boundary edges or surfaces of internal structures are encountered by the sound waves, they are reflected back to the trans-ducer, which acts alternately as a transmitter or receptor.

Rem term used to describe radiologic dose equivalent in traditional units; sievert in SI units. 1 rem = 0.01 Sv.

Repeat analysis a review of the conditions that require a repeat of a radiographic image or study.

Resistance the impedance effect of conductor atoms to the flow of electrons; there is resistance to the electron flow in all circuits with some absorption and, thus, loss of energy.

Resolution recorded detail; the appearance of well-defined structural edges of the radiographic image; affected by sharpness and contrast.

Rheostat an electrical control (resistor) used to vary the amount of current entering a circuit; used to control current to the primary of the step-down transformer.

Roentgen see *Ray.*

Safelight lights and filters designed for use in the darkroom to minimize fogging of medical imaging films.

Schematic usually a drawing of an electrical circuit; can be an abstract or conceptual outline or plan.

Screen see *Fluoroscope* and *Intensifying screen.*

Secondary radiation see *Radiation.*

Section, body section see *Tomography.*

Semiconductor a silicon or selenium device that has inherent low resistance to the flow of current in one direction; used in modern rectifying systems.

Sensitometer a device used to expose a radiograph to produce a stepwedge of photographic densities used to make qualitative measurements of the response of the film to exposure and development; the exposed stepwedge is evaluated by the use of a densitometer, and sensitometric curves are generated.

Sensitometric curve a graphic representation used to describe the photographic characteristics (e.g., speed, contrast, latitude) of a radiographic film product; also referred to as a characteristic curve or H & D curve (after Hurter and Driffield).

Sensitometry a qualitative measurement of the response of film to exposure and development.

Shield a protective device such as lead sheeting, gonadal coverings, and eye lens shields used to protect patient and/or operator from unnecessary exposure to ionizing radiation.

SI units the refined modern version of the metric system known as the International System of Measure, introduced as a means of providing a common language for communications between nations and the sciences.

Siemens the SI unit of electrical conductivity.

Sinewave an oscillating curve that is used to diagram the flow of alternating current or the change in electrical and magnetic fields of electromagnetic radiations.

Slit camera a quality assurance test tool used to measure the size of the projected focal spot in a specified direction; resulting in the effective focal spot.

Solenoid a coil of wire with current flowing through it.

Solid state electronic devices such as silicon diode rectifiers used to rectify alternating current; see *Semiconductor*.

Solution liquid-containing substances with water used as a solvent; these include developer, fixer, and replenishments solutions.

Source often substituted for focal spot; known as source image receptor distance (SID).

Spatial pertaining to an extension in space; as in scatter radiation emanating in all directions.

Spectrum electromagnetic radiations arranged in the order of their wavelengths.

Spinning top a rotating metallic disk used to check the timer of single-phase x-ray equipment.

Star pattern a pattern of alternating radiopaque spokes and radiolucent spaces, used to determine focal spot size.

Static (1) at rest, not moving; in a fixed or stationary position; (2) a form of artifact seen on a radiograph, caused by a discharge of electricity caused by friction.

Stem radiation see *Radiation, extrafocal*.

Stepwedge increasing thickness of aluminum of equal size steps; a quality control tool for room output comparison, processor integrity, and so on.

Stereo shift a predetermined change in the location of the x-ray tube in relation to the part under study for the purpose of producing a three-dimensional effect on a radiographic image.

Stereoradiography the use of two separate exposures on two films to produce a three-dimensional image when viewed in a stereoscopic viewer.

Subtraction photographic or electronic process of removing overlying structures from a radiographic image.

Technique chart a guide for the selection of exposure factors needed to produce a radiographic image; formulated after consideration for radiographic image, radiographic equipment calibration and limitations, automatic processor control, use of radiographic accessories, patient habitus, positioning, and pathology.

Teleroentgenogram a radiograph obtained using an extended FFD (usually 6 feet, as with a chest radiograph) to overcome image enlargement.

Thermionic emission the "boiling off" of free electrons by the heating of a filament within the vacuum of a glass tube.

Thermoluminescent dosimeter (TLD) a personal monitoring device that stores energy caused by x-radiation; when the crystals in the device are heated, the stored radiation can be measured, since the thermal luminescent crystals give off light proportional to the radiation exposure received by the TLD.

Timer (1) a mechanism used to initiate and terminate an exposure of a predetermined time; (2) automatic exposure device—an automatic timer in which the exposure is initiated by the radiographer, but the length of the exposure is automatically terminated after a preselected density has been reached; can be either a phototimer or ionization chamber; (3) cumulative—indicates the lapsed times of a fluoroscopic examination; usually a preset time that shuts off the machine automatically; must be reset before fluoroscopy can begin again; (4) impulse—a conventional electronic timer, usually reliable to 1/120th of a second; (5) synchronous— a conventional motor-driven timer, not reliable for exposure shorter than 1/20th of a second.

Tomography the generic term selected by the International Commission of Units and Standards to designate all systems of body section radiography; includes planigraphy, stratigraphy, ordography, and laminagraphy.

Transformer an induction apparatus used to change electrical energy at one voltage and current to electrical energy at another voltage and current through magnetic induction.

Transmittance the percentage of incident light that is transmitted through a radiograph.

Umbra geometric sharpness at the edges of a structure on a radiograph; true or sharply defined as opposed to penumbra.

Unit smallest standardized measure of size, weight, or other quality.

Valve tube a vacuum tube rectification device used to change alternating current into direct current.

Variable kilovoltage technique see *Kilovoltage.*

Video disk recorder a recorder that uses a rigid disk coated with magnetic material.

Video tape recorder a recorder that uses magnetically sensitive plastic tape.

View the body part as seen on a radiograph or other recording media; refers to the actual radiograph or medical image.

Viewbox an illuminator used to view radiographs. It contains fluorescent tubes and is covered with white glass or plastic to diffuse the transmitted light.

Vignetting a lower intensity of light at the periphery of the field than at the center of the fluoroscopic image on an image intensifier.

Volt unit of electrical pressure.

Voltage the electromotive force or difference in potential when a current of one ampere flows through a conductor that has a potential difference of one volt; the power consumed equals one watt.

Watt unit of electrical power; measured in ohms.

Wavelength the distance from a given point on a wave to the same point on the next wave.

Workstation an electronic device consisting of one or more television monitors to display, manipulate, and evaluate text and medical images.

X-ray tube (1) a vacuum tube (diode) designed especially for the purpose of producing x-rays; (2) grid-controlled—an x-ray tube with a third electrode near the filament; the potential may be varied to turn the x-rays on or off for precision x-ray exposure timing.

Zero potential having neither positive nor negative voltage or pressure.

Zonography a type of tomography that uses exposure angles of 10 degrees or less to produce images approximately 1-cm thick.

Abbreviations, Symbols, and Professional Organizations

Abbreviations

A	atomic mass number
A	atomic weight
A	ampere
Å	Angstrom
ABC	automatic brightness control
AC	alternating current
AEC	automatic exposure control
AED	automatic exposure device
Ag	silver
Al Eq	aluminum equivalent
ALARA	as low as reasonably achievable
AP	anteroposterior
BE	barium enema
Bq	Becquerel
c	constant velocity
C	Celsius
C	Centigrade
Ca	cancer
Ci	Curie
CIF	contrast improvement factor
C/kg	coulomb per kilogram
Cm	centimeter
CR	central ray
CRT	cathode ray tube
CT	computed tomography
D	distance
D	dose (absorbed)
DC	direct current
DE	dose equivalent
DSA	digital subtraction angiography
e	electron
ESE	entrance skin exposure
eV	effective voltage
eV	electron volt
F	Fahrenheit
FB	foreign body
FFD	focal film distance
FOD	focal object distance
F/s	frames per second
FS	focal spot
Gy	Gray
H & D	Hurter and Driffield
HU	heat unit
HVL	half-value layer
Hz	Hertz
I	electrical current; amperage
ID	identification
IF	intensification factor
K	contrast improvement factor (grid)
K	Kelvin
k	kilo
keV	effective kilovoltage
kg	kilogram
kHz	kilohertz
kV	kilovoltage
kVp	kilovoltage peak
L	logarithm to the base 10
LAT	lateral
LAO	left anterior oblique
LET	linear energy transfer
lp/mm	lines per millimeter
LPO	left posterior oblique
LSF	line spread function
M	meter
m	milli
mA	milliampere
mAs	milliampere second
MG	minification gain
MKS	meter/kilogram/second
mm	millimeter

Angeline M. Cullinan and John E. Cullinan:
PRODUCING QUALITY RADIOGRAPHS, 2ND ED.
© 1987, 1994 J. B. Lippincott Company.

Mo	molybdenum		Be	beryllium
MPD	maximal permissible dose		Br	bromine
MRI	magnetic resonance imaging		C	carbon
ms	millisecond		Ca	calcium
MTF	modulation transfer function		CaWo$_4$	calcium tungstate
N	newton		Cd	cadmium
Ni	nickel		Ce	cesium
OFD	object film distance		CsI	cesium iodide
OID	object image distance		Cu	copper
P	penumbra		Er	erbium
PA	posteroanterior		Fe	iron
PACS	picture archiving communication system		Gd	gadolinium
			Gd$_2$O$_2$S	gadolinium oxysulfide
Pb	lead		I	iodine
pV	peak voltage		Ho	holmium
QA	quality assurance		La	lanthanum
QC	quality control		LaOBr	lanthanum oxybromide
QDE	quantum detection efficiency		Mo	molybdenum
R	resistance		Pb	lead
R	roentgen		Ra	radium
Ra	radium		Se	selenium
Rad	radiation-absorbed dose		Si	silicon
RAO	right anterior oblique		Sn	tin
RBE	radiation biologic effect		Tb	terbium
Rem	dose equivalent		U	uranium
RPM	revolutions per minute		W	tungsten
RPO	right posterior oblique		Y	yttrium
s	second		Y$_2$O$_2$S	yttrium oxysulfide
Se	selenium		ZnCdS	zinc cadmium sulfide
Sec	seconds			
SI	International System			
Si	silicon			
SID	source image detector distance			
SOD	source object distance			
SSD	source skin distance			
Sv	sievert			
T	time			
TFD	target film distance			
TOD	target object distance			
TLD	thermoluminescent dosimeter			
US	ultrasound			
V	volt; potential			
V	electromotive force; voltage			
W	watt			
Z	atomic number			
Z	impedance			

Symbols

α	alpha particle
β	beta particle
τ	gamma ray
λ	lambda
μ	micro-; micron
μm	micrometer
ν	nu
Ω	ohm
P	resistivity (rho)
Σ	selectivity (grid)
Σ	sigma
λ	wavelength
X	x-ray

Chemical Symbols

Ag	silver
Al	aluminum
Au	gold
Ba	barium
BaSo$_4$	barium sulfate

Professional Organizations and Societies

ACR	American College of Radiology 1891 Preston White Drive Reston, VA 22091

AERS   Association of Educators in
Radiological Sciences
2021 Spring Road
Suite 600
Oak Brook, IL 60521

AHRA   American Health Care Radiology
Administrators
PO Box 334
Sudbury, MA 01776

AMA   American Medical Association
Division of Allied Health Education
and Accreditation
535 N Dearborn Street
Chicago, IL 60610

ARRS   American Roentgen Ray Society
1891 Preston White Drive
Reston, VA 22091

ARRT   American Registry of Radiologic
Technologists
1255 Northland Drive
Mendota Heights, MN 55120

ASRT   American Society of Radiologic
Technologists
15000 Central Avenue SE
Albuquerque, NM 87023

HHS   Health and Human Services,
Department of
200 Independence Avenue, SW
Washington, DC 20201

ISRRT   International Society of Radiographers
and Radiologic Technologists
52 Addison Crescent
Don Mills, Ontario, Canada M3B 1K8

NEMA   National Electrical Manufacturers
Association
2101 L Street NW
Suite 300
Washington, DC 20037

OSHA   Occupational Safety and Health
Administration
200 Constitution Avenue NW
Washington, DC 20210

RSNA   Radiological Society of North America
2021 Spring Road
Suite 600
Oak Brook, IL 60521

WHO   World Health Organization
Avenue Attpa
CH-1211
Geneva 27, Switzerland

Technical Formulas and Related Data

Technical information and related data such as mathematics, formulas, and examples, when applicable, are grouped together so that the reader can appreciate the interactive effect they have, one on the other.

The material presented in this chapter should provide an understanding of the basic mathematics and geometry needed to modify technical factors. Included in this chapter are tables that describe the International System of Measurement (SI units); formulas showing the relation of electrical current, power, resistance, and tranformer operation; and other commonly used principles of exposure.

In practice, it is not usually necessary to mathematically calculate every change in exposure factors.

Basic Mathematics

Mathematics and algebraic functions are performed in terms of their expressed symbols: addition $(+)$, subtraction $(-)$, division $(\div, :)$, and multiplication $(\times, \cdot, [\times], [exponential notations]^\times$, and placement of letters $[ab])$.

Decimals and fractions are often used in technical conversions, and some radiologic principles can be stated as ratios, proportions, or percentages. Exponential notations are used to make mathematic operations easier. Formulas relating to image geometry and the measurement of points, surfaces, and angles produced by the ob-

ject and the x-ray beam can be applied to radiologic principles.

Decimals

Decimals are expressed as follows:

1	= units
0.1	= tens
0.01	= hundreds
0.001	= thousands
0.0001	= ten thousands

Changing Decimals to Fractions

Decimals can also be expressed as fractions. A decimal is expressed as a fraction whose denominator is indicated by 10 or some higher power of 10. The number of places to the right of the decimal point indicates the number of zeros in the denominator when the decimal is changed to a fraction.

Examples:

$$0.1 = \frac{1}{10} \quad 0.07 = \frac{7}{100} \quad 0.004 = \frac{4}{1000}$$

Changing Fractions to Decimals

It is sometimes easier to use the decimal equivalent of a fraction when computing technical changes.

A fraction can be changed into a decimal by dividing the numerator by the denominator.

Example:

$$\frac{1}{2} = 2\overline{)1.0}^{\,0.5} = 0.5$$

$$\frac{1}{20} = 20\overline{)1.00}^{\,0.05} = 0.05$$

Fractions

If the numerator and denominator of a fraction are both multiplied or divided by the same factor, the value of the fraction is not affected.

Example: In the fraction $^{20}/_{25}$, the numerator and denominator can be reduced by dividing each by 5. The value of the fraction $^4/_5$ is the same as the fraction $^{20}/_{25}$.

If two similar numbers or letters (not being added or subtracted) are found in the numerator and denominator, the similar items may be cancelled without affecting the value of the fraction.

Example:

$$\frac{AB}{AC} = \frac{\cancel{A}B}{\cancel{A}C} = \frac{B}{C}$$

or

$$\frac{(4)(5)}{(4)(4)} = \frac{(\cancel{4})(5)}{(\cancel{4})(4)} = \frac{5}{4}$$

Note that if the fractions were stated as

$$\frac{A - B}{AC} \quad \text{or} \quad \frac{5 - 4}{4}$$

the similar items (A or 4) could not be cancelled.

If two fractions have the same denominator, the one with the larger numerator is the greater fraction.

Example: In the fractions $^1/_5$ and $^3/_5$, $^3/_5$ is the greater fraction.

If two fractions have the same numerator, the one with the larger denominator is the smaller fraction.

Example: In the fractions $^3/_9$ and $^3/_{12}$, $^3/_{12}$ is the smaller fraction.

In order to add or subtract fractions, a common denominator must be found.

Example:

$$\frac{3}{4} + \frac{5}{8} =$$

$$\frac{6}{8} + \frac{5}{8} = \frac{11}{8}$$

Example:

$$\frac{5}{9} - \frac{1}{3} =$$

$$\frac{5}{9} - \frac{3}{9} = \frac{2}{9}$$

To divide fractions, invert the second fraction and multiply.

Example:

$$\frac{A}{B} \div \frac{C}{D} = \frac{A}{B} \times \frac{D}{C} = \frac{AD}{BC}$$

Proof: Assign an arbitrary numerical value to A, B, C, and D.

$$A = 2, B = 3, C = 4, D = 5$$

Step 1 $\quad \dfrac{2}{3} \div \dfrac{4}{5}$

Step 2 $\quad \dfrac{2}{3} \times \dfrac{5}{4}$

Step 3 $\quad \dfrac{10}{12} = \dfrac{AD}{BC}$

Ratios and Proportions

Ratios

A ratio indicates a relation of one quantity or term to another. It can be expressed with the symbol : or as a fraction. The symbol : is read "is to" or "to."

In determining the efficiency of a grid (its ability to limit the amount of scatter radiation reaching the image detector), it is important that the radiographer know the grid ratio. When a grid is rated at 5:1, it is understood that the height of the lead lines are five times greater than the width of the interspacing material.

Proportions

Proportions indicate two or more equal ratios that are separated by the symbols = or ∷. Proportions can be either directly or inversely related. In a direct proportion, if the factors in the first ratio are changed, a similar change occurs in the second ratio. In an inverse proportion, if the factors in the first ratio are changed, an inverse change occurs in the second ratio.

The symbol ∷ used to indicate a proportion, is read "equal to."

Example:

A:B∷C:D is read
A to B is equal to C to D

or

A is to B as C is to D

Radiographers must often calculate for an unknown in a proportion when changing technical factors. When three factors are known, it is easy to solve for the unknown fourth factor. For example, if it is necessary to change the distance at which a radiograph may be taken, the radiographer can determine how the distance change will affect the density on the radiographic image, the intensity of the beam in relation to patient dosage and exposure, and the amount of mAs needed to maintain the original intensity or film density. The formulas needed to make the above technical adjustments will be presented later in this chapter.

Equations

Equations are mathematical expressions of equality. Two sides of an equation remain equal if similar mathematic or algebraic functions are performed on both sides of the equation at the same time.

Example:

Given: $3X = 54$. To solve for X, divide each side of the equation by 3.
$X = 18$.

Given: $X + 3 = 21$. To solve for X, subtract 3 from each side of the equation.
$X = 18$.

Given: $X - 6 = 12$. To solve for X, add 6 to each side of the equation.
$X - 6 + 6 = 12$
$+ 6$
$X = 18$

Given: $\dfrac{X}{6} = 3$. To solve for X, multiply each side of the equation by 6.

$$(6)\left(\frac{X}{6}\right) = (3)(6)$$
$$\frac{6X}{6} = 18$$
$$X = 18$$

Percent

Percent can be expressed as a decimal or a fraction.

Example:

$$5\% = 0.05 \text{ or } \frac{5}{100} = \frac{1}{20}$$

To add a percent sign to a number, multiply the number by 100.

Example:

$3 = 300\%$.

To remove a percent sign from a number, divide by 100.

Example:

$100\% = 1$
$10\% = 0.10$

Exponents

Scientific or exponential notation is used to write very large or very small numbers.

Exponents indicate the number of times a base number (usually 10) has been multiplied by itself.

Example:

$$10^1 = 10$$
$$10^2 = 10 \times 10 = 100$$
$$10^3 = 10 \times 10 \times 10 = 1000$$
$$10^4 = 10 \times 10 \times 10 \times 10 = 10,000$$
$$10^5 = 10 \times 10 \times 10 \times 10 \times 10 = 100,000$$

The number of zeros placed to the right of the base number indicates the exponent when scientific notation is used to write a number. A minus exponent indicates a fraction. The $(-)$ exponent indicates the number of zeros placed to the right of the decimal point of the base number.

Example:

$$10^{-5} = \frac{1}{100000} \text{ or } 0.000001$$

$$10^{-3} = \frac{1}{1000} \text{ or } 0.0001$$

To multiply numbers using scientific notation, add the exponents.

Example:

$$10^3 \times 10^5 = 10^8$$

To divide numbers using scientific notation, subtract the exponents.

Example:

$$10^6 \div 10^3 = 10^3$$

To raise a number to a higher power using scientific notation, multiply the exponents.

Example:

$$(10^3)^2 = 10^6$$

Similar Triangles

Similar triangles are triangles whose sides and angles are similar in shape. A line drawn parallel to the base of a triangle will produce a similar triangle. The similar sides of similar triangles are proportional to each other.

In radiologic technology, the radiographer uses the principle of similar triangles to solve problems dealing with magnification (enlargement). The relation of collimator opening to field size can also be calculated in this manner. Radiologists use the principle of similar triangles to determine the actual size and location of an object compared to the image (e.g., for fetal maternal measurements or foreign body localization).

Problems can be easier to solve if a rough sketch is drawn and labeled. The information from the sketch can then be stated as a proportion (Figs. A-1 and A-2).

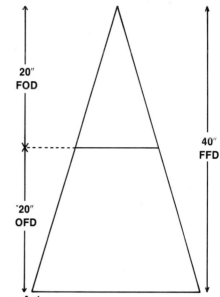

Figure A-1
Principle of Similar Triangles
The principle of similar triangles can be used to calculate measurements in radiology. The letters used to label the schematic in Figure A-2 are arbitrary and do not have to be memorized if the principle is understood. These letters do not constitute a formula for field size dimensions but are used for this illustration to identify the relationship of similar triangles to each other.

It is suggested that when confronted with a problem dealing with a distance-to-size relationship, a rough sketch be made of the stated dimensions. The sketch should be labeled, and the dimensions of the similar triangle should be stated as a proportion.

Using similar triangles, the degree of enlargement of an object can be predicted in its linear as well as area measurements. If all distances, that is, 20-inch FOD, 20-inch OFD = 40-inch FFD are known, the true size of an object recorded on a radiograph can be calculated. The geometric relationship just stated would yield a 2× linear enlargement, 4× area enlargement. See Figure A-2 for an example of collimator field size determination.

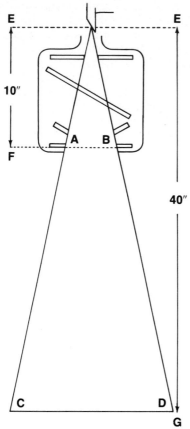

Figure A-2
Collimator/Field Size Determination

The principle of similar triangles can be used to predict one or both dimensions of a projected field size if the size of the collimator exit shutter opening is known. Conversely, the collimator exit shutter size can be determined if the field size is known.

The height of the first triangle is measured from the focal spot (E) to the base of the triangle (F) at the level of the exit shutter opening in the collimator (AB).

The height of the second triangle represents the FFD (EG) measured from the focal spot (E) to the base of the triangle (G) at the level of the field size opening (CD).

Example:

$$\frac{AB}{CD} = \frac{EF}{EG}$$

Temperature Conversion

F	0	10	20	30	40	50	60	70	80	90	100
C	-18	-12	-7	-1	4	10	16	21	27	32	38

To convert from Fahrenheit to Celsius (Centigrade) temperature, use the following formula:

$$C = \frac{5}{9}(F - 32)$$

I M P O R T A N T

Remember to subtract 32 from the Fahrenheit temperature before ⅝ F is calculated in the Celsius to Fahrenheit formulas.

Example:

70°F to °C
$$C = \frac{5}{9}(F - 32)$$

$$\frac{5}{9}(70 - 32)$$

$$\frac{5}{9}(38)$$

$$\frac{190}{9} = 21.1$$

To convert from Celsius to Fahrenheit temperature, use the formula:

$$F = \frac{9}{5}C + 32$$

I M P O R T A N T

Remember to calculate ⅗ C before 32 is added in the Celsius to Fahrenheit conversion.

Example:

21.1°C to °F
$$F = \frac{9}{5}C + 32$$

$$\frac{9}{5}(C) + 32$$

$$\frac{9(21.1)}{5} + 32$$

$$\frac{189.9}{5} + 32$$

$$37.98 + 32 = 69.98$$

$$F = 70°$$

The Kelvin scale, in which absolute zero equals 0°, is the unit of measure for temperature in the International System of Measurements.

Systems of Measure

The three systems of measure used by radiographers in the United States are:

1. The traditional English system
2. The MKS metric system (meter-kilogram-second)
3. The refined modern version of the metric system, known as the International System of Units (SI)

Measurements in the metric system have been used in science, industry, and medicine for many years (Tables A-1 and A-2). SI units were introduced as a means of providing a common language for international communications between nations and the sciences. In the 1970s, the International Commission on Radiation Units and Measurements (ICRU) introduced the SI units for measurement of radiation units and suggested replacing the traditional units with the SI units (Table A-3) over a 10-year period. An understanding of SI radiation units of measure is important to radiographers.

In the metric system the prefixes of milli-, centi-, and deci-, when placed in front of the basic units, indicate a lesser amount. When deca-, hecto-, and kilo- are placed in front of the basic units, they indicate a greater amount.

Size Relations in Units of Measure

The seven basic units of measure—weight, length, time, current, temperature, substance, and luminescence (Table A-4)—can be further expanded into many other units (Table A-5) to measure parameters such as area, volume, density, velocity, mass, electrical force, conductance, and resistance. For example, using the measurement for length, area and volume can be derived. Area is equal to the product of two sides of a surface. This measurement can be expressed in English or metric units such as square inches or square centimeters (cm^2).

The area of a square is calculated by squaring one side.

$$A = a^2$$

Table A-1. Wavelength Relationships

Energy	Measured in	Approximate Wavelength
Commercial alternating current	Meters (M)	$\pm 10^6$ M 1,000,000 M
Radio	Meters (M)	$\pm$ 100 M
Television	Meters (M)	$\pm$ 1 M
Visible light	Angstrom units (Å)	$\pm 10^4$ Å
Medical x-radiation	Angstrom units (Å)	$\pm$ 0.1 to 0.5 Å

I M P O R T A N T: *The waveform remains the same (~) in all of the above; however, the penetrating ability of the wave increases as the wavelength becomes shorter. Photon energy is not all of the same wavelength; the x-ray beam is heterogeneous, having many wavelengths and energies within the range of medical x-radiation.*

39.3 in. = 1 meter
2.54 cm = 1 in.
1 cm = 1/100th meter
1 mm = 1/1000 meter
1 micron (μ) = 1/1000 mm
1 Angstrom unit (Å) = 1/10,000 μ (0.1 nm, 1/100,000,000, 10^{-8} cm, 10^{-10} m, or 0.1 nm)
1 nm = 10^{-9} m

Table A-2. English and Metric Corresponding Units

English			Metric				Power				
Weight	*Length*	*Time*	*Weight*	*Length*	*Time*	*Fraction*	*of 10*	*Decimal*	*English*	*Metric*
							10^3	1000	thousands	kilo
							10^2	100	hundreds	hecto
							10^1	10	tens	deka
pound	yard	second	gram	meter	second		1	1	unit	
ounce	foot		liter							
	inch									
						1/10	10^{-1}	0.1	tenths	deci
						1/100	10^{-2}	0.01	hundredths	centi
						1/1000	10^{-3}	0.001	thousandths	milli

Table A-3. Radiation Units of Measure*

Traditional Unit	Symbol	Measure of	SI Unit	Symbol	Relation
rad	rad	Absorbed dose	Gray	Gy	1 rad = 0.01 Gy Gy/0.01 = 1 rad
rem	rem	Dose equivalent	Sievert	Sv	1 rem = 0.01 Sv Sv/0.01 = 1 rem
Curie	Ci	Radioactivity	Becquerel	Bq	1 Ci = 3.7×10^{10} Bq Bq/3.7×10^{10} = 1 Ci
Roentgen	R	Exposure		C/kg	Measured in Coulomb per kilogram (C/kg) 1 R = 2.58×10^{-4} C/kg C/kg/2.58×10^{-4} = 1 R

For practical purposes, in radiologic technology, exposure, absorbed dose, and dose equivalent are said to be equal. Exposure is the quantity most easily understood. In diagnostic radiology, however, there is concern for the absorbed dose (the energy transferred per unit mass of matter by the ionizing radiation).

In the SI system, the Gray (Gy), the unit for absorbed dose, has been received when 1 joule (J) of energy has been transferred to 1 kg of mass.

Table A-4. Seven Basic Units of Measure

Quantity	Unit	SI Symbol
Length	meter	m
Mass	kilogram	kg
Time	second	s
Electric current	ampere	A
Thermodynamic temperature	Kelvin	K
Amount of substance	mole	mol
Luminous intensity	candela	cd

Table A-5. Some Units Derived from the Seven Basic Units

Quantity	Unit	SI Symbol	Other Units
Acceleration	meter per second squared	—	m/s²
Density	kilogram per cubic meter	—	kg/m³
Electrical capacitance	farad	F	C/V
Electrical conductance	siemens	S	A/V
Electrical potential difference	volt	V	W/A
Electromotive force	volt	V	W/A
Electrical resistance	ohm	Ω	V/A
Energy	joule	J	N · m
Force	newton	N	kg · m/s²
Frequency	hertz	Hz	cycle/sec
Illuminance	lux	lx	lm/m²
Luminance	candela per square meter	—	cd/m²
Power	watt	W	J/s
Quantity of electricity	coulomb	C	A · s
Quantity of heat	joule	J	N · m
Velocity	meter per second	—	m/s
Voltage	volt	V	W/A
Volume	cubic meter	—	m³
Work	joule	J	N/m

Example: If a square has the dimension of 3 × 3 inches, the area of the square will be 3², or 9 square inches.

The area of a rectangle can be calculated by multiplying base times height.

Example: If the base of a rectangle were 5 inches and the height of a rectangle were 4 inches, the area of the rectangle would be 20 square inches.

The area of a circle is equal to

$$\pi r^2$$

$$\pi = \frac{22}{7} \text{ or } 3.14$$

r   = radius of the circle

Example: If the radius of a circle were equal to 5 inches, the area of the circle would be

$$\pi(5)^2 =$$
$$\pi(25) = 3.14(25) = 78.5 \text{ sq in}$$

When volume is to be measured, a third dimension must be added.

Example: In a cube, volume is the product of three sides and is expressed in cubic units (e.g., cubic inches, cubic centimeters).

Density can be derived by dividing the mass (weight) of an object by its volume. This relation is often expressed in radiologic technology in reference to tissue density as the mass or amount of tissue per unit of volume.

IMPORTANT

Mass density should not be confused with optical density.

Velocity can be derived from length and time (wavelength and frequency).

Basic Physics and Electrical Formulas

An awareness of basic physics and electrical formulas is helpful in the appreciation of the physical principles of radiography.

Basic Atomic Structure
(See Chapter 1)

The number of protons and neutrons in an atom determines the mass number (A) of the atom. The number of protons in an atom indicates the atomic number of an atom (Z). When represented symbolically, the atomic weight is written in superscript, the atomic number in subscript $_Z^A X$.

In a stable (non-ionized) atom, the number of protons (+ charges) equals the number of electrons (− charges).

Electrons are arranged in energy shells according to a complex system derived from quantum theory. The relation of the electron shell number to the maximal number of electrons permissible in a given shell can be expressed by the formula $2(N)^2$ (Fig. A-3; Table A-6).

The closer the electron shells are to the nucleus, the greater the binding power and the greater the energy required to dislodge the electron from its shell. Matter and energy are closely related and are interchangeable, as stated in Albert Einstein's theory:

$E = MC^2$
$E = \text{mass} \times \text{speed of light}^2$

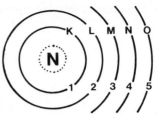

Figure A-3

Electrical Power

Power, expressed in watts (W), is equal to the electromotive force, expressed in voltage (V), times the current, expressed in amperes (I):

$P = VI$

Resistance

There is a relation between voltage (V), current (I), and resistance (R) as stated in Ohm's law. When resistance opposes the flow of electrical current, the current (I) is equal to the voltage (V) divided by the resistance (R):

$$I = \frac{V}{R}$$

or voltage (V) is equal to current (I) times resistance (R):

$V = IR$

or resistance (R) is equal to voltage (V) divided by current (I):

$$R = \frac{V}{I}$$

The resistance will depend on the material offering the resistance, the length and cross-sectional area, and its temperature.

Table A-6. Electron Shell Arrangement

Spectroscopic Designation	Shell Number	Example $2(N)^2$	Number of Electrons
K	1	$2(1)^2$	2
L	2	$2(2)^2$	8
M	3	$2(3)^2$	18
N	4	$2(4)^2$	32
O	5	$2(5)^2$	50

Resistance in a wire is directly proportional to the length of the wire. Resistance is inversely proportional to the cross-sectional area of a wire and is increased as temperature increases.

Power Loss or Power Used

To compute for power loss or the amount of power used in an electrical circuit, we must first consider the formula for power

$$P = VI$$

Resistance in a circuit results in some loss of power; therefore, a formula that shows the relation to voltage and amperage must also be considered. Such a relation exists in Ohm's law, where $V = IR$. By substituting IR for V in the power formula, power loss can be stated

$$Power = VI$$
$$Power\ Loss = IR \cdot I$$
$$Power\ Loss = I^2R$$

Since alternating current permits greater power (wattage) to be transmitted over a given distance with less power loss, power companies usually deliver electrical current in the form of alternating current. The x-ray tube, however, requires direct current for efficient operation. The current is changed from alternating current to direct current by rectification.

With full-wave rectification, both cycles of the alternating current are used.

The terms *power*, *work*, and *energy* are closely related but should not be used interchangeably. Work is equal to force times distance:

$$W = F \times D$$

Rectification

If a test tool (spinning top) is used to check the timer on a single-phase, full-wave rectified unit, for each $\frac{1}{120}$ of a second that the disk revolves, a small black image (dot) will be registered on the film (Fig. A-4).

Example:
If $\frac{1}{10}$ of a second were used to expose the film using the spinning top, the number of black dots that should be present on the radiograph could be determined by dividing $\frac{1}{10}$ of a second by $\frac{1}{120}$ of a second.

$$\frac{1}{10} \div \frac{1}{120} =$$
$$\frac{1}{10} \times \frac{120}{1} = \frac{120}{10} = 12\ (dots)$$

If the rectification system failed or if the equipment were not rectified, there would be half the number of dots, because a dot would be recorded every $\frac{1}{60}$ of a second.

$$\frac{1}{10} \div \frac{1}{60} =$$
$$\frac{1}{10} \times \frac{60}{1} = 6\ (dots)$$

If the time of exposure is not known, by counting the number of dots on the image (e.g., 12 dots), the time of exposure can be calculated by multiplying the dots by $\frac{1}{120}$ of a second (full-wave rectified), since there would be one dot for each $\frac{1}{120}$ of a second.

$$12 \times \frac{1}{120} = \frac{12}{120} = \frac{1}{10}th\ second$$

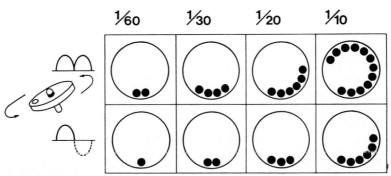

Figure A-4

If the equipment is 3Ø rectified equipment, a template test tool is necessary to measure the arc produced by the almost constant voltage.

Voltage, Current, and Resistance

The voltage measured across a resistor can be calculated if the current flowing through the circuit and the resistance in the circuit are known.

$$V = IR$$

If a series of resistors are connected in a circuit, each resistor lowers the voltage a fraction of the total voltage. There would be only one path for the current flow, and current would be equal at all points.

In a parallel circuit, there are several paths available for current flow to follow. In this situation, each resistor has the full voltage applied to it.

The term *resistance* is used in reference to simple direct current. *Impedance* denotes resistance in alternating current.

Resistance in a Series Circuit

In a series circuit, the total resistance (R) is equal to the sum of all resistances (r) in the circuit (Table A-7).

$$R = r_1 + r_2 + r_3 \text{ (and so on)}$$

Example:
If three resistors were wired in series in a circuit with $r_1 = 5$ ohms, $r_2 = 10$ ohms, and $r_3 = 15$ ohms, the total resistance (R) in the circuit would be 30 ohms.

Table A-7. Relation of Current–Voltage–Resistance in Circuits*

Series	Parallel
$R = r_1 + r_2 + r_3$	$\dfrac{1}{R} = \dfrac{1}{r_1} + \dfrac{1}{r_2} + \dfrac{1}{r_3}$
$I = i_1 = i_2 = i_3$	$I = i_1 + i_2 + i_3$
$V = v_1 + v_2 + v_3$	$V = v_1 = v_2 = v_3$

*In a series circuit, the connections are in a line along the same conductor. In a parallel series, the connections bridge the conductor.

Resistance in a Parallel Series

When resistors are wired in parallel in a circuit, the total resistance (R) will be less than the resistance (r) of any single resistor in the circuit, since the current is divided among several branches or paths (Table A-7).

There is a reciprocal relation between the resistance in a parallel series and the total resistance.

$$\frac{1}{R} = \frac{1}{r_1} + \frac{1}{r_2} + \frac{1}{r_3} \text{ (and so on)}$$

Example:
If two 8-ohm resistors are wired in parallel in a circuit, the total resistance would be

$$\frac{1}{R_T} = \frac{1}{8} + \frac{1}{8} = \frac{2}{8}$$

$$R_T = \frac{8}{2} = 4 \text{ ohms}$$

Total Voltage in a Series Circuit

The total voltage (V) in a series circuit can be calculated by adding the voltage input at each terminal junction.

$$V = v_1 + v_2 + v_3$$

Current in a Parallel Series

In a parallel series, the current flowing through the main branch (1) is equal to the sum of the current in all other branches (i).

$$I = i_1 + i_2 + i_3$$

Current in a parallel circuit follows several paths and is divided among the paths. The voltage applied in the parallel circuit is equal at all points (Table A-7).

IMPORTANT

Total resistance takes into consideration several forms of resistance (inductive, capacitive, and electrical) and is known as *impedance*.

Transformer Principles

A transformer is used to step up or step down voltage in an electrical circuit.

Transformers require alternating current for their operation and operate on the principle of mutual induction.

The electromotive force (voltage) induced in the secondary coils of the transformer is directly proportional to the number of turns in the coils in the secondary side of the transformer. If the turn ratio is increased on the secondary side, the transformer will step up voltage. If the turn ratio is decreased on the secondary side, the voltage will be decreased.

V_S = secondary voltage
V_P = primary voltage
N_S = number of turns in secondary
N_P = number of turns in primary

$$\frac{V_P}{V_S} = \frac{N_P}{N_S}$$

Example:

If the primary coil of a transformer has 10 turns and a potential of 100 volts and the secondary coil has 5000 turns, the potential in the secondary can be calculated.

$$\frac{100}{V_S} = \frac{10}{5000}$$
$$10V_S = 500,000$$
$$V_S = 50,000 \text{ or } 50 \text{ kVp}$$

This would be a step-up transformer. The current (amperage) induced in the secondary coils of a transformer is inversely proportional to the voltage applied to the primary coils of the transformer. As voltage in the secondary is increased, amperage decreases; as amperage is increased, voltage decreases.

$$\frac{I_P}{I_S} = \frac{V_S}{V_P}$$

The efficiency of a transformer is determined by the ratio of outgoing power to incoming power.

$$\text{Transformer efficiency} = \frac{\text{power out}}{\text{power in}}$$
$$\begin{array}{l}\text{Percentage of} \\ \text{efficiency of} \\ \text{transformer}\end{array} = \frac{\text{power out}}{\text{power in}} \times 100$$

Formulas as Applied to Principles of Exposure

X-Ray Tube Heat Units

Heat units generated for a single exposure with single-phase equipment are the product of mA · time · kVp. The heat units generated by three-phase, six-pulse equipment can be determined by multiplying the single $\emptyset$ heat units by the factor 1.35. For 3$\emptyset$ 12-pulse equipment, the 3$\emptyset$ multiplication factor is changed to 1.41.

Example:

$$\text{HU (3}\emptyset\text{, 6-pulse)} = \text{mA} \cdot \text{time} \cdot \text{kVp} \cdot 1.35$$
$$\text{HU (3}\emptyset\text{, 12-pulse)} = \text{mA} \cdot \text{time} \cdot \text{kVp} \cdot 1.41$$

To determine total heat units (when multiple exposures are made in sequence), multiply the heat units per single exposure by the number of exposures in the series.

Grids

Grid Ratio

Grid ratio is expressed as the relation of the height of the lead grid lines (h) to the distance between the lead lines (d).

$$\text{Grid ratio} = \frac{h}{d}$$

Grid Selectivity

Grid selectivity is the relation of the amount of primary radiation to the amount of secondary radiation transmitted through a grid.

$$\Sigma(\text{grid selectivity}) = \frac{\text{primary transmitted}}{\text{secondary transmitted}}$$

Grid Frequency

Grid frequency indicates the number of lead lines per inch in the grid. If efficiency is to be maintained, as grid frequency increases, the grid ratio also increases.

Radiographic Contrast with a Grid

The relation of contrast achieved with a grid to contrast without a grid can be expressed as the contrast improvement factor (CIF).

$$CIF = \frac{contrast \ with \ grid}{contrast \ without \ grid}$$

mAs and Grids

A change in mAs can be made to compensate for changes in grid ratio.

1. List the grid ratio from a non-grid to 16:1 grid and assign a correction factor value to each grid:

$$
\begin{aligned}
non \ grid &= 1 \\
5{:}1 &= 2 \\
6{:}1 &= 3 \\
8{:}1 &= 4 \\
12{:}1 &= 5 \\
16{:}1 &= 6
\end{aligned}
$$

2. Find the grid correction factor of a new grid.
3. Find the grid correction factor of original grid.
4. Divide the new grid correction factor by the original grid correction factor.
5. Multiply the result by the original mAs to determine the new mAs needed to maintain a given density.

Example: If 100 mAs is required for a given technique using a 5:1 grid, the exposure required for use with an 8:1 grid can be determined by dividing the grid correction factor assigned to the 8:1 grid (4) by the grid correction factor assigned to the 5:1 grid (2) and arriving at a correction factor

of 2. When the correction factor is multiplied by the original mAs (100), the new mAs is obtained.

$$2(100) = 200 \ mAs$$

kVp and Grids

Since the relation of kVp to density is not linear, changes made with kilovoltage to compensate for grid conversions are approximations (Table A-8).

Radiographers rarely change technique from non-grid to a high-ratio grid; however, it may be necessary to perform one part of an examination without a grid and another part of the series with a low- to moderate-ratio grid.

Radiographic Density

Density is determined by the log of the light incident to the radiograph (from the viewbox) to the light transmitted through the radiograph (from the viewbox).

$$D = \log \frac{incident \ light}{transmitted \ light}$$

Since radiographs are transparencies, a density of 1 indicates that for every 10 units of light that fall on the film, only 1 unit, or 10%, is transmitted through the film.

An area on the radiograph with a density of 2 would permit only $\frac{1}{100}$th, or 1%, of the incident light to be transmitted through the film.

Relation of mA to Time

$$mA \cdot T = mAs$$

The product of milliamperage and the time factor expressed in seconds results in mAs (milliampere seconds).

Example:

$$\left. \begin{array}{l} 100 \ mA \ at \ 0.1 \ sec = \\ 100 \ (0.1) = \end{array} \right\} 10 \ mAs$$

Relation of mAs to Time

mA is inversely proportional to time. If a given density is to be maintained, an inverse amount of

Table A-8. kVp/Grid Conversions*

Grid Ratio	Add
5:1	8 kVp
6:1	8 kVp
8:1	15 kVp
12:1	20–25 kVp
16:1	20–25 kVp

*The kilovoltage values listed above are theoretical. In practice, conversion from a non-grid technique to a grid technique rarely occurs.

mA is required as the length of exposure (time) is changed.

$$\frac{mA_1}{mA_2} = \frac{T_2}{T_1}$$

Example: If 100 mA is used for $\frac{1}{10}$ (0.1) of a second to produce an acceptable radiographic density, 50 mA would be required to produce the same density at $\frac{1}{5}$ of a second (0.2).

$$\frac{mA_1}{mA_2} = \frac{T_2}{T_1}$$
$$\frac{100}{X} = \frac{0.2}{0.1}$$
$$0.2X = 100\,(0.1)$$
$$0.2X = 10$$
$$X = \frac{10}{0.2} = 50 \text{ mA}$$

mAs_1 (100) = mAs_2 (100); therefore, density remains unchanged.

mAs and Density

Radiographic density is directly proportional to mAs. This relationship is linear. A doubling of the mAs factor results in a doubling of radiographic density. Since mAs is the product of mA and time (mA · T = mAs), an increase or decrease in either factor results in a corresponding density change on the radiograph.

IMPORTANT

At least a 30% change in mAs is required for a change in density to be perceived on a radiograph.

Density and Distance

Changes in focal film distance produce changes in radiographic density (Fig. A-5).

The Inverse Square Law is used to compute the intensity of the beam (amount of radiation that will cause exposure to the patient or film blackening). The change in beam intensity or radiographic density varies inversely with the square of the distance.

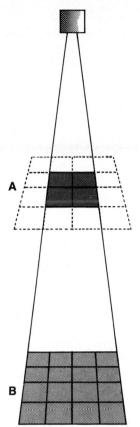

Figure A-5
The Effect of Focal Film Distance on the Radiographic Image

Changes in focal film distance will produce visible changes in radiographic density and the size of the field covered by the beam. The intensity of the x-ray beam (relative to the exposure to the image receptor film blackening and dosage to the patient) will also be affected by changes in distance.

A 36-inch FFD is shown (A) compared with a 72-inch FFD (B). Note the size of the x-ray field at 36 inches (A) compared with that at 72 inches (B). There is a 2× linear, 4× area enlargement, with the x-ray intensity of B reduced to one fourth the intensity of A.

When a change in the FFD is made, the change in radiographic density and beam intensity varies inversely with the square of the distance.

$$\frac{I_1}{I_2} = \frac{D_2^2}{D_1^2}$$

I = intensity of beam
D = focal film distance

Example:

If the amount of radiation reaching a patient at 40 inches is 3 R and the distance were increased to 60 inches, the dosage would be reduced to 1.33 R.

$$\frac{3R}{X} = \frac{60^2}{40^2}$$
$$\frac{3R}{X} = \frac{3600}{1600}$$
$$3R(1600) = 3600X$$
$$X = \frac{4800}{3600}$$
$$X = 1.33 \text{ R}$$

This same reasoning can be applied to the amount of radiation that will cause a film to exhibit a radiographic density. As distance is increased, radiographic density decreases in proportion to D^2.

mAs and Distance and Density

The amount of milliamperage and time needed to produce a given radiographic density varies directly with the square of the distance.

$$\frac{mAs_1}{mAs_2} = \frac{D_1^2}{D_2^2}$$

Since $mA \cdot T = mAs$, the relation of mA or time to distance is also directly proportional.

$$\frac{mA_1}{mA_2} = \frac{D_1^2}{D_2^2}$$

and

$$\frac{T_1}{T_2} = \frac{D_1^2}{D_2^2}$$

Example:

If 100 mA were used at a 40-inch FFD and it were necessary to decrease the FFD to 36 inches, 81 mA would be needed to maintain density.

$$\frac{100}{X} = \frac{40^2}{36^2}$$
$$\frac{100}{X} = \frac{1600}{1296}$$
$$1600X = 129,600$$
$$X = 81 \text{ mA}$$

If 0.5 second were used at a 40-inch FFD and it were necessary to increase the FFD to 48 inches,

0.72 of a second would be required to maintain density.

Example:

$$\frac{T_1}{T_2} = \frac{D_1^2}{D_2^2}$$
$$\frac{0.5}{X} = \frac{(40)^2}{(48)^2}$$
$$1600X = 1152$$
$$X = 0.72$$

A short formula can be used to calculate changes in mAs (mA or time) and distance. If the new distance is divided by the old distance and the resultant conversion factor is then squared, this factor multiplied times the original mAs will yield the new mAs required at the new distance. This method permits the radiographer to work with smaller numbers, since only one factor will be squared.

Example 1:

Using the factors in the previous example:

Step 1 $\dfrac{36 \text{ (new distance)}}{40 \text{ (old distance)}} = 0.9$

Step 2 $(0.9)^2 = 0.81$
Step 3 $0.81 \times 100 \text{ mA} = 81 \text{ mA}$

Example 2:

Step 1 $\dfrac{48 \text{ in (new distance)}}{40 \text{ in (old distance)}} = 1.2$

Step 2 $(1.2)^2 = 1.44$
Step 3 $1.44 \times 0.5 \text{ sec} = 0.72 \text{ sec}$

Reciprocity Law (mAs–Density Relation)

When equal products of mA and time are used to produce two radiographs (e.g., 100 mA at 1 sec or 200 mA at 0.5 sec) and all other factors remain unchanged, the radiographic density should be equal, since $mAs_1 = mAs_2$.

In theory, reciprocity may fail when using intensifying screens at extremely long or extremely short exposure times. In practice, reciprocity law failure can occur with exposures such as those used for the posteroanterior chest (10 msec or less) and pluridirectional tomographic studies (6–9 sec).

Photographic Effect

Milliamperage, time (in seconds), kilovoltage, and distance produce a photographic effect on the radiograph. This relationship can be stated in the formula

$$PE = \frac{mA \times T \cdot kV^2}{D^2}$$

kVp and Density

Changes in kVp are not linear in their effect on radiographic density. Changes in the lower and higher kilovoltage ranges have a greater effect on density than changes at moderate kilovoltages.

If a 15% change (increase or decrease) in kVp is made at any kilovoltage range, the effect should be a doubling or halving, respectively, of the radiographic density if all other factors remain unchanged (Fig. A-6).
Example:
To reduce density to ½ *given 40 kVp:*

40 × 0.15 = 6.00
40 − 6 = 34 kVp = ½ density of image produced at 40 kVp

To increase density:

40 + 6 = 46 kVp = double density of image produced at 40 kVp

Example:
To reduce density to ½ *given 100 kVp:*

100 × 0.15 = 15 kVp
100 − 15 = 85 kVp = ½ density of image produced at 100 kVp

To double density:

100 + 15 = 115 kVp = double density of image produced at 100 kVp

Radiographers often substitute ± 10 kVp in the 60 to 70 kVp range to change density, since 60 kVp at 0.15 = 9 kVp and 70 kVp at 0.15 = 10.5 kVp. A ± 10 kVp change is not acceptable across the entire kilovoltage range used for medical radiography.

Kilovoltage and Milliamperage Compensations

If a change in kVp is required but density must remain the same, the mAs must also be simulta-

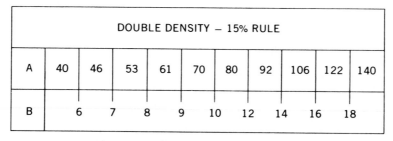

	DOUBLE DENSITY — 15% RULE									
A	40	46	53	61	70	80	92	106	122	140
B		6	7	8	9	10	12	14	16	18

A. Original Kilovoltage Value
B. Increase in kVp Needed to Double Density

Figure A-6
The 15% Rule Versus "Rule of Thumb" for Density Changes
Kilovoltage values ranging from 40 kVp to 140 kVp are shown (A) with a 15% increase in kilovoltage (B) to double radiographic density. A "rule of thumb" adjustment of kVp is sometimes substituted for the 15% kilovoltage change. This rule states that radiographic density can be maintained if an adjustment of one half mAs is accompanied by an increase of 10 kVp. The reduction of 10 kVp and the doubling of mAs has the same effect on density. In the typical kilovoltage range (60 kVp to 80 kVp) used for most medical radiographs, this "rule of thumb" approximates the 15% calculation. As kilovoltage is lowered to the 40 kVp range or elevated to 125 kVp or greater, the 10 kVp adjustment no longer approximates the 15% change.

neously adjusted. Since a 15% change (increase) in kVp results in a two times increase in density, by adjusting the mAs factor to half the original mAs, radiographic density can be maintained. If kilovoltage must be decreased by 15%, a doubling of the mAs will produce a radiograph of comparable density.

Intensifying Screens

Effect on Density

When a change in intensifying screen speed is made, the effect on radiographic density can be predicted if each screen speed is assigned a conversion factor. Medium or average speed screens are assigned a value of 1. Faster or slower systems are assigned numbers relative to the average screen (Table A-9).

Intensification Factor (IF) and Intensifying Screens

The difference in radiation needed to obtain the same film blackening with and without intensifying screens is the intensification factor (IF), and it can be expressed in the following manner:

$$IF = \frac{\text{exposure without screens}}{\text{exposure with screens}}$$

The Contrast Improvement Factor

The contrast on a radiograph obtained with intensifying screens compared to a direct exposure radiograph is known as the contrast improvement factor (CIF).

$$CIF = \frac{\text{contrast with screens}}{\text{contrast without screens}}$$

Table A-9. mAs/Screen Conversions

Screen Type	Conversion Factor
Direct exposure (medical film)	50 × mAs
Detail or slow	2–4 × mAs
Medium	1
High speed (fast)	½ × mAs
Rare earth (2 × fast)	¼ mAs

Intensifying Screens—Absorption Conversion Ratio

Intensifying screen effectiveness relies on the absorption of radiation by the screens and the conversion of the absorbed energy into light (fluorescence), which is capable of exposing radiographic film (Fig. A-7).

Image-Intensified Brightness Gain (Intensification)

With the image intensifier, the intensification factor depends on the relation of the gain in light achieved by the reduction in size of the output phosphor from the input phosphor size (minification factor) and the gain achieved by acceleration of the photons to the output phosphor (flux gain).

brightness gain = minification × flux

Flux gain occurs from the acceleration of electrons striking the output phosphor. Minification gain (MG) is achieved by electronically focusing the light of the input phosphor to a smaller area (output phosphor).

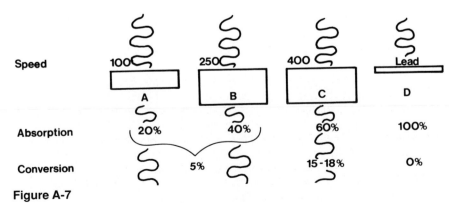

Figure A-7

$$MG = \left(\frac{\text{diameter of input phosphor}}{\text{diameter of output phosphor}} \right)^2$$

Example: The minification achieved with an input phosphor of 6 inches on an output phosphor of 1 inch would be $(\frac{6}{1})^2 = 36$. If the flux gain for each electron ejected from the photocathode surface produced 50 light photons for each electron accelerated, the brightness gain on the 6-inch intensifier would be

50×36, or a gain of 1800

For a 9-inch input phosphor with a flux gain of 50 and a minification gain of 9^2, a brightness gain of 4050 would be achieved:

50×81, or a gain of 4050

Collimation and Field Size

It is possible to determine field size of a collimated area by using the principles of similar triangles. The sides of similar triangles (equal in shape, but not size) have a direct relation to each other (see Fig. A-2).

Example:
Determine the collimator opening size required to cover a 10×12-inch field size if the collimator opening is 10 inches from the source.

$$\frac{AB}{CD} = \frac{EF}{EG}$$

Side 1) $\dfrac{X}{12} = \dfrac{10}{40}$ Side 2) $\dfrac{X}{10} = \dfrac{10}{40}$

$X = 3$ in $X = 2.5$ in

The collimator opening should be 2.5×3 inches to cover a 10×12 inch field.

Recorded Detail

Geometric principles influence the edge sharpness on an image.

Focus Film Distance; Object Film Distance; Focal Spot Size; and Detail

The smaller the focal spot size, the sharper the geometric detail.

P = penumbra (area lacking sharpness)
FS = focal spot size
FOD = focal object distance
OFD = object film distance
FFD = focal film distance

$$\text{Penumbra (P)} = \frac{\text{effective FS} \times \text{OFD}}{\text{FOD}}$$

Geometric detail is increased whenever unsharpness can be decreased.

Example: If a 0.6-mm focal spot is substituted for a 1.2-mm focal spot for an examination made at a 40-inch FFD with a 10-inch OFD, 30-inch FOD, the image will be significantly sharper.

$$P = \frac{1.2 \times 10}{30} = 0.4$$

$$P = \frac{0.6 \times 10}{30} = 0.2$$

IMPORTANT

Remember that FOD = FFD − OFD.

Example: When the focal film distance is increased from 40 inches to 72 inches as in bedside radiography compared with conventional chest radiography, the unsharp quality of the image approximates the image made at the shortened FFD using the same factors except for the FOD.

$$P = \frac{1.2 \times 10}{62} = 0.193$$

Geometric blur caused by penumbra is diminished, and the sharpness of the small focal spot is approximated.

The location of the source and the body part in relation to the image detector greatly influences the degree of penumbra on the image (Fig. A-8). If the OFD could be reduced, image blur would also decrease.

Example: Using the same factors as stated in the original example except for the OFD, which was reduced to 5 inches,

$$P = \frac{0.6 \times 5}{35} = 0.085$$

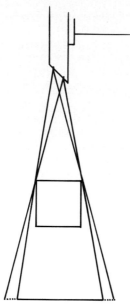

Figure A-8
The Effect of Focal Spot Size on Image Sharpness

Ideally, radiation should originate from a point source for optimal sharpness (recorded detail). Since x-radiation arises from a focal area on the target, greater than a point source, structural edges may appear unsharp. The widened divergent beam passing over the edges of the structure produces a penumbral effect immediately adjacent to the sharp umbral shadow. The degree of unsharpness is dependent upon the size of the focal spot and the distance that the object is placed from the recording media. As the object is brought closer to the detector, or if the focal film distance is increased, recorded detail improves. The optimal image would be generated by increased focal film distance, minimal object film distance, and the smallest possible focal spot size.

In this illustration, the object is positioned approximately two thirds of the distance from the focal spot and one third of the distance from the image detector. This results in approximately a 50% enlargement of the part. In practice, this relationship would not be acceptable unless a fractional focal spot (0.3 mm or less) were used for enlargement techniques.

In the best situation, the smallest focal spot, the shortest OFD, and the longest FOD would result in the least amount of image blur:

$$P = \frac{0.6 \times 5}{67} = 0.045$$

IMPORTANT

These examples do not take into consideration other influences on image blur, such as motion or the use of intensifying screens.

IMPORTANT

Although the formula stated for unsharpness is universally accepted, it must be noted that in the examples given, the factors are expressed in millimeters and inches and have not been converted to a common unit of measure, such as millimeters. Most textbooks use this conceptual approach when explaining how to calculate geometric blur.

Magnification

Magnification and Object Film Distance

Geometric principles can be used to solve problems of magnification and distance or determine the size of an object or the size of the resultant image. The width of the image and the width of the object are related to the distance of the image and the distance of the object from the source. In radiography, the FFD is the distance from the focal spot to the film, and the FOD is the distance from the focal spot to the object.

Magnification (M)

$$M = \frac{FFD}{FOD}$$

Percentage of Magnification

To compute the degree to which an object is magnified, subtract the object width from the image width, divide by the object width, and multiply by 100.

$$\% \text{ of mag} = \frac{\text{image width} - \text{object width}}{\text{object width}} \times 100$$

Area Enlargement

Enlargement (magnification) occurs in linear and area dimensions. In enlargement techniques, a distance that produces a 2× linear enlargement pro-

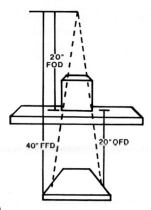

Figure A-9

duces a $4\times$ area, since the area of a square or rectangle is the product of two sides (base $\times$ height) (Fig. A-9).

Stereo Shift

The interpupillary distance and the distance at which stereo images are viewed are directly related to the degree of stereo shift and the FFD.

$$\frac{\text{interpupillary distance}}{\text{viewing distance}} = \frac{\text{tube shift}}{\text{FFD}}$$

The distance between the pupils of the eyes is approximately 2.5 inches; the viewing distance for stereo radiography is usually about 25 inches. This is a 1:10 ratio.

Example: If a 40-inch FFD were used, the total tube shift required to produce stereo images would be 4 inches. Each exposure must be made 2 inches either side of midline:

$$\frac{1}{10} = \frac{X}{40}$$
$$10X = 40$$
$$X = 4$$

IMPORTANT

The tube shift must be in the direction of the grid lines to avoid grid cutoff; there must be no change in the position of the part or degree of inspiration between images; and the collimator shutter pattern must be open to a greater degree in the dimensions of the tube shifts to avoid image cutoff.

Technical Conversion Exercises

The radiographer can predict the outcome of radiographs made with various exposure factors under given conditions. This type of problem is usually presented as an exercise to determine whether the application of the principles of radiographic exposure are understood. In practice, problems of this type will not be encountered, since it is not advisable to simultaneously make several changes in technical factors.

Problems should be written with significant differences in mAs, kVp, time, or distance to make the mathematical operations meaningful.

Contributing Factors

Facts to remember about *density:*

The highest mAs = greatest density
The fastest screen–film combination = greatest density
The lowest grid ratio = greatest density
Direct exposure techniques – least density
The shortest distance = greatest density
The longest time = greatest density
The highest kVp = greatest density
The smallest area of collimation = the least density (conventional techniques)

Facts to remember about *contrast:*

The lowest kVp = greatest contrast (short scale)
The highest grid ratio = greatest contrast (short scale)
The smallest area of collimation = the greatest contrast (short scale)

Facts to remember about *detail* (geometric):

The smallest focal spot = greatest detail
The shortest object film distance = greatest detail
The greatest focal film distance = greatest detail
The shortest time = greatest detail if motion is a consideration
The slowest screen–film system = the greatest detail (when comparing the same phosphor type)
Direct exposure technique = the greatest detail

To determine the effect of technical changes:

1. Evaluate and determine the number of distractor groups in each item, for example,
   a. 100 mAs
   b. 200 mAs
   c. 150 mAs

    d. 50 mAs
    e. 75 mAs
    number of distractor groups = 5

2. Consider each similar factor in the groups and evaluate against other factors; determine which factor would produce the greatest density; and assign a number value to that factor. For example, 200 mAs would produce the greatest density; therefore, it would be assigned the highest number value (5), 150 mAs (4), 100 mAs (3), 75 mAs (2), 50 mAs (1).
    a. 100 mAs (3)
    b. 200 mAs (5)
    c. 150 mAs (4)
    d. 50 mAs (1)
    e. 75 mAs (2)

3. If two or more factors in the group are similar, assign them the same numerical value starting with the number of distractor groups in the problem, for example,
    a. 100 mAs (5)
    b. 100 mAs (5)
    c. 50 mAs (3)
    d. 75 mAs (4)
    e. 100 mAs (5)
    The greatest density would be achieved with

100 mAs; therefore, a, b, and e would be assigned the number 5; d should be assigned number 4; and c should be assigned number 3.

4. Proceed to the next factor group and, using the same procedure, assign numerical factors.

5. Add the assigned values *across* each distractor group.

6. The distractor group with the highest total will be the option that will produce the greatest density.

7. If two distractor groups have the same total reevaluate them using the procedure described above.

See examples below.

I M P O R T A N T

This same logic can be used to determine the greatest detail, contrast, and so on. Consider only those factors that have a noticeable effect on the result being evaluated. It is not necessary to consider focal spot size when evaluating contrast or density; however, it certainly must be considered when evaluating detail.

Example:

mA		Time	kVp	Screens	FFD	mAs	kVp	Screens		
A.	100	⅓ sec	100	Medium	30 in	33 (3)	100 (3)	Medium (3)	30 in (4) = 13
B.	200	⅛ sec	85	High	45 in	25 (2)	85 (2)	High (4)	45 in (1) = 9
C.	50	1 sec	115	Medium	36 in	50 (4)	115 (4)	Medium (3)	36 in (3) = 14
D.	400	¹⁄₂₀ sec	100	High	40 in	20 (1)	100 (3)	High (4)	40 in (2) = 10

C = greatest density

Example: Consider the factors listed below. Which radiograph would exhibit the shortest scale of contrast?

mA		Time	kVp	Grid	FFD
A.	600	⅕ sec	80	8:1	30 in
B.	200	½ sec	92	6:1	50 in
C.	500	¼ sec	80	12:1	30 in
D.	300	⅕ sec	116	5:1	72 in

Remember to assign the highest value to the shortest scale of contrast achieved with each factor.

A.	80 kVp = (4)	8:1 grid	(3) = 7
B.	92 kVp = (3)	6:1 grid	(2) = 5
C.	80 kVp = (4)	12:1 grid	(4) = 8
D.	116 kVp = (2)	5:1 grid	(1) = 3

80 kVp with 12:1 grid will produce the shortest scale of contrast.

Index

The letter f *following a page number indicates a figure; the letter* t *following a page number indicates a table.*